# INSULIN RESISTANCE IN CHILDREN AND ADOLESCENTS

# INSULIN RESISTANCE IN CHILDREN AND ADOLESCENTS

DENIS DANEMAN AND JILL HAMILTON
EDITORS

**Nova Science Publishers, Inc.**
*New York*

For permission to use material from this book please contact us:
Telephone 631-231-7269; Fax 631-231-8175
Web Site: http://www.novapublishers.com



**Library of Congress Cataloging-in-Publication Data**

Daneman, Denis.
Insulin resistance in children and adolescents / Denis Daneman and Jill Hamilton.
p. ; cm.
Includes bibliographical references and index.
ISBN 1-59454-215-5 (hardcover)
1. Diabetes in children. 2. Diabetes in adolescence. 3. Insulin resistance--Pathophysiology.
[DNLM: 1. Insulin Resistance--physiology--Adolescent. 2. Insulin Resistance--physiology--Child. 3. Diabetes Mellitus--physiopathology--Adolescent. 4. Diabetes Mellitus--physiopathology--Child. WK 820 D179i 2004] I. Hamilton, Jill, 1966- II. Title.
RJ420.D5D36 2004
618.92'462--dc22 2004023065

*Published by Nova Science Publishers, Inc. ✦ New York*

# CONTENTS

# PREFACE

Insulin resistance is a simple concept with complex ramifications. The notion that insulin action differs in different people and under different circumstances has been known for a considerable period of time. For example, it has long been recognized that young children with type 1 diabetes are "sensitive" to small changes in insulin dosage, while obese adults with type 2 diabetes may require huge doses of insulin to establish metabolic control. What is more recent is the finding that insulin action differs in a number of different and very common conditions and may in fact be a central contributor to the pathogenesis of some or all of these, including obesity, atherogenesis, type 2 diabetes, the metabolic syndrome, hypertension, hyperandrogenism, polycystic ovarian syndrome and perhaps some types of malignancy.

The increasing burden of obesity and its ramifications has firmly and increasingly focused the spotlight on insulin resistance in recent years. Yet most of this attention has been paid to adults and much less to the consequences and causes of insulin resistance in children and teens. This is despite the fact that many of the adult diseases associated with insulin resistance, such as obesity, type 2 diabetes, atherosclerosis, have their origins in childhood. Furthermore, insulin resistance has long been documented in certain circumstances in children and teens with type 1 diabetes (e.g. at disease onset, with episodes of ketoacidosis or poor metabolic control), and is likely an adaptive response contributing to the growth spurt of puberty. More recently, in utero contributions to programming of insulin resistance and its consequences have been brought to light, initially by Barker and his colleagues who have championed the field of 'fetal origins of adult disease.'

Given the rapid explosion in research in insulin resistance and its increasing importance throughout the life span, we felt it timely to bring together in one place a thorough analysis of the field. The objectives of this book are two-fold: first, to educate the reader about the importance and spectrum of insulin resistance in the childhood population, and, second, to help stimulate and focus further investigation in this exciting area.

We have attempted to gather the contributions of leaders in the field of insulin resistance in the pediatric population. The sequence of the chapters moves from basic mechanisms, to measurement of insulin sensitivity, to description of specific disorders, to prevention and management. Huang, Huang and Klip have contributed a detailed review of the cellular and molecular mechanisms at play in the insulin action pathway and describe how circulating factors and pathologic conditions interfere with normal insulin signaling. These incredibly complex pathways provide the targets for the development of agents which may interfere with the development and progression of diseases related to insulin resistance. The hunt is clearly on for safe and effective medications to accomplish this: the biguanides, specifically metformin, and the glitazones are the early runners in a long line of exciting developments in this field.

Arslanian and her colleagues have contributed greatly to the field of insulin resistance in childhood across a broad spectrum of disorders. For this book, her group provides a path through the morass of methods for measuring insulin resistance: what do they all mean and how should we interpret the findings? This is the first step from the bench to the bedside, and should allow the reader the ability to critically review the data presented in all of the other chapters, which focus on both physiological responses (e.g. puberty, intrauterine growth retardation) and specific disease states (e.g both type 1 and 2 diabetes, obesity, PCOS).

Jefferies, Hofman and Cutfield have made important contributions to the field of the fetal origins of adult disease. There is increasing evidence that glucose homeostasis is fundamentally changed in the situations of both increased and reduced fetal nutrition. In the case of reduced nutrition, the physiologic changes of the fetus are adaptive to the reality of the intrauterine environment and lead to a cascade of events, including reduced fetal growth immediately with programmed insulin resistance and its ramifications years later.

Moran and Rosenberg review the changes in insulin action during adolescent development and highlight how these are, in fact, an adaptive mechanism that is part of normal human development. This group has demonstrated that while glucose metabolism is resistant to insulin action during puberty, insulin-mediated protein metabolism remains normal. The compensatory hyperinsulinism that is required during puberty to maintain glucose homeostasis therefore stimulates increased protein deposition, an essential element of the pubertal growth spurt. This adaptive role of insulin resistance becomes maladaptive in the presence of type 1 diabetes as pointed out in the chapter by Simoneau-Roy and colleagues.

Weiss, Caprio and colleagues provide insights into how the metabolic correlates of obesity are closely coupled with the presence of insulin resistance and hyperinsulinemia. This group has reported that insulin resistance is the best predictor of both impaired glucose tolerance and type 2 diabetes in obese children and adolescents and that both increased visceral adiposity and intramyocellular lipid content were found in youth with impaired glucose tolerance and diabetes. Thus it appears one of the important risk factors for progression of insulin resistance to diabetes is altered partitioning of fat in adipose tissue and muscle. The staggering increase in childhood obesity ensures that this will be a most fertile field for ongoing research.

Phillips, Dewan and Jones address the issue of type 2 diabetes in youth. While much of the knowledge about type 2 diabetes and its management is derived from studies in adults, there is a rapidly evolving pediatric literature. Furthermore, this is seen as a wake-up call to health care researchers, providers and public policy developers that the obesity epidemic in childhood has consequences of potentially enormous magnitude.

DiMartino-Nardi and Garcia review the relationship between insulin resistance and the spectrum of disorders associated with hyperandrogenism in children and teens: specifically, premature adrenarche and polycystic ovarian syndrome. This is another example of the link between early metabolic abnormalities in childhood evolving into other conditions associated with insulin resistance. Interestingly therapeutic manipulations aimed at improving insulin sensitivity appear to have beneficial effects on other aspects of the condition, such as restoring spontaneous menses in PCOS. Very early data suggest that prevention or delay of PCOS may be possible through insulin sensitization, and further studies are warranted.

Our group, Simoneau-Roy, Daneman and Hamilton, has attempted to provide some insights into the role of insulin resistance in a host of conditions, most particularly type 1 diabetes, but also in other disorders including cystic fibrosis, β-thalassemia major, cancer survivors, lipodystrophic and genetic disorders of insulin action, and with the use of specific therapeutic agents. In all of these, insulin resistance either contributes to or leads to disordered glucose metabolism.

Finally, Freemark discusses what we know about treating insulin resistance, emphasizing the successes and challenges of both lifestyle and pharmacological therapies. There has been a major increase in the range of agents available to treat the syndromes associated with insulin resistance in adults, and some are beginning to be explored in children and adolescents. Of particular note, is the emphasis on the desperate need for preventive measures to halt the progression of the obesity epidemic.

Of necessity, much of the work described in each chapter comes from the experience in adults with the spectrum of insulin resistance-related conditions. There is far less research conducted in the pediatric age group, but the knowledge base is expanding rapidly. Where gaps exist, opportunities for research abound. We hope that this book will help to raise awareness of the importance of insulin resistance not only among health care professionals involved in the care of the childhood and adolescent populations, but also researchers, other health professionals and public health authorities who may have an impact on improving insulin resistance and its myriad consequences.

So where do we go from here? Clearly there is much new knowledge yet to be gained: further insight into mechanisms of how insulin resistance develops and in particular identifying genetic factors which predispose individuals to the development of insulin resistance and its pathologic consequences; study of the adipocyte as an endocrine organ and how adipocytokine pathways integrate with insulin signaling pathways to impact on insulin resistance; treatment of insulin resistance with new agents targeted at different parts of these signaling pathways; and the development and testing of strategies to prevent insulin resistance in at-risk pediatric populations. The future of this field of research and clinical endeavors promises to be rich indeed.

*Denis Daneman MB BCh FRCPC*
Professor of Pediatrics
*Jill K. Hamilton MD FRCPC*
Assistant Professor of Pediatrics
University of Toronto and The Hospital for Sick Children,
Toronto, Canada.
July 2004.

# ACKNOWLEDGEMENTS

We wish to thank the authors of all of the chapters for their superb contributions. We greatly appreciate their efforts. We also acknowledge the efforts of Mira Milne for administrative support in the editing of the chapters. Finally, we thank the publishers, Nova Science, for their willingness to publish this book.

In: Insulin Resistance in Children and Adolescents ISBN 1-59454-215-5
Editors: D. Daneman and J. Hamilton, pp. 1-30 

*Chapter 1*

# CELLULAR AND MOLECULAR MECHANISMS OF INSULIN RESISTANCE

***Carol Huang, Xudong Huang and Amira Klip***
The Hospital for Sick Children, Toronto

## ABSTRACT

Insulin resistance is emerging as a significant health risk in children. Currently, our understanding of the mechanisms underlying insulin resistance is far from complete. Insulin regulates glucose disposal via the increase of glucose uptake into fat and skeletal muscles, with the glucose transporter GLUT4 being the main port of entry for glucose. The components of the insulin signalling pathway that regulate this crucial process include the insulin receptor (IR), insulin receptor substrates (IRS), phosphoinositol-3-kinase (PI3K), Akt/PKB, and possibly atypical protein kinase C (aPKC). Various defects along this signalling pathway have been found in insulin resistant patients as well as in both *in vivo* and *in vitro* models of insulin resistance. These defects include alterations in the protein expression, activity, or localization within the cell. As well, the expression, activation, and traffic of GLUT4 appear to be altered. In pathological conditions that contribute to the development of insulin resistance such as obesity, excess glucocorticoid or growth hormone, and increased oxidative stress, abnormal modifications of the insulin signalling molecules have been observed. These conditions serve as models to understand the mechanisms of insulin resistance, and also suggest that targeting these alterations early on may provide an effective strategy in preventing the progression of insulin resistance to diabetes.

## INTRODUCTION

Glucose homeostasis is in great part maintained through the impact of the hormone insulin on several tissues (most particularly the liver, muscle and adipose tissues) and on diverse pathways, including glucose, protein and fat metabolism. In the liver, insulin reduces glucose production via inhibition of gluconeogenesis and glycogenolysis. Insulin also promotes lipid storage in liver and adipocytes, and attenuates lipolysis in fat and muscle. One of the most important metabolic endpoints of insulin signalling is enhancement of glucose uptake into peripheral tissues, namely skeletal muscles and adipocytes, to facilitate processing of the glucose through glycolysis or glycogen synthesis.

Glucose entry into cells is mediated through a family of transmembrane proteins, the glucose transporters (GLUT). The main insulin responsive glucose transporter is GLUT4, which is also the main GLUT expressed in muscles and adipose cells [1]. Although GLUT1 is also present in these tissues, its contribution to insulin-stimulated glucose disposal is minor in comparison to that of GLUT4 [2]. Work from several groups using diverse biochemical approaches has shown that 90% of GLUT4 resides in intracellular compartments of unstimulated muscle and fat cells [3-5]. Upon insulin stimulation, there is a redistribution of GLUT4 towards the plasma membrane, a process termed translocation [3, 4, 6, 7]. In several animal models of insulin resistance and in humans with type 2 diabetes, insulin-stimulated GLUT4 translocation is impaired [1, 8, 9]. Of note, the *acquired* insulin resistance observed in rats made diabetic by pancreatic ablation with streptozocin also involves diminished GLUT4 translocation [10].

In states of insulin resistance, normal levels of insulin fail to appropriately suppress hepatic glucose production and lipolysis, or to fully stimulate insulin-mediated GLUT4 translocation and glucose disposal [1, 11]. Type 2 diabetes is characterized by insulin resistance, but resistance to the hormone also develops in individuals with poorly controlled type 1 diabetes (see Chapter 9). Since skeletal muscles are responsible for greater than 80% of insulin-stimulated glucose clearance *in vivo*, we will focus this review on insulin-mediated regulation of glucose uptake into skeletal muscles.

## The Insulin Signalling Pathway

Insulin action in target tissues begins with binding of the hormone to its receptor on the plasma membrane (Figure 1). The insulin receptor (IR) is a transmembrane protein consisting of two α- and two β- subunits linked by disulfide bonds. After insulin binds to the α-subunits, the β-subunits undergo intramolecular transphosphorylation, whereby one β-subunit phosphorylates its adjacent β-subunit on tyrosine residues. In addition to tyrosine phosphorylation, the insulin receptor can also be phosphorylated at serine/threonine sites. This is most likely a negative regulatory step, as serine/threonine phosphorylation decreases tyrosine kinase activity of the insulin receptor [12-14].

Tyrosine phosphorylation of the juxtamembrane domain of the insulin receptor allows it to bind and subsequently phosphorylate tyrosine residues on a number of important proteins such as the insulin receptor substrates (IRS-1/2/3/4), SHC, Grb-1, Gab-1, Cbl, and APS. A PH (pleckstrin homology) domain at the $NH_2$ terminus of IRS-1 mediates binding to charged headgroups of specific phosphatidylinositides, targeting IRS-1 to membrane structures. A PTB (phosphotyrosine binding) domain is located just adjacent to the PH domain, and is critical in recognizing the phosphotyrosine in the amino acid sequence NPXpY (asparagine-proline-any amino acid-phosphotyrosine) motif of the insulin receptor [15]. Tyrosine-phosphorylated IRS-1 has many docking sites for substrates containing SH2 domains, such as the p85 regulatory subunit of type 1A phosphatidylinositide-3 kinase (PI3-kinase), p50, small adapter proteins Grb-2 and Nck, and SHP2 protein tyrosine phosphatase [16, 17]. Therefore, IRS serves as a divergent point in the insulin signalling pathway, allowing insulin to regulate multiple functions including carbohydrate, lipid and protein metabolism, as well as gene expression, cell growth, proliferation and differentiation.

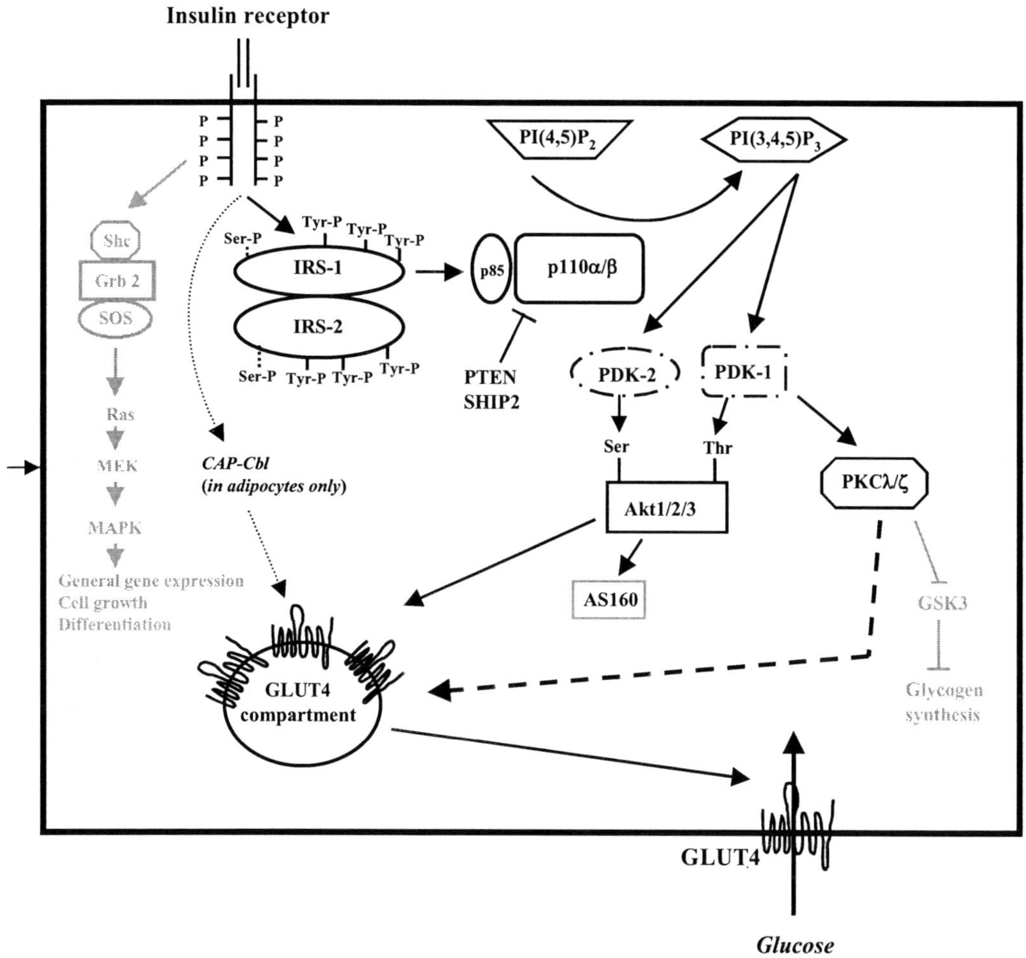


Figure 1. Insulin signalling pathway in muscles and adipocytes

Insulin stimulation increases the association of PI3-kinase with IRS, and *in vivo* and *in vitro* studies support an essential role for PI3-kinase in regulating movement of GLUT4 from intracellular compartments to the plasma membrane, facilitating glucose uptake [18-21]. PI3-kinase consists of a regulatory subunit that interacts with IRSs, and a catalytic subunit that phosphorylates phosphatidylinositols in cellular membranes. There are at least eight different isoforms of the regulatory subunits including p85α, p55α, and p50α, all of which are spliced from the p85α gene. The p85β and $p55^{PIK}$ isoforms are derived from separate genes. p85α is ubiquitous and is important in mediating ligand-dependent PI3-kinase signallingv [22]. In response to insulin, PI3-kinase translocates from the cytosol to intracellular and plasma membranes, where it generates the lipids phosphatidylinositol-3-phosphate ($PI_3P$), phosphatidylinositol-3,4-bisphosphate ($PI3,4P_2$) and phosphatidylinositol 3,4,5 triphosphate ($PIP_3$) [23]. These lipids interact with PH-domain-containing proteins that are thereby recruited to the membranes, such as protein kinase PDK-1, which activates the serine/threonine kinase Akt (also known as protein kinase B, PKB) and the atypical protein kinase C isoforms ζ and λ [24].

Three isoforms of Akt (1, 2, 3) have been identified to date. In response to insulin stimulation, Akt1 is phosphorylated at threonine 308 and serine 473. Dual phosphorylation of Akt at these sites is required for its full activation. PDK-1 phosphorylates Akt at threonine 308 in the activation loop, and serine 473 is thought to be phosphorylated by PDK-2, but the identity of PDK-2 is still being debated [25]. There is evidence suggesting that Akt autophosphorylates on serine 473 because a kinase-inactive mutant fails to be phosphorylated on serine 473. However, in PDK-1-null embryonic stem cells, where Akt is not phosphorylated at threonine 308 and therefore has very low Akt activity, serine 473 phosphorylation can still occur in response to insulin, suggesting that there is an autonomous PDK-2 [26].

Until recently, the role of Akt/PKB in insulin-stimulated GLUT4 translocation has been controversial. In 3T3-L1 adipocytes expression of a constitutively active Akt increased GLUT4 translocation and glucose transport, and this effect was additive to that of insulin [27]. In rat adipocytes, introduction of an excess wild-type Akt or constitutively active Akt led to insulin-independent translocation of GLUT4, and presence of an Akt mutant (Akt-179A) inhibited insulin-stimulated GLUT4 translocation [28]. However, a later study using a different Akt mutant (Akt-AA) in 3T3-L1 adipocytes showed that the mutant inhibited insulin-stimulated protein synthesis but not glucose transport [29]. In a rat skeletal muscle cell line (L6 myoblast), expression of a more stringent dominant inhibiting mutant Akt (AAA-Akt) blocked insulin-stimulated GLUT4 translocation, which was rescued by over-expression of wild-type Akt [30]. Most recently, using RNA-interference to reduce expression of Akt in 3T3-L1 adipocytes, it was shown that both Akt1 and Akt2 were important mediators of insulin-stimulated GLUT4 translocation, with the latter playing a more significant role [31]. Consistent with the above results, the Akt2-null mice were insulin resistant, displaying fed and fasting hyperglycaemia, hyperinsulinemia, glucose intolerance, and impaired muscle glucose uptake [32]. Therefore, Akt seems to be involved in regulation of glucose homeostasis in several tissues.

PDK-1 also directly phosphorylates and activates atypical PKCs (aPKCs), PKCζ and PKCλ. The aPKCs exist in a folded, auto-inhibitory state such that the pseudosubstrate sequence in the $NH_2$-terminal regulatory domain lies in the substrate-binding site of the carboxy-terminal catalytic domain, preventing its phosphorylation and activation. Binding of $PIP_3$ to the regulatory domains of the aPKC leads to unfolding of the protein and increases in enzyme activity. Activation of aPKCs by insulin is decreased in skeletal muscles from patients with type 2 diabetes and animal models of insulin resistance [33], and may contribute to the defect in insulin-stimulated glucose uptake in diabetes.

The downstream targets of Akt/PKB and aPKCs in insulin-mediated glucose transport are beginning to be identified. AS160, a 160-kDa protein found in adipocytes, is phosphorylated by Akt and contains GTPase-activating domain (GAP) for Rabs, which are small G proteins that regulate protein traffic. AS160 is phosphorylated by Akt after insulin stimulation, and a non-phosphorylatable mutant AS160 inhibits insulin-stimulated GLUT4 translocation in 3T3-L1 adipocytes [34].

Precisely how insulin regulates the traffic of GLUT4 through the various intracellular compartments, and the identities of these compartments are under intense investigation. Like other transmembrane proteins, GLUT4 continuously cycles between the cell surface and its intracellular compartments, including early endosomes and recycling endosomes. Insulin accelerates the inter-endosomal traffic and exocytosis of GLUT4 in myoblasts [35]. An understanding of how GLUT4 traffic is altered in insulin resistance will offer new targets for therapeutic intervention.

## DEFECTS IN THE INSULIN SIGNAL TRANSDUCTION PATHWAY

Insulin resistance is a characteristic feature of type 2 diabetes and plays a major role in the development of the disease. The evidence for this comes from (1) the presence of insulin resistance in first-degree relatives of patients with type 2 diabetes 10-20 years before the onset of the disease [36, 37]; (2) cross-sectional studies demonstrating that insulin resistance is a consistent finding in patients with type 2 diabetes [38, 39]; and (3) prospective studies demonstrating that insulin resistance is the best predictor of whether or not an individual will later develop diabetes [36, 38]. Insulin resistance can be defined as an impaired biological response to either exogenous or endogenous insulin. The biological responses could, in theory, include metabolic processes, namely changes in glucose, lipid or protein metabolism, and/or mitogenic processes, namely alterations in growth, differentiation and gene expression. In general, however, insulin resistance refers to primarily decreased insulin-mediated glucose uptake. For the measurement of insulin resistance, the most widely accepted research method is the euglycemic insulin clamp technique [40], as measurements are performed at a steady state of both insulin and glucose concentrations.

The main site of insulin resistance in type 2 diabetes is skeletal muscle, since 70-80% of the decrease in whole body glucose metabolism in patients with type 2 diabetes can be accounted for by decreased muscle glucose uptake [41]. Although insulin stimulated glucose oxidation can be impaired in type 2 diabetes, this represents a relatively late event, whether measured using indirect calorimetry [41] or as glycolytic flux using the tritiated water technique [42]. Reduced glucose-induced thermogenesis and reduced maximal aerobic capacity have also been demonstrated in patients with type 2 diabetes and their nondiabetic offspring [43]. Nevertheless, the major manifestation of peripheral insulin resistance in individuals with type 2 diabetes is the decreased rate of muscle glycogen synthesis, as determined by subtracting the rate of glucose oxidation from total glucose uptake [42, 44] or by *in vivo* NMR analysis of glycogen [45].

The decrease in insulin-stimulated glycogen synthesis could result from impaired glucose transport/phosphorylation [46] or glycogen synthesis [47, 48]. Which defect may be more important in insulin resistance is still being debated. Intracellular glucose-6-phosphate is an intermediary metabolite between glucose transport and glycogen synthesis, so its intracellular concentration will respond to the relative activities of these two steps. In the event of decreased activity of glycogen synthase in diabetes, glucose-6-phosphate concentrations in patients with diabetes would be expected to increase relative to those of normal individuals. Since no change in muscle glucose-6-phosphate was observed in patients with type 2 diabetes, and an increase in this metabolite was seen in healthy individuals during a hyperinsulinemic/hyperglycemic clamp, Shulman et al. suggested that impaired glucose transport is the rate limiting step responsible for decreased insulin-stimulated muscle glucose metabolism in type 2 diabetes [49]. However, when absolute glucose disposal rates were matched in diabetic patients during a hyperglycemic insulin clamp with those in control subjects during a euglycemic insulin clamp, increased muscle glucose-6-phosphate levels were comparable in type 2 diabetic patients and healthy control subjects [50]. These results point at the muscle glycogen synthase as the primary site of muscle insulin resistance. In accordance with this, muscle glucose-6-phosphate levels were higher in diabetic rats compared to normal rats matched for absolute glucose disposal rates [51]. Further, defects in glucose uptake and glycogen synthesis are evident in human skeletal muscle cultures when glycogen synthase gene expression was inactivated with antisense oligonucleotides [52].

Taken together, defects in both glucose transport and glycogen synthesis can be demonstrated in patients with type 2 diabetes. Thus, it is likely that both defects may exist independently or simultaneously. It has also been suggested that glucose transport is more important in glucose disposal at low insulin levels whereas glycogen synthesis predominates at high insulin levels [53]. These dual defects could point to the existence of diverse upstream defects in insulin signalling. Indeed, insulin signalling to PI 3-kinase is reduced by about 50-60% in skeletal muscle of patients with type 2 diabetes [9]. Little is known about the mechanism(s) of insulin resistance in type 1 diabetes. Given the presence of insulin resistance in individuals at risk before and after the onset of type 1 diabetes (see Chapter 9) and the curvilinear relationship between insulin secretion and insulin action [54], one would speculate that improvement in insulin sensitivity would be beneficial in the treatment of type 1 diabetes.

## Molecular Mechanisms of Muscle Insulin Resistance

The metabolic defects leading to insulin resistance are the consequence of changes in gene sequences, gene expression and/or protein modification. Thus, identification of specific changes affecting insulin action and glucose metabolism in patients with insulin resistance and type 2 diabetes and in diabetic animal models would provide the opportunity to understand the pathophysiology of the disease.

### Insulin Receptor

As the first step in insulin action, the insulin receptor was considered a plausible candidate gene for insulin resistance. A number of point mutations in the insulin-receptor gene have been identified in patients with genetic syndromes of extreme insulin resistance such as leprechaunism or the Type A syndrome of insulin resistance. Some of these point mutations had functional consequences and cause different forms of receptor defects of decreased receptor mRNA levels, impaired transport of the receptor to the cell surface and truncated receptor lacking a transmembrane domain [55]. However, these naturally occurring mutations of the insulin receptor are rare, and hence do not appear to play a major role in the development of common type 2 diabetes. The insulin receptor exists as two alternative splicing isoforms which differ by the absence (HIR-A or $Ex11^-$) or presence (HIR-B or $Ex11^+$) of 12 amino acids at the COOH-terminus of the α-subunit [56, 57]. Whereas $Ex11^+$ has lower binding affinity for insulin and IGF-II, and lower rates of internalization and recycling, it has higher tyrosine kinase activity compared to Ex11[-58]. Some studies showed increased mRNA and protein levels of $Ex11^+$ in muscle or fat tissue of patients with type 2 diabetes [59] and in skeletal muscle and cultured muscle cells from insulin resistant patients with myotonic dystrophy [60], while others showed no difference in $Ex11^+$ mRNA levels between control and diabetic subjects [59]. Thus, the specific role of each isoform of the insulin receptor in the development of insulin resistance remains to be defined.

## Insulin Receptor Substrate-1/-2 and PI 3-Kinase

A Gly972→Arg polymorphism (G972R) of the IRS-1 gene was reported to be associated with type 2 diabetes [61], and was implicated in reduced insulin signalling [62] as well as in β-cell dysfunction [63]. Apart from this, no consistent mutations have been found in IRS-2, Shc or PI3-kinase genes responsible for muscle insulin resistance in type 2 diabetes [64-66]. The G972R polymorphism of IRS-1 lies between two potential tyrosine phosphorylation sites involved in binding of the p85 subunit of PI3-kinase to IRS-1, and potentially influences such binding. Indeed, expression of the G972R variant of IRS-1 causes a defect in p85 binding to IRS-1 and a decrease in IRS-1-associated PI3-kinase activity [62].

Other potentially important sites of IRS-1 include Ser(307), Ser(612), Ser(632), Ser(662), Ser(731), and Ser(789), which may mediate an inhibitory effect on insulin signalling. Ser(307) is adjacent to the PTB domain of IRS-1, which lies C-terminally to the PH domain in the N terminus of IRS-1. The PH domain targets IRS-1 to the plasma membrane and allows the PTB domain to bind to a phosphorylated Tyr in the JM domain of the insulin receptor to form functional contact between the two proteins [67]. It is possible that phosphorylation of Ser(307) impairs this functional interaction and thus inhibits insulin signalling [68]. In keeping with this view, it has been suggested that the TNFα-mediated inhibition of IRS-1 tyrosine phosphorylation involves, at least in part, Ser(307) phosphorylation through activation of JNK [69]. Similarly, since Ser(612), Ser(632), Ser(662), Ser(731) and Ser(789) are located close to the major tyrosine phosphorylation sites of IRS-1 involved in the PI 3-kinase binding, phosphorylation of these serine residues could affect IRS-1 binding to and/or activation of PI 3-kinase and impair insulin action [70]. Indeed, increased Ser(789) phosphorylation of IRS-1 has been observed in livers of genetically insulin-resistant rats [71]. However, not all IRS-1 serine phosphorylation is inhibitory. To the contrary, phosphorylation of Ser(265), Ser(302), Ser(325), and Ser(358) by protein kinase B protects IRS-1 from the action of Tyr phosphatases and maintains the substrate in its Tyr-phosphorylated, signalling-active form [72]. Together, these studies suggest that increased phosphorylation of some but not all serine residues of IRS-1 could represent a mechanism for the development of insulin resistance, and may provide a pharmaceutical target for treatment of the disease.

Decreased protein levels of IRS-1 and IRS-2 have been reported in muscle from obese humans and insulin resistant animals [73]. The decrease in IRS-1/-2 proteins may not be the result of reduced gene expression, because no significant difference was seen in mRNA levels of IRS-1, IRS-2 or Shc in skeletal muscle of people with type 2 diabetes relative to control subjects, despite the ability of insulin to downregulate mRNA expression of these substrates [74]. Therefore, changes in protein degradation but not gene expression may be the underlying mechanism for the decrease in IRS proteins in the diabetic state. Given the recent identification of calpain 10 as a putative candidate gene for type 2 diabetes [75], it is interesting to note that calpains have been ascribed a role in insulin-mediated breakdown of the IRS protein [76]. Nevertheless, a causal relationship between decreased IRS protein content and the development of insulin resistance remains to be established.

## Other Genes with Altered Expression in Type 2 Diabetes

There is a growing list of abnormally expressed genes in muscle of patients with insulin resistance and type 2 diabetes. The genes with increased expression include PED/PEA-15, PC1 and Rad. The increased gene expression of PED/PEA-15 has been reported in fibroblasts and skeletal muscle from people with type 2 diabetes [77]. In vitro overexpression of the PED/PEA-15 gene showed an inhibitory effect on insulin-stimulated glucose uptake and GLUT 4 translocaton in L6 muscle cells [77]. PC-1 is a membrane glycoportein with pyrophosphatase activity that seems to act as an intrinsic inhibitor of insulin receptor tyrosin kinase activity [78]. Rad belongs to a Ras superfamily of GTPases and in vitro has a GTP-hydrolyzing activity [79]. Overexpression of Rad in cultured myotubes and adipocytes decreases insulin-mediated glucose uptake [80].

Among genes with decreased expression in skeletal muscle of individuals with type 2 diabetes are PI3-kinase, GLUT 4, Hexokinase II and glycogen synthase [81-83]. More recently, a decrease in gene expression of the cysteine proteinase cathepsin L was observed in muscle in type 2 diabetes [84]. Although the functional consequence of altered cathepsin L gene expression remains to be defined, it is interesting to note that the recently cloned type 2 diabetes candidate gene calpain 10 is also a cysteine proteinase, and that the lower muscle calpain 10 mRNA level was associated with lower rate of 24 h carbohydrate oxidation in humans with normal glucose tolerance [75]. These results could suggest a possible role for cysteine proteinases in glucose metabolism.

## Glycogen Synthase

It is well known that muscle glycogen synthase activity is impaired in patients with type 2 diabetes; however, it is not known whether this defect is inherited or acquired. The evidence for a genetic defect comes from: (1) impaired muscle glycogen synthase activity in first-degree relatives of patients with type 2 diabetes [50];[47]; (2) an association of a XbaI polymorphism in the skeletal muscle glycogen synthase gene with type 2 diabetes and features of insulin resistance [85]; (3) the genetic linkage between the development of glucose intolerance in response to high fat feeding and the glycogen synthase region on chromosome 7 in C57BL/6J mice [86]; and (4) decreased expression of the glycogen synthase gene in cultured skeletal muscle cells [87]. Environmental factors may also play a role in impaired glycogen synthesis in patients with type 2 diabetes. In keeping with this view, chronic exposure of cultured human skeletal muscle cells from normal subjects to high insulin and/or glucose impaired glycogen synthase activity [87]. Further, high fat-feeding of mice and rats is known to induce insulin resistance which includes changes in glycogen synthase activity [84]. A twin study showed that glycogen synthase activity and gene expression were increased by insulin in muscle after an insulin clamp of healthy control subjects, and these responses were diminished in muscle of twins with type 2 diabetes but not in their nondiabetic monozygotic co-twins compared to the control subjects [82]. These results suggest that impaired stimulation of glycogen synthase activity and mRNA expression by insulin is most likely an acquired defect secondary to the derangement of glucose metabolism in type 2 diabetes.

## GLUT4

Decreased GLUT4 translocation to cell surface has also been demonstrated in skeletal muscle of patients with type 2 diabetes [8, 9, 88], as well as in cultured L6 muscle cells under high glucose and insulin conditions [89]. This defect may not result from pretranslational changes of the GLUT 4 gene, because no changes in either GLUT4 gene expression [90] or its gene sequence [91, 92] were seen in skeletal muscle of patients with insulin resistance and type 2 diabetes. In line with this, overexpression of the GLUT4 transgene in skeletal muscle of obese mice improves glucose tolerance but does not prevent insulin resistance [93]. Thus, it is more likely that the observed defect of GLUT4 translocation results from altered insulin signalling cascades as discussed above and/or abnormal GLUT4 traffic machinery. To support this view, Garvey et al. reported abnormal accumulation of GLUT4 protein in a dense membrane fraction in the basal state, and an abnormal subcellular distribution of GLUT4 in response to insulin in skeletal muscle of insulin-resistant patients with or without type 2 diabetes [8]. The observation of this translocation defect in muscle of diabetic and nondiabetic patients would suggest that it may represent an early and perhaps a primary defect. A similar defect has also been seen in adipocytes of patients with type 2 diabetes [94]. The underlying mechanism for GLUT4 translocation defect may include those molecules that are part of the GLUT4 traffic machinery such as soluble N-ethylmaleimide attachment protein receptors (SNAREs) and their accessory proteins. Indeed, altered expression of the vesicle-associated membrane protein-2 (VAMP-2), t-SNARE syntaxin 4 and accessory protein Munc18c was observed with muscle insulin resistance in animal studies [95, 96]. The recently identified protein TUG as a GLUT4 tether that retains GLUT4 in the intracelluar space also represents a interesting candidate for a GLUT 4 traffic defect [97]. Nevertheless, the exact molecular mechansim for muscle insulin resistance remains unclear.

In addition to insulin resistance of skeletal muscle and fat, “insulin resistance” may also occur in the β cell of the pancreas. The BIRKO (β cell insulin receptor knockout) mice clearly demonstrated that insulin is required for the normal functioning of pancreatic β cells. These mice selectively lose glucose-stimulated insulin secretion with progressive impairment of glucose tolerance [98]. Components of the insulin signalling pathway, i.e. IRS-1/2[99, 100], and Akt [101]are present in the β cells and plays an important role in regulating their growth and differentiation [102]. Furthmore, recent studies have implicated polymorphism of transcription factors, which are known to cause monogenetic forms of diabetes such as MODY, in the pathogenesis of insulin resistance of the β cells and development of type 2 diabetes. MODY 1 is caused by mutations in hepatocyte nuclear factor-4α (HNF4α), and interestingly, single nucleotide polymorphism (SNP) near the promoter of HNF4α is associated with increased risk of developing type 2 diabetes in the Finnish population [103], and a loss-of-function mutation in the HNF4α gene is associated with type 2 diabetes in a Japanese population [104]. The homeodomain-containing protein, insulin promoter factor-1 (IPF-1), also known as PDX1, is a transcription factor that is critical for development of the pancreas, and dominant negative mutation of PDX1 causes MODY 4 [105]. Several mutations in PDX1 that are not associated with MODY have been shown to increase the risk of developing type 2 diabetes [106, 107]. These mutations lead to decreased binding activity to the human insulin gene promoter. Heterozygous mutations of these transcription factors can also interact in a synergistic fashion to cause type 2 diabetes [108]. Recent studies have began to shed light on the network of transcription factors that participate in the " regulatory circuits" in the pancreas. Taking advantage of microarray technology, Odom et al has recently found that HNF1α, HNF4α, and HNF6, which were known to function cooperatively in liver, also form a network of multicomponent and feedforward regulatory loop in the pancreas [109]. Consistent with previous studies, it was found that HNF1α and HNF4 regulate each other's expression [108, 109]. Based on the regulatory network in liver, a model that integrates the activities of insulin and transcription factors in regulation of pancreatic β cell function has been proposed by Kulkarni and Kahn: insulin can regulate the activity of HNF3β, which controls HNF4α, HNF1α, and PDX-1 expression [110]. HNF1β also regulates PDX-1 and HNF4α. Therefore, similar circuitry is operating in both the liver and the pancreas, linking hepatic insulin resistance to defective insulin secretion and type 2 diabetes [111].

## In Vitro and In Vivo Models of Insulin Resistance

### High Glucose and/or High Insulin and Insulin Resistance

In insulin resistant individuals, the failure to increase glucose disposal into peripheral tissues in response to insulin leads to chronic (albeit subclinical) elevation in glucose followed by a compensatory rise in insulin [36, 112]. A striking correlation between hyperglycaemia and exacerbation of insulin resistance has been demonstrated [113, 114]. In patients with type 1 and type 2 diabetes, improvements in blood glucose control also enhance insulin sensitivity [115]. In pancreatectomized diabetic animals, reversal of hyperglycaemia by phlorizin (an inhibitor of renal glucose re-uptake) improves insulin sensitivity [116, 117]. In ZDF rats (an obese, hyperinsulinemic diabetic animal model) amelioration of hyperglycaemia by another renal glucose transporter inhibitor (T-1095) induced partial recovery of the defects in glucose uptake into adipocytes and hepatic glucose production rate, without significant improvement of muscle glucose utilization. This suggests that in ZDF rats, hyperglycaemia has significant contribution to insulin resistance of the liver and adipocytes but not muscles [118]. These studies illustrate that hyperglycaemia can reduce insulin action in diverse tissues. In control rats, prolonged glucose infusion led to translocation of PKC–βI, βII, α, and θ to the plasma membrane [119]. Translocation of PKC θ has been linked to serine phosphorylation of IRS-1, which would down regulate IRS-1 tyrosine phosphorylation and its ability to recruit downstream signalling molecules [120]. Whether these molecular events are sufficient to explain the hyperglycaemia-induced insulin resistance remains to be determined.

Isolated rat muscles treated with high glucose and high insulin *in vitro* display reduced insulin-stimulated glucose uptake, glycogen synthesis, and Akt phosphorylation but not PI3 kinase activity. The defect in Akt also occurred in muscles incubated only with high glucose. It is possible that hyperglycaemia-mediated impairment of insulin action in the muscle may be related to inhibition of Akt but independent of PI3-kinase [121].

In L6 myotubes pretreated with high glucose and insulin *in vitro*, the effects on the insulin signalling pathways and regulation of GLUT4 translocation were also examined [89, 122]. In the presence of high glucose and insulin, there was a significant reduction of insulin receptor and IRS-1 protein expression and insulin-stimulated tyrosine phosphorylation. There was also impaired insulin-stimulated PI3-kinase activity and Akt activation. Interestingly, high glucose and insulin interfered with insulin-mediated actin remodeling, which participates in insulin-mediated GLUT4 translocation to the plasma membrane, and a corresponding reduction in GLUT4 translocation was observed. Consistent with the study in isolated rat muscles [121], exposure of L6 myotubes to high glucose alone did not affect insulin-stimulated glucose transport (Huang, C. and Klip, A., unpublished data). Similarly, in 3T3-L1 adipocytes and primary cultured rat adipocytes, pretreatment with high glucose and insulin diminished insulin stimulated glucose transport, GLUT4 translocation to the plasma membrane, IRS-1 tyrosine phosphorylation and PI3-kinase activity [123]. Of note, however, GLUT4 protein expression was also reduced as observed in mature adipocytes, but not in muscle of patients with type 2 diabetes.

## Circulating Factors Contributing to Insulin Resistance

***Free Fatty Acids***

Elevation in serum FFAs is a common feature of obesity and type 2 diabetes, and it is strongly associated with decreased insulin sensitivity. In some cases, elevated FFA levels are predictive of progression from glucose intolerance to type 2 diabetes [45].

Both animal and human studies show that an acute elevation of serum FFA levels (as induced by a lipid infusion) can decrease insulin-stimulated glucose uptake in 2-4 h [124-126]. In healthy human volunteers, acute elevation of FFAs induced by a lipid infusion led to a biphasic defect: first, inhibition of insulin-stimulated glucose uptake or phosphorylation occurs within 3-4 h of lipid infusion while glycogen synthase activity is still normal; and second, prolonging the lipid infusion to 6 h resulted in inhibition of glycogen synthase activity [127].

The possible mechanistic link between elevated FFAs and insulin resistance was first proposed by Randle, who hypothesized that increased FFA oxidation caused elevation of the intra-mitochondrial acetyl-CoA/CoA and $NADH/NAD^+$ ratios leading to inactivation of pyruvate dehydrogenase [128]. This is followed by an increase in citrate, which inhibits phosphofructokinase, resulting in accumulation of glucose-6-phosphate. Elevated glucose-6-phosphate inhibits hexokinase, consequently lowering net glucose uptake. This hypothesis has been challenged recently because in muscle, intracellular glucose-6-phosphate level drop rather than rise during lipid infusion [45].

Defects along the insulin signalling pathway have been observed in obesity, lipid- infused healthy volunteers, fat fed or lipid-infused animals, and FFA-treated cell culture systems. In vitro studies using either muscle or adipose cell lines have provided some insight into the cross-talk between FFA and insulin signalling [129-132]. Pretreatment of C2C12 (mouse) myotubes with palmitate for 16-18 hours diminished insulin-stimulated glycogen synthesis and Akt/PKB activation, with no effect on insulin-mediated IRS-1 tyrosine phosphorylation and PI3-K activation. Ceramide reproduced all of these effects, suggesting that palmitate exert its effects through ceramide [130]. In contrast, pretreatment with unsaturated FFA led to a small inhibition of PI3-K activity, with no effect on either insulin-stimulated Akt/PKB activation or glycogen synthesis. A proposed mechanism is that palmitate increases the activity of PP2A family serine/threonine phosphatase, causing dephosphorylation of Akt/PKB, which manifested in a decrease in glycogen synthesis [133].

Lipid species can also function as signalling intermediates. Palmitate, oleate and linoleate are converted to long-chain acyl-CoAs in the cytosol, transported into the mitochondria, and metabolized either through β oxidation or used to form triglycerides, phospholipids, and second messengers such as diacylglycerol (DAG). FFA can activate PKC directly or via DAG, leading to translocation of these enzymes to the plasma membrane. Most studies suggest that activation of conventional (PKCα, β, and σ) and novel PKCs (PKCδ, ε, θ, and η) is primarily associated with insulin resistance, most likely via increasing the serine/threonine phosphorylation of IR and/or IRS-1, which inhibit propagation of insulin signalling [126]. Furthermore, atypical PKCs (PKCζ and PKCλ) may participate in positive regulation of insulin-stimulated glucose metabolism [33].

In conclusion, there is strong evidence for interactions and perhaps causalities between obesity, elevated free fatty acid level, insulin resistance, and type 2 diabetes. The precise role if any of PKCs and PP2A as mediators of high-fat-induced insulin resistance provide awaits further clarification.

### *TNFα*

TNFα is a cytokine with various biological actions including induction of anorexia and weight loss. There is growing evidence that it plays a significant role in insulin resistance. TNFα interacts with two cell-surface receptors, p55 and p75 (p60 and p80 in human). Some, but not all studies, have found an elevation in both TNFα and TNFα-receptor expression in obese subjects, which decreases following weight loss [134]. TNFα is also expressed at higher levels in muscles of insulin resistant and diabetic patients, where an inverse linear relationship between maximal glucose disposal rate and muscle TNF levels was observed [135]. Antibodies to TNF receptor infused into ZDF rats improved insulin-stimulated glucose disposal, tyrosine phosphorylation of the insulin receptor and IRS-1 [136]. TNFα$^{-/-}$ mice are more resistant to high fat diet-induced weight gain and hyperinsulinemia compared to TNFα$^{+/+}$ obese mice, and have significantly higher insulin sensitivity and insulin receptor autophosphorylation. These results suggest that in the absence of TNFα, the insulin receptor is protected from the negative effects of obesity [137]. TNFα receptor (p55$^{-/-}$/p75$^{-/-}$) knockout in ob/ob (leptin knockout) mice also caused improved insulin sensitivity compared to p55$^{+/+}$/p75$^{+/+}$ mice [137]. However, these results were not reproduced in a second study with p55$^{-/-}$/p75$^{-/-}$ mice [138]. In human cultured adipocytes, both receptors can independently mediate inhibition of insulin-stimulated glucose transport [139]. Taken together, these findings suggest that both TNFα and its receptors may be involved in the development of insulin resistance, but it is not known if they participate directly in insulin resistance observed in diabetes in human.

Despite the controversy, several possible mechanisms for TNFα induced insulin resistance have been proposed. In adipocytes and hepatocytes in culture, TNFα elevated the serine phosphorylation of IRS-1 [131], which may in turn negatively regulate insulin signalling pathway by inhibition of tyrosine phosphorylation of IRS-1 and/or induction of a proteasome-mediated degradation of IRS-1. TNFα also activates JNK, IKK, Akt, and mTOR, which are all serine kinases that can directly or indirectly phosphorylate IRS-1 [14, 69, 140].

Inhibition of JNK activity can reduce the TNFα induced IRS-1 serine phosphorylation [141]. In both diet-induced and genetic models of obesity-associated insulin resistance, there is abnormally elevated JNK activity, and the absence of JNK1 provided protection from obesity-induced insulin resistance. Importantly, obese $JNK^{+/+}$ mice have markedly increased IRS-1 serine 307 phosphorylation, and such increase was not observed in the obese $JNK^{-/-}$ mice, indicating that serine 307 of IRS-1 is a target of JNK *in vivo*[142]. Therefore, JNK-1 may be an attractive therapeutic target for obesity-induced insulin resistance.

Another link between TNFα and insulin resistance maybe IKKβ. TNFα activates, and salicylate and aspirin inhibit IKKβ activity [143]. It has been shown that in two genetically obese animals (*ob/ob* mice and *ZDF* rats) basal IKKβ activity was elevated, and after 3-4 weeks of high dose salicylate, glucose tolerance and triglyceride levels improved and serum FFA levels dropped. In *ZDF* rats, salicylate treatment reversed the decrease in insulin-mediated insulin receptor and Akt phosphorylation in the muscle. Activation or over-expression of IKKβ decreased insulin signalling, which was reversed by salicylate, and heterozygous deletion of *Ikk*β protected against the development of high-fat feeding induced insulin resistance [144]. In 3T3-L1 adipocytes, TNFα pretreatment lowered insulin-stimulated tyrosine phosphorylation of the IR and IRS, an effect reversed by prior treatment with salicylate [144]. A potential link between IKKβ and insulin resistance is PKC$\theta$. Animals rendered insulin resistant by FFA infusion have high PKC$\theta$ activity [120, 145], and PKC$\theta$ activates IKK/NF-κB in certain cells [146]. In rats, the FFA induced reduction in insulin-stimulated glucose uptake and activation of IRS-1 associated PI 3-kinase activity of skeletal muscle was prevented by pretreatment with salicylate. Furthermore, heterozygous IKKβ knockout mice protected from developing the lipid infusion-induced insulin resistance [147]. These studies support a strong association between elevation in fatty acids and TNFα to activation of PKC$\theta$ and IKKβ and subsequent down-regulation of the insulin signalling pathway.

In humans, recent studies suggest that obesity-related type 2 diabetes is a low-grade chronic inflammatory state, with elevated levels of TNFα and other cytokines, both of which can increase nitric oxide (NO) production through increase expression of iNOS in cultured myocytes, rat muscles, and adipocytes [148, 149]. In animal models of obesity, iNOS expression is elevated in muscle and fat. The iNOS2 knockout ($Nos2^{-/-}$) mice are protected from developing high fat-induced insulin resistance [150]. High fat feeding induced iNOS production in obese wild-type mice, which was associated with impaired insulin mediated activation of PI3-K and Akt. These defects did not occur in high-fat-fed $Nos2^{-/-}$ mice, suggesting that iNOS may be involved in diet-induced obesity associated insulin resistance. The mechanism of regulation and interaction between other inflammatory cytokines, iNOS, and the insulin signalling pathway is yet to be determined.

***Oxidative Stress***

Both FFA and hyperglycaemia have been associated with an increase in reactive oxygen species (ROS) and oxidative stress, although the exact source(s) of ROS production is not known [151]. Oxidative stress is defined as an imbalance between the production of reactive oxygen and nitrogen species and antioxidant, leading to damage to DNA, protein, and lipids, which have been observed in diabetic patients [152]. More interestingly, increased oxidative stress impairs the insulin signalling pathway as follows: exposure of 3T3-L1 adipocytes to low concentrations of $H_2O_2$ -inhibited insulin-stimulated GLUT4 translocation and glucose uptake [153]. Although IRS-1 tyrosine phosphorylation and association of IRS-1 with PI3-K was not impaired, oxidative stress prevented the insulin-mediated increase of IRS-1-associated PI3-K activity in intracellular membranes as well as Akt phosphorylation, suggesting that a mis-targeting of PI3-K molecules had occurred and prevented down-stream signalling [154].

***Growth Hormone***

Growth hormone (GH) has a wide spectrum of metabolic effects, including stimulation of lipolysis, protein synthesis, and hepatic glucose production and reduction of insulin-stimulated glucose utilization. Chronic elevation of GH can promote insulin resistance and may contribute to the development of diabetes [155, 156].

Interestingly, GH has both insulin mimetic and anti-insulin effects. Acute stimulation with GH increases GLUT4 translocation and glucose uptake into adipocytes in culture. Furthermore, GH potentiates tyrosine phosphorylation of IRS-1 in a time and dose-dependent manner, and elevates IRS-1 associated PI3-kinase activity by 4-fold [156, 157]. However, activation of PI3-kinase may not be required for GH-mediated glucose uptake, since over-expression of a inactive regulatory subunit of PI3-kinase or treatment with the PI3-kinase inhibitor wortmannin, had no effect on GH-induced GLUT4 translocation and glucose uptake [158].

Details on the molecular mechanisms of GH-induced insulin resistance are emerging. In rats chronically treated with GH, there is a reduction in insulin-stimulated tyrosine phosphorylation of IR, IRS-1 and IRS-2, as well as a reduction in the interaction between PI3-kinase and the IRS proteins in liver and muscle[159]. In skeletal muscle of transgenic mice overexpressing GH, there is a drop in IR content, and tyrosine phosphorylation of IR, IRS-1, and PI3-kinase activity[160]. In 3T3-L1 adipocytes, chronic exposure to GH diminished insulin-stimulated glucose transport, Akt phosphorylation and Akt membrane targeting. Surprisingly, pretreatment with GH enhanced tyrosine phosphorylation of IRS-1, association of IRS-1 with the p85 subunit of PI3-kinase, and IRS-1 associated PI3-kinase activity. Specifically, GH induced an increase in the association of p85 with IRS-1 in the cytosol. Therefore, in GH-treated 3T3-L1 adipocytes, there seems to be an uncoupling of the PI3-kinase from its downstream signals as well as an alteration in distribution of the signalling molecules [161]. The discrepancy between the results from whole animal study versus those of adipocytes in culture may stem from secondary changes in the metabolic state associated with GH-induced insulin resistance *in vivo*.

***Glucocorticoids***

The prevalence of diabetes in patients exposed to excessive exogenous and endogenous glucocorticoids has been reported at 20-25% and 80-90%, respectively. In animal models, resistance occurs at the level of the muscle, adipocytes, liver, and pancreatic β cells.

Muscles from rats treated with dexamethasone (DEX) had decreased basal and insulin-stimulated glucose uptake, reduced GLUT4 translocation, and no change in total GLUT4 protein levels. These muscles had impaired IGF-1- and hypoxia-mediated glucose uptake as well, suggesting that DEX-induced defect is not restricted to the insulin signalling pathway, but generalized to intracellular traffic (including that of GLUT4) [162]. In DEX-treated 3T3-L1 adipocytes, the GLUT1 but not GLUT4 protein content was decreased, as well as reduced insulin-stimulated GLUT4 translocation. This was accompanied by a drop in IRS-1 and a rise in IRS-2 protein content and tyrosine phosphorylation. When IRS-1 protein content was normalized using an adenovirus infection system, there was no restoration of insulin-induced glucose uptake. Furthermore, glucose uptake induced by over-expression of PI3-kinase, constitutively active Akt, oxidative stress, AICAR, or osmotic shock were all reduced after dexamethasone treatment [163]. These results suggest that dexamethasone-induced insulin resistance resides beyond the early insulin signalling pathway, possibly at the final steps regulating GLUT4 translocation or fusion with the plasma membrane.

Excessive glucocorticoid interferes with insulin-mediated suppression of hepatic glucose production, in part by increasing the expression of gluconeogenic enzymes (phosphoenolpyruvate carboxykinase and glucose 6-phosphatase) [164]. Furthermore, hepatic expression of PPAR-α may contribute to DEX-induced insulin resistance [165].

***Adipokines and Insulin Resistance***

Adipocytes secrete several factors that participate in regulation of energy homeostatsis and possibly insulin signalling in the periphery. Most notably are adiponectin [166] and leptin. Adiponectin, also known as Acrp30, is a 30 kDa complement-related protein synthesized exclusively by adipocytes [167]. Serum concentrations of adiponectin correlate inversely with BMI, insulin sensitivity, and fasting insulin levels [168, 169]. Furthermore, the presence of coronary artery disease is associated with even lower serum adiponectin levels [170]. Animal studies have shown that recombinant adiponectin can increase muscle fatty acid oxidation, decrease serum FFA, glucose, triglycerides, suppress hepatic glucose production, and ameliorate insulin resistance in mice [171-174]. Furthermore, adiponectin-deficient transgenic mice has elevated serum level of TNFα and become severely insulin resistant when challenged with a high-fat and high-sucrose diet [175], and exhibited more neointimal formation in response to external vascular injury, supporting an anti-atherogenic role of adiponectin [176]. The mechanism of adiponectin action seems to be via activation of 5'-AMP-activated protein kinase (AMPK) and increase fatty-acid oxidation in liver and skeletal muscles [177]. Adiponectin receptors were recently identified; receptor 1 (AdipoR1) is mainly expressed in skeletal muscle and receptor 2 (AdipoR2) is predominantly expressed in the liver [178]. This study found that in addition to activation of AMPK, adiponectin also activates p38 mitogen-activated protein kinase (p38MAPK). Adiponectin stimulated fatty-acid oxidation and glucose uptake in myocytes were partially reduced by dominant negative mutants of AMPK or specific inhibitor of p38MAPK, suggesting that both AMPK and p38MAPK participate in adiponectin-stimulated fatty-acid oxidation and glucose uptake in muscles. Interestingly, expression of the AdipoR1/2 receptors in insulin resistant ob/ob mice was significantly decreased in skeletal muscles and adipocytes, point to the possibility of "adiponectin resistance" in insulin resistance [179].

Whether a causal relationship exists between adiponectin and insulin sensitivity is unclear. A majority of studies have found good predictive value between adiponectin gene polymorphism and serum adiponectin levels, as well as strong association of low adiponectin levels with development of insulin resistance and type 2 diabetes [180-183]. But there is no direct proof that polymorphism of the adiponectin gene predicts type 2 diabetes [175, 182, 184].

Another important adipokine is leptin. Since cloning of the leptin gene in 1994, a huge body of literature has devoted to the understanding its physiological functions. Leptin regulates appetite and energy expenditure and its main biological function is to maintain energy homeostasis when caloric intake is reduced [185]. There is no unifying conclusion about the relationship between leptin and insulin resistance, since most *in vivo* studies suggest that leptin improves insulin sensitivity while studies in vitro suggest that it attenuates insulin activity [186]. Cross sectional studies in human have shown that patients with lower leptin levels gained more weight over time, and it has been estimated that 5-10% of obese patients are "hypoleptinemic" [187]. However, most obese patients have high serum leptin levels, suggesting that obesity might be associated with "leptin resistance" [188]. Studies in isolated rat skeletal muscles showed that exposure to leptin ex vivo had no effect on glucose uptake [189], but in vivo (both intravenous [IV] and intracerebroventricular [ICV]) administration of leptin in mice increased glucose flux in muscles [190], suggesting that the effect of leptin on glucose flux is through central nervous system. Indeed, leptin can inhibit AMPK activity in arcuate and paraventricular hypothalamus, and inhibition of AMPK activity in hypothalamus by leptin, insulin, or refeeding reduces appetite [191]. The same group showed that leptin can increase fatty-acid oxidation when administered either IV or ICV, through activation of AMPK in the skeletal muscles [192], and activation of AMPK by a variety of mechanism can increase glucose flux into muscles [193].

There are several potential points of cross-talk between the insulin signalling pathway and leptin signalling, since both hormones recruits some of the same signalling molecules, such as IRS protein, PI3-kinase [194, 195], Akt, and glycogen synthase kinase [196]. Leptin has been found to attenuate insulin signalling in hepatocyte [197], fibroblasts, and skeletal muscle [198] cells in culture. Conversely, chronic hyperinsulinemia can impair leptin action by inhibiting leptin-induced insulin secretion [199].

In summary, adipokines can function at several levels: first, they have direct effect on glucose metabolism in liver and muscles, most likely via its regulation on AMPK activity and fatty-acid oxidation. Second, they act centrally on the hypothalamus to regulate appetite and energy metabolism, interestingly, also through modulation of AMPK activity centrally. Although there is no direct evidence at the present time that primary deficiency of either adiponectin or leptin can cause polygenetic type 2 diabetes, maintenance of adipokines within "normal" or "physiological" range by pharmacological means have shown to improve insulin sensitivity. A better understanding of the interaction between adipokine and the insulin signalling pathway both in the CNS and the peripheral will provide novel targets for modulation of whole body glucose homeostasis.

## CONCLUSIONS

Insulin resistance is defined as the failure of insulin to increase glucose disposal appropriately. Insulin regulates glucose disposal via increasing glucose uptake into fat and skeletal muscles, mainly through GLUT4. Studies over the past decade have shown that insulin receptor, insulin receptor substrates (IRS-1/2), PI3-K, Akt/PKB, and possibly, atypical PKC, all play significant roles in the regulation of glucose uptake. Furthermore, in insulin resistant conditions, the protein levels, intracellular localization, or activities of these molecules are reduced. Emerging "new players" in insulin resistance include JNK, IKKβ, and PKCθ.

Circulating factors contributing to insulin resistance include FFA, TNFα, GH, and glucocorticoids. TNFα and other inflammatory cytokines can activate PKCθ, JNK, IKKβ, and Akt, all of which can potentially increase serine phosphorylation of insulin receptor and IRS-1, therefore reducing the activities of these molecules and resulting in decreased glucose uptake. Elevated FFA can induce insulin resistance via similar mechanisms. Excessive GH causes a reduction in the activities of IR/IRS-1/PI 3-kinase/Akt, but the mechanism(s) mediating these changes has yet to be identified. Lastly, glucocorticoid-induced insulin resistance may have its main culprit at the level of hepatic glucose production via PPARα. Understanding the interactions among these factors, and their contribution to deteriorating glucose homeostasis, will lead to development of effective preventive and therapeutic strategies against insulin resistance and type 2 diabetes.

## References

[1] Klip A MA. Regulation of glucose transporters by insulin and exercise: cellular effects and implications for diabetes. Handbook of physiology - *The endocrine pancreas and regulation of metabolism,* 2002:451-494.

[2] Rudich A, Konrad D, Torok D, et al. Indinavir uncovers different contributions of GLUT4 and GLUT1 towards glucose uptake in muscle and fat cells and tissues. *Diabetologia* 2003; 46:649-58.

[3] Mitsumoto Y, Klip A. Development regulation of the subcellular distribution and glycosylation of GLUT1 and GLUT4 glucose transporters during myogenesis of L6 muscle cells. *J Biol Chem* 1992; 267:4957-62.

[4] Marette A, Richardson JM, Ramlal T, et al. Abundance, localization, and insulin-induced translocation of glucose transporters in red and white muscle. *Am J Physiol* 1992; 263:C443-52.

[5] Cushman S, Wardzala L. Potential mechanism of insulin action on glucose transport in the isolated rat adipose cell. Apparent translocation of intracellular transport systems to the plasma membrane. *J. Biol. Chem.* 1980; 255:4758-4762.

[6] Satoh S, Nishimura H, Clark A, et al. Use of bismannose photolabel to elucidate insulin-regulated GLUT4 subcellular trafficking kinetics in rat adipose cells. Evidence that exocytosis is a critical site of hormone action. *J. Biol. Chem.* 1993; 268:17820-17829.

[7] Ueyama A, Yaworsky KL, Wang Q, Ebina Y, Klip A. GLUT-4myc ectopic expression in L6 myoblasts generates a GLUT-4- specific pool conferring insulin sensitivity. *Am J Physiol* 1999; 277:E572-8.

[8] Garvey WT, Maianu L, Zhu JH, Brechtel-Hook G, Wallace P, Baron AD. Evidence for defects in the trafficking and translocation of GLUT4 glucose transporters in skeletal muscle as a cause of human insulin resistance. *J Clin Invest* 1998; 101:2377-86.

[9] Zierath JR, He L, Guma A, Odegoard Wahlstrom E, Klip A, Wallberg-Henriksson H. Insulin action on glucose transport and plasma membrane GLUT4 content in skeletal muscle from patients with NIDDM. *Diabetologia* 1996; 39:1180-9.

[10] Klip A, Ramlal T, Bilan PJ, Cartee GD, Gulve EA, Holloszy JO. Recruitment of GLUT-4 glucose transporters by insulin in diabetic rat skeletal muscle. *Biochem Biophys Res Commun* 1990; 172:728-36.

[11] Saltiel AR. New perspectives into the molecular pathogenesis and treatment of type 2 diabetes. *Cell* 2001; 104:517-29.

[12] Takayama S, White MF, Kahn CR. Phorbol ester-induced serine phosphorylation of the insulin receptor decreases its tyrosine kinase activity. *J Biol Chem* 1988; 263:3440-7.

[13] Strack V, Stoyanov B, Bossenmaier B, Mosthaf L, Kellerer M, Haring HU. Impact of mutations at different serine residues on the tyrosine kinase activity of the insulin receptor. *Biochem Biophys Res Commun* 1997; 239:235-9.

[14] Le Marchand-Brustel Y, Gual P, Gremeaux T, Gonzalez T, Barres R, Tanti JF. Fatty acid-induced insulin resistance: role of insulin receptor substrate 1 serine phosphorylation in the retroregulation of insulin signalling. *Biochem Soc Trans* 2003; 31:1152-6.

[15] Backer JM, Shoelson SE, Weiss MA, et al. The insulin receptor juxtamembrane region contains two independent tyrosine/beta-turn internalization signals. *J Cell Biol* 1992; 118:831-9.

[16] Patti ME, Virkamaki A, Landaker EJ, Kahn CR, Yki-Jarvinen H. Activation of the hexosamine pathway by glucosamine in vivo induces insulin resistance of early postreceptor insulin signaling events in skeletal muscle. *Diabetes* 1999; 48:1562-71.

[17] Sun XJ, Rothenberg P, Kahn CR, et al. Structure of the insulin receptor substrate IRS-1 defines a unique signal transduction protein. *Nature* 1991; 352:73-7.

[18] Backer JM, Schroeder GG, Kahn CR, et al. Insulin stimulation of phosphatidylinositol 3-kinase activity maps to insulin receptor regions required for endogenous substrate phosphorylation. *J Biol Chem* 1992; 267:1367-74.

[19] Cheatham B, Vlahos CJ, Cheatham L, Wang L, Blenis J, Kahn CR. Phosphatidylinositol 3-kinase activation is required for insulin stimulation of pp70 S6 kinase, DNA synthesis, and glucose transporter translocation. *Mol Cell Biol* 1994; 14:4902-11.

[20] Tanti JF, Gremeaux T, Grillo S, et al. Overexpression of a constitutively active form of phosphatidylinositol 3-kinase is sufficient to promote Glut 4 translocation in adipocytes. *J Biol Chem* 1996; 271:25227-32.

[21] Tsakiridis T, McDowell HE, Walker T, et al. Multiple roles of phosphatidylinositol 3-kinase in regulation of glucose transport, amino acid transport, and glucose transporters in L6 skeletal muscle cells. *Endocrinology* 1995; 136:4315-22.

[22] Vanhaesebroeck B, Waterfield MD. Signaling by distinct classes of phosphoinositide 3-kinases. *Exp Cell Res* 1999; 253:239-54.

[23] Corvera S, Czech MP. Direct targets of phosphoinositide 3-kinase products in membrane traffic and signal transduction. *Trends Cell Biol* 1998; 8:442-6.

[24] Cohen P. The Croonian Lecture 1998. Identification of a protein kinase cascade of major importance in insulin signal transduction. *Philos Trans R Soc Lond B Biol Sci* 1999; 354:485-95.

[25] Whiteman EL, Cho H, Birnbaum MJ. Role of Akt/protein kinase B in metabolism. *Trends Endocrinol Metab* 2002; 13:444-51.

[26] Scheid MP, Woodgett JR. PKB/AKT: functional insights from genetic models. *Nat Rev Mol Cell Biol* 2001; 2:760-8.

[27] Kohn AD, Summers SA, Birnbaum MJ, Roth RA. Expression of a constitutively active Akt Ser/Thr kinase in 3T3-L1 adipocytes stimulates glucose uptake and glucose transporter 4 translocation. *J Biol Chem* 1996; 271:31372-8.
[28] Cong LN, Chen H, Li Y, et al. Physiological role of Akt in insulin-stimulated translocation of GLUT4 in transfected rat adipose cells. *Mol Endocrinol* 1997; 11:1881-90.
[29] Kitamura T, Ogawa W, Sakaue H, et al. Requirement for activation of the serine-threonine kinase Akt (protein kinase B) in insulin stimulation of protein synthesis but not of glucose transport. *Mol Cell Biol* 1998; 18:3708-17.
[30] Wang Q, Somwar R, Bilan PJ, et al. Protein kinase B/Akt participates in GLUT4 translocation by insulin in L6 myoblasts. *Mol Cell Biol* 1999; 19:4008-18.
[31] Katome T, Obata T, Matsushima R, et al. Use of RNA interference-mediated gene silencing and adenoviral overexpression to elucidate the roles of AKT/protein kinase B isoforms in insulin actions. *J Biol Chem* 2003; 278:28312-23.
[32] Garofalo RS, Orena SJ, Rafidi K, et al. Severe diabetes, age-dependent loss of adipose tissue, and mild growth deficiency in mice lacking Akt2/PKB beta. *J Clin Invest* 2003; 112:197-208.
[33] Farese RV. Function and dysfunction of aPKC isoforms for glucose transport in insulin-sensitive and insulin-resistant states. *Am J Physiol Endocrinol Metab* 2002; 283:E1-11.
[34] Sano H, Kane S, Sano E, et al. Insulin-stimulated phosphorylation of a Rab GTPase-activating protein regulates GLUT4 translocation. *J Biol Chem* 2003; 278:14599-602.
[35] Foster LJ, Li D, Randhawa VK, Klip A. Insulin accelerates inter-endosomal GLUT4 traffic via phosphatidylinositol 3-kinase and protein kinase B. *J Biol Chem* 2001; 276:44212-21.
[36] Warram JH, Martin BC, Krolewski AS, Soeldner JS, Kahn CR. Slow glucose removal rate and hyperinsulinemia precede the development of type II diabetes in the offspring of diabetic parents. *Ann Intern Med* 1990; 113:909-15.
[37] Eriksson J, Franssila-Kallunki A, Ekstrand A, et al. Early metabolic defects in persons at increased risk for non-insulin-dependent diabetes mellitus. *N Engl J Med* 1989; 321:337-43.
[38] Lillioja S, Mott DM, Howard BV, et al. Impaired glucose tolerance as a disorder of insulin action. Longitudinal and cross-sectional studies in Pima Indians. *N Engl J Med* 1988; 318:1217-25.
[39] Reaven GM, Bernstein R, Davis B, Olefsky JM. Nonketotic diabetes mellitus: insulin deficiency or insulin resistance? *Am J Med* 1976; 60:80-8.
[40] Scheen AJ, Paquot N, Castillo MJ, Lefebvre PJ. How to measure insulin action in vivo. *Diabetes Metab Rev* 1994; 10:151-88.
[41] DeFronzo RA, Jacot E, Jequier E, Maeder E, Wahren J, Felber JP. The effect of insulin on the disposal of intravenous glucose. Results from indirect calorimetry and hepatic and femoral venous catheterization. *Diabetes* 1981; 30:1000-7.
[42] Vaag A, Alford F, Henriksen FL, Christopher M, Beck-Nielsen H. Multiple defects of both hepatic and peripheral intracellular glucose processing contribute to the hyperglycaemia of NIDDM. *Diabetologia* 1995; 38:326-36.
[43] Groop L, Forsblom C, Lehtovirta M, et al. Metabolic consequences of a family history of NIDDM (the Botnia study): evidence for sex-specific parental effects. *Diabetes* 1996; 45:1585-93.

[44] DeFronzo RA, Bonadonna RC, Ferrannini E. Pathogenesis of NIDDM. A balanced overview. *Diabetes Care* 1992; 15:318-68.

[45] Shulman GI. Cellular mechanisms of insulin resistance. *J Clin Invest* 2000; 106:171-6.

[46] Vestergaard H, Bjorbaek C, Hansen T, Larsen FS, Granner DK, Pedersen O. Impaired activity and gene expression of hexokinase II in muscle from non-insulin-dependent diabetes mellitus patients. *J Clin Invest* 1995; 96:2639-45.

[47] Schalin-Jantti C, Harkonen M, Groop LC. Impaired activation of glycogen synthase in people at increased risk for developing NIDDM. *Diabetes* 1992; 41:598-604.

[48] Bak JF, Moller N, Schmitz O, Saaek A, Pedersen O. In vivo insulin action and muscle glycogen synthase activity in type 2 (non-insulin-dependent) diabetes mellitus: effects of diet treatment. *Diabetologia* 1992; 35:777-84.

[49] Magnusson I, Rothman DL, Katz LD, Shulman RG, Shulman GI. Increased rate of gluconeogenesis in type II diabetes mellitus. A 13C nuclear magnetic resonance study. *J Clin Invest* 1992; 90:1323-7.

[50] Beck-Nielsen H, Vaag A, Damsbo P, et al. Insulin resistance in skeletal muscles in patients with NIDDM. *Diabetes Care* 1992; 15:418-29.

[51] Rossetti L, Giaccari A. Relative contribution of glycogen synthesis and glycolysis to insulin-mediated glucose uptake. A dose-response euglycemic clamp study in normal and diabetic rats. *J Clin Invest* 1990; 85:1785-92.

[52] Park KS, Ciaraldi TP, Carter L, et al. Induction of insulin resistance in human skeletal muscle cells by downregulation of glycogen synthase protein expression. *Metabolism* 2000; 49:962-8.

[53] Yki-Jarvinen H, Young AA, Lamkin C, Foley JE. Kinetics of glucose disposal in whole body and across the forearm in man. *J Clin Invest* 1987; 79:1713-9.

[54] Greenbaum CJ. Insulin resistance in type 1 diabetes. *Diabetes Metab Res Rev* 2002; 18:192-200.

[55] Taylor SI, Kadowaki T, Kadowaki H, Accili D, Cama A, McKeon C. Mutations in insulin-receptor gene in insulin-resistant patients. *Diabetes Care* 1990; 13:257-79.

[56] Ullrich A, Bell JR, Chen EY, et al. Human insulin receptor and its relationship to the tyrosine kinase family of oncogenes. *Nature* 1985; 313:756-61.

[57] Ebina Y, Ellis L, Jarnagin K, et al. The human insulin receptor cDNA: the structural basis for hormone-activated transmembrane signalling. *Cell* 1985; 40:747-58.

[58] Sesti G, Federici M, Lauro D, Sbraccia P, Lauro R. Molecular mechanism of insulin resistance in type 2 diabetes mellitus: role of the insulin receptor variant forms. *Diabetes Metab Res Rev* 2001; 17:363-73.

[59] Haring HU, Mehnert H. Pathogenesis of type 2 (non-insulin-dependent) diabetes mellitus: candidates for a signal transmitter defect causing insulin resistance of the skeletal muscle. Diabetologia 1993; 36:176-82.

[60] Savkur RS, Philips AV, Cooper TA. Aberrant regulation of insulin receptor alternative splicing is associated with insulin resistance in myotonic dystrophy. *Nat Genet* 2001; 29:40-7.

[61] Laakso M, Malkki M, Kekalainen P, Kuusisto J, Deeb SS. Insulin receptor substrate-1 variants in non-insulin-dependent diabetes. *J Clin Invest* 1994; 94:1141-6.

[62] Almind K, Inoue G, Pedersen O, Kahn CR. A common amino acid polymorphism in insulin receptor substrate-1 causes impaired insulin signaling. Evidence from transfection studies. *J Clin Invest* 1996; 97:2569-75.

[63] Porzio O, Federici M, Hribal ML, et al. The Gly972-->Arg amino acid polymorphism in IRS-1 impairs insulin secretion in pancreatic beta cells. *J Clin Invest* 1999; 104:357-64.

[64] Bernal D, Almind K, Yenush L, et al. Insulin receptor substrate-2 amino acid polymorphisms are not associated with random type 2 diabetes among Caucasians. *Diabetes* 1998; 47:976-9.

[65] Almind K, Ahlgren MG, Hansen T, Urhammer SA, Clausen JO, Pedersen O. Discovery of a Met300Val variant in Shc and studies of its relationship to birth weight and length, impaired insulin secretion, insulin resistance, and type 2 diabetes mellitus. *J Clin Endocrinol Metab* 1999; 84:2241-4.

[66] Hansen T, Andersen CB, Echwald SM, et al. Identification of a common amino acid polymorphism in the p85alpha regulatory subunit of phosphatidylinositol 3-kinase: effects on glucose disappearance constant, glucose effectiveness, and the insulin sensitivity index. *Diabetes* 1997; 46:494-501.

[67] Withers DJ, White M. Perspective: The insulin signaling system--a common link in the pathogenesis of type 2 diabetes. *Endocrinology* 2000; 141:1917-21.

[68] Paz K, Hemi R, LeRoith D, et al. A molecular basis for insulin resistance. Elevated serine/threonine phosphorylation of IRS-1 and IRS-2 inhibits their binding to the juxtamembrane region of the insulin receptor and impairs their ability to undergo insulin-induced tyrosine phosphorylation. *J Biol Chem* 1997; 272:29911-8.

[69] Aguirre V, Uchida T, Yenush L, Davis R, White MF. The c-Jun NH(2)-terminal kinase promotes insulin resistance during association with insulin receptor substrate-1 and phosphorylation of Ser(307). *J Biol Chem* 2000; 275:9047-54.

[70] Mothe I, Van Obberghen E. Phosphorylation of insulin receptor substrate-1 on multiple serine residues, 612, 632, 662, and 731, modulates insulin action. *J Biol Chem* 1996; 271:11222-7.

[71] Qiao LY, Zhande R, Jetton TL, Zhou G, Sun XJ. In vivo phosphorylation of insulin receptor substrate 1 at serine 789 by a novel serine kinase in insulin-resistant rodents. *J Biol Chem* 2002; 277:26530-9.

[72] Paz K, Liu YF, Shorer H, et al. Phosphorylation of insulin receptor substrate-1 (IRS-1) by protein kinase B positively regulates IRS-1 function. *J Biol Chem* 1999; 274:28816-22.

[73] Virkamaki A, Ueki K, Kahn CR. Protein-protein interaction in insulin signaling and the molecular mechanisms of insulin resistance. *J Clin Invest* 1999; 103:931-43.

[74] Huang X, Vaag A, Hansson M, Groop L. Down-regulation of insulin receptor substrates (IRS)-1 and IRS-2 and Src homologous and collagen-like protein Shc gene expression by insulin in skeletal muscle is not associated with insulin resistance or type 2 diabetes. *J Clin Endocrinol Metab* 2002; 87:255-9.

[75] Baier LJ, Permana PA, Yang X, et al. A calpain-10 gene polymorphism is associated with reduced muscle mRNA levels and insulin resistance. *J Clin Invest* 2000; 106:R69-73.

[76] Smith LK, Rice KM, Garner CW. The insulin-induced down-regulation of IRS-1 in 3T3-L1 adipocytes is mediated by a calcium-dependent thiol protease. *Mol Cell Endocrinol* 1996; 122:81-92.

[77] Condorelli G, Vigliotta G, Iavarone C, et al. PED/PEA-15 gene controls glucose transport and is overexpressed in type 2 diabetes mellitus. *Embo J* 1998; 17:3858-66.

[78] Maddux BA, Sbraccia P, Kumakura S, et al. Membrane glycoprotein PC-1 and insulin resistance in non-insulin-dependent diabetes mellitus. *Nature* 1995; 373:448-51.

[79] Reynet C, Kahn CR. Rad: a member of the Ras family overexpressed in muscle of type II diabetic humans. *Science* 1993; 262:1441-4.

[80] Moyers JS, Bilan PJ, Reynet C, Kahn CR. Overexpression of Rad inhibits glucose uptake in cultured muscle and fat cells. *J Biol Chem* 1996; 271:23111-6.

[81] Andreelli F, Laville M, Ducluzeau PH, et al. Defective regulation of phosphatidylinositol-3-kinase gene expression in skeletal muscle and adipose tissue of non-insulin-dependent diabetes mellitus patients. *Diabetologia* 1999; 42:358-64.

[82] Huang X, Vaag A, Hansson M, Weng J, Laurila E, Groop L. Impaired insulin-stimulated expression of the glycogen synthase gene in skeletal muscle of type 2 diabetic patients is acquired rather than inherited. *J Clin Endocrinol Metab* 2000; 85:1584-90.

[83] Pendergrass M, Koval J, Vogt C, et al. Insulin-induced hexokinase II expression is reduced in obesity and NIDDM. *Diabetes* 1998; 47:387-94.

[84] Huang X, Hansson M, Laurila E, Ahren B, Groop L. Fat feeding impairs glycogen synthase activity in mice without effects on its gene expression. *Metabolism* 2003; 52:535-9.

[85] Groop LC, Kankuri M, Schalin-Jantti C, et al. Association between polymorphism of the glycogen synthase gene and non-insulin-dependent diabetes mellitus. *N Engl J Med* 1993; 328:10-4.

[86] Seldin MF, Mott D, Bhat D, et al. Glycogen synthase: a putative locus for diet-induced hyperglycaemia. *J Clin Invest* 1994; 94:269-76.

[87] Henry RR, Ciaraldi TP, Abrams-Carter L, Mudaliar S, Park KS, Nikoulina SE. Glycogen synthase activity is reduced in cultured skeletal muscle cells of non-insulin-dependent diabetes mellitus subjects. Biochemical and molecular mechanisms. *J Clin Invest* 1996; 98:1231-6.

[88] Koistinen HA, Galuska D, Chibalin AV, et al. 5-amino-imidazole carboxamide riboside increases glucose transport and cell-surface GLUT4 content in skeletal muscle from subjects with type 2 diabetes. *Diabetes* 2003; 52:1066-72.

[89] Huang C, Somwar R, Patel N, Niu W, Torok D, Klip A. Sustained exposure of L6 myotubes to high glucose and insulin decreases insulin-stimulated GLUT4 translocation but upregulates GLUT4 activity. *Diabetes* 2002; 51:2090-8.

[90] Pedersen O, Bak JF, Andersen PH, et al. Evidence against altered expression of GLUT1 or GLUT4 in skeletal muscle of patients with obesity or NIDDM. *Diabetes* 1990; 39:865-70.

[91] Pontiroli AE, Capra F, Veglia F, et al. Genetic contribution of polymorphism of the GLUT1 and GLUT4 genes to the susceptibility to type 2 (non-insulin-dependent) diabetes mellitus in different populations. *Acta Diabetol* 1996; 33:193-7.

[92] Bjorbaek C, Echwald SM, Hubricht P, et al. Genetic variants in promoters and coding regions of the muscle glycogen synthase and the insulin-responsive GLUT4 genes in NIDDM. *Diabetes* 1994; 43:976-83.

[93] Marshall BA, Hansen PA, Ensor NJ, Ogden MA, Mueckler M. GLUT-1 or GLUT-4 transgenes in obese mice improve glucose tolerance but do not prevent insulin resistance. *Am J Physiol* 1999; 276:E390-400.

[94] Maianu L, Keller SR, Garvey WT. Adipocytes Exhibit Abnormal Subcellular Distribution and Translocation of Vesicles Containing Glucose Transporter 4 and Insulin-Regulated Aminopeptidase in Type 2 Diabetes Mellitus: Implications Regarding Defects in Vesicle Trafficking. *J Clin Endocrinol Metab* 2001; 86:5450-5456.

[95] Spurlin BA, Thomas RM, Nevins AK, et al. Insulin resistance in tetracycline-repressible Munc18c transgenic mice. *Diabetes* 2003; 52:1910-7.

[96] Maier VH, Gould GW. Long-term insulin treatment of 3T3-L1 adipocytes results in mis- targeting of GLUT4: implications for insulin-stimulated glucose transport. *Diabetologia* 2000; 43:1273-81.

[97] Bogan JS, Hendon N, McKee AE, Tsao TS, Lodish HF. Functional cloning of TUG as a regulator of GLUT4 glucose transporter trafficking. Nature 2003; 425:727-33.

[98] Kulkarni RN, Bruning JC, Winnay JN, Postic C, Magnuson MA, Kahn CR. Tissue-specific knockout of the insulin receptor in pancreatic beta cells creates an insulin secretory defect similar to that in type 2 diabetes. *Cell* 1999; 96:329-39.

[99] Withers DJ, Burks DJ, Towery HH, Altamuro SL, Flint CL, White MF. Irs-2 coordinates Igf-1 receptor-mediated beta-cell development and peripheral insulin signalling. *Nat Genet* 1999; 23:32-40.

[100] Kido Y, Burks DJ, Withers D, et al. Tissue-specific insulin resistance in mice with mutations in the insulin receptor, IRS-1, and IRS-2. *J Clin Invest* 2000; 105:199-205.

[101] Bernal-Mizrachi E, Wen W, Stahlhut S, Welling CM, Permutt MA. Islet beta cell expression of constitutively active Aktl/PKB alpha induces striking hypertrophy, hyperplasia, and hyperinsulinemia. *J Clin Invest* 2001; 108:1631-8.

[102] Kulkarni RN. Receptors for insulin and insulin-like growth factor-1 and insulin receptor substrate-1 mediate pathways that regulate islet function. *Biochem Soc Trans* 2002; 30:317-22.

[103] Silander K, Mohlke KL, Scott LJ, et al. Genetic variation near the hepatocyte nuclear factor-4 alpha gene predicts susceptibility to type 2 diabetes. *Diabetes* 2004; 53:1141-9.

[104] Zhu Q, Yamagata K, Miura A, et al. T130I mutation in HNF-4alpha gene is a loss-of-function mutation in hepatocytes and is associated with late-onset Type 2 diabetes mellitus in Japanese subjects. *Diabetologia* 2003; 46:567-73.

[105] Hui H, Perfetti R. Pancreas duodenum homeobox-1 regulates pancreas development during embryogenesis and islet cell function in adulthood. *Eur J Endocrinol* 2002; 146:129-41.

[106] Hani EH, Stoffers DA, Chevre JC, et al. Defective mutations in the insulin promoter factor-1 (IPF-1) gene in late-onset type 2 diabetes mellitus. *J Clin Invest* 1999; 104:R41-8.

[107] Macfarlane WM, Frayling TM, Ellard S, et al. Missense mutations in the insulin promoter factor-1 gene predispose to type 2 diabetes. *J Clin Invest* 1999; 104:R33-9.

[108] Shih DQ, Heimesaat M, Kuwajima S, Stein R, Wright CV, Stoffel M. Profound defects in pancreatic beta-cell function in mice with combined heterozygous mutations in Pdx-1, Hnf-1alpha, and Hnf-3beta. *Proc Natl Acad Sci U S A* 2002; 99:3818-23.

[109] Odom DT, Zizlsperger N, Gordon DB, et al. Control of pancreas and liver gene expression by HNF transcription factors. *Science* 2004; 303:1378-81.

[110] Sund NJ, Vatamaniuk MZ, Casey M, et al. Tissue-specific deletion of Foxa2 in pancreatic beta cells results in hyperinsulinemic hypoglycaemia. *Genes Dev* 2001; 15:1706-15.

[111] Kulkarni RN, Kahn CR. Molecular biology. HNFs--linking the liver and pancreatic islets in diabetes. *Science* 2004; 303:1311-2.

[112] Martin BC, Warram JH, Krolewski AS, Bergman RN, Soeldner JS, Kahn CR. Role of glucose and insulin resistance in development of type 2 diabetes mellitus: results of a 25-year follow-up study. *Lancet* 1992; 340:925-9.

[113] DeFronzo RA, Simonson D, Ferrannini E. Hepatic and peripheral insulin resistance: a common feature of type 2 (non-insulin-dependent) and type 1 (insulin-dependent) diabetes mellitus. *Diabetologia* 1982; 23:313-9.

[114] Klip A, Tsakiridis T, Marette A, Ortiz PA. Regulation of expression of glucose transporters by glucose: a review of studies in vivo and in cell cultures. *Faseb J* 1994; 8:43-53.

[115] Pratipanawatr T, Cusi K, Ngo P, Pratipanawatr W, Mandarino LJ, DeFronzo RA. Normalization of plasma glucose concentration by insulin therapy improves insulin-stimulated glycogen synthesis in type 2 diabetes. *Diabetes* 2002; 51:462-8.

[116] Rossetti L, Smith D, Shulman GI, Papachristou D, DeFronzo RA. Correction of hyperglycaemia with phlorizin normalizes tissue sensitivity to insulin in diabetic rats. *J Clin Invest* 1987; 79:1510-5.

[117] Hetenyi G, Jr., Gauthier C, Byers M, Vranic M. Phlorizin-induced normoglycaemia partially restores glucoregulation in diabetic dogs. *Am J Physiol* 1989; 256:E277-83.

[118] Nawano M, Oku A, Ueta K, et al. Hyperglycaemia contributes insulin resistance in hepatic and adipose tissue but not skeletal muscle of ZDF rats. *Am J Physiol Endocrinol Metab* 2000; 278:E535-43.

[119] Houdali B, Nguyen V, Ammon HP, et al. Prolonged glucose infusion into conscious rats inhibits early steps in insulin signalling and induces translocation of GLUT4 and protein kinase C in skeletal muscle. *Diabetologia* 2002; 45:356-68.

[120] Yu C, Chen Y, Cline GW, et al. Mechanism by which fatty acids inhibit insulin activation of insulin receptor substrate-1 (IRS-1)-associated phosphatidylinositol 3-kinase activity in muscle. *J Biol Chem* 2002; 277:50230-6.

[121] Kurowski TG, Lin Y, Luo Z, et al. Hyperglycaemia inhibits insulin activation of Akt/protein kinase B but not phosphatidylinositol 3-kinase in rat skeletal muscle. *Diabetes* 1999; 48:658-63.

[122] Tong P, Khayat ZA, Huang C, Patel N, Ueyama A, Klip A. Insulin-induced cortical actin remodeling promotes GLUT4 insertion at muscle cell membrane ruffles. *J Clin Invest* 2001; 108:371-81.

[123] Ricort JM, Tanti JF, Van Obberghen E, Le Marchand-Brustel Y. Alterations in insulin signalling pathway induced by prolonged insulin treatment of 3T3-L1 adipocytes. *Diabetologia* 1995; 38:1148-56.

[124] Boden G, Jadali F. Effects of lipid on basal carbohydrate metabolism in normal men. *Diabetes* 1991; 40:686-92.

[125] Roden M, Price TB, Perseghin G, et al. Mechanism of free fatty acid-induced insulin resistance in humans. *J Clin Invest* 1996; 97:2859-65.

[126] Dresner A, Laurent D, Marcucci M, et al. Effects of free fatty acids on glucose transport and IRS-1-associated phosphatidylinositol 3-kinase activity. *J Clin Invest* 1999; 103:253-9.

[127] Boden G, Chen X, Ruiz J, White JV, Rossetti L. Mechanisms of fatty acid-induced inhibition of glucose uptake. *J Clin Invest* 1994; 93:2438-46.

[128] Randle PJ, Garland PB, Newsholme EA, Hales CN. The glucose fatty acid cycle in obesity and maturity onset diabetes mellitus. *Ann N Y Acad Sci* 1965; 131:324-33.

[129] Summers SA, Garza LA, Zhou H, Birnbaum MJ. Regulation of insulin-stimulated glucose transporter GLUT4 translocation and Akt kinase activity by ceramide. *Mol Cell Biol* 1998; 18:5457-64.

[130] Schmitz-Peiffer C, Craig DL, Biden TJ. Ceramide generation is sufficient to account for the inhibition of the insulin-stimulated PKB pathway in C2C12 skeletal muscle cells pretreated with palmitate. J Biol Chem 1999; 274:24202-10.

[131] Hajduch E, Balendran A, Batty IH, et al. Ceramide impairs the insulin-dependent membrane recruitment of protein kinase B leading to a loss in downstream signalling in L6 skeletal muscle cells. *Diabetologia* 2001; 44:173-83.

[132] Powell DJ, Hajduch E, Kular G, Hundal HS. Ceramide disables 3-phosphoinositide binding to the pleckstrin homology domain of protein kinase B (PKB)/Akt by a PKCzeta-dependent mechanism. *Mol Cell Biol* 2003; 23:7794-808.

[133] Cazzolli R, Carpenter L, Biden TJ, Schmitz-Peiffer C. A role for protein phosphatase 2A-like activity, but not atypical protein kinase Czeta, in the inhibition of protein kinase B/Akt and glycogen synthesis by palmitate. *Diabetes* 2001; 50:2210-8.

[134] Hotamisligil GS, Arner P, Caro JF, Atkinson RL, Spiegelman BM. Increased adipose tissue expression of tumor necrosis factor-alpha in human obesity and insulin resistance. *J Clin Invest* 1995; 95:2409-15.

[135] Saghizadeh M, Ong JM, Garvey WT, Henry RR, Kern PA. The expression of TNF alpha by human muscle. Relationship to insulin resistance. *J Clin Invest* 1996; 97:1111-6.

[136] Hotamisligil GS, Shargill NS, Spiegelman BM. Adipose expression of tumor necrosis factor-alpha: direct role in obesity-linked insulin resistance. *Science* 1993; 259:87-91.

[137] Uysal KT, Wiesbrock SM, Marino MW, Hotamisligil GS. Protection from obesity-induced insulin resistance in mice lacking TNF-alpha function. *Nature* 1997; 389:610-4.

[138] Schreyer SA, Chua SC, Jr., LeBoeuf RC. Obesity and diabetes in TNF-alpha receptor-deficient mice. *J Clin Invest* 1998; 102:402-11.

[139] Liu L, Spelleken M, Rohrig K, Hauner H, Eckel J. Tumor necrosis factor-alpha acutely inhibits insulin signaling in human adipocytes: implication of the p80 tumor necrosis factor receptor. *Diabetes* 1998; 47:515-522.

[140] Ozes ON, Akca H, Mayo LD, et al. A phosphatidylinositol 3-kinase/Akt/mTOR pathway mediates and PTEN antagonizes tumor necrosis factor inhibition of insulin signaling through insulin receptor substrate-1. *PNAS* 2001; 98:4640-4645.

[141] Gao Z, Zuberi A, Quon MJ, Dong Z, Ye J. Aspirin inhibits serine phosphorylation of insulin receptor substrate 1 in tumor necrosis factor-treated cells through targeting multiple serine kinases. *J Biol Chem* 2003; 278:24944-50.

[142] Hirosumi J, Tuncman G, Chang L, et al. A central role for JNK in obesity and insulin resistance. *Nature* 2002; 420:333-6.

[143] Yin MJ, Yamamoto Y, Gaynor RB. The anti-inflammatory agents aspirin and salicylate inhibit the activity of I(kappa)B kinase-beta. *Nature* 1998; 396:77-80.

[144] Yuan M, Konstantopoulos N, Lee J, et al. Reversal of obesity- and diet-induced insulin resistance with salicylates or targeted disruption of Ikkbeta. *Science* 2001; 293:1673-7.

[145] Griffin ME, Marcucci MJ, Cline GW, et al. Free fatty acid-induced insulin resistance is associated with activation of protein kinase C theta and alterations in the insulin signaling cascade. *Diabetes* 1999; 48:1270-4.

[146] Sun Z, Arendt CW, Ellmeier W, et al. PKC-theta is required for TCR-induced NF-kappaB activation in mature but not immature T lymphocytes. *Nature* 2000; 404:402-7.

[147] Kim JK, Kim YJ, Fillmore JJ, et al. Prevention of fat-induced insulin resistance by salicylate. *J Clin Invest* 2001; 108:437-46.

[148] Bedard S, Marcotte B, Marette A. Cytokines modulate glucose transport in skeletal muscle by inducing the expression of inducible nitric oxide synthase. *Biochem J* 1997; 325 ( Pt 2):487-93.

[149] Kapur S, Marcotte B, Marette A. Mechanism of adipose tissue iNOS induction in endotoxemia. *Am J Physiol* 1999; 276:E635-41.

[150] Perreault M, Marette A. Targeted disruption of inducible nitric oxide synthase protects against obesity-linked insulin resistance in muscle. *Nat Med* 2001; 7:1138-43.

[151] Evans JL, Goldfine ID, Maddux BA, Grodsky GM. Are Oxidative Stress-Activated Signaling Pathways Mediators of Insulin Resistance and {beta}-Cell Dysfunction? *Diabetes* 2003; 52:1-8.

[152] West IC. Radicals and oxidative stress in diabetes. *Diabet Med* 2000; 17:171-80.

[153] Tirosh A, Potashnik R, Bashan N, Rudich A. Oxidative stress disrupts insulin-induced cellular redistribution of insulin receptor substrate-1 and phosphatidylinositol 3-kinase in 3T3- L1 adipocytes. A putative cellular mechanism for impaired protein kinase B activation and GLUT4 translocation. *J Biol Chem* 1999; 274:10595-602.

[154] Rudich A, Tirosh A, Potashnik R, Hemi R, Kanety H, Bashan N. Prolonged oxidative stress impairs insulin-induced GLUT4 translocation in 3T3-L1 adipocytes. *Diabetes* 1998; 47:1562-9.

[155] Cutfield WS, Wilton P, Bennmarker H, et al. Incidence of diabetes mellitus and impaired glucose tolerance in children and adolescents receiving growth-hormone treatment. *Lancet* 2000; 355:610-3.

[156] Herrington J, Carter-Su C. Signaling pathways activated by the growth hormone receptor. *Trends Endocrinol Metab* 2001; 12:252-7.

[157] Ridderstrale M, Degerman E, Tornqvist H. Growth hormone stimulates the tyrosine phosphorylation of the insulin receptor substrate-1 and its association with phosphatidylinositol 3-kinase in primary adipocytes. *J Biol Chem* 1995; 270:3471-4.

[158] Sakaue H, Ogawa W, Takata M, et al. Phosphoinositide 3-kinase is required for insulin-induced but not for growth hormone- or hyperosmolarity-induced glucose uptake in 3T3-L1 adipocytes. *Mol Endocrinol* 1997; 11:1552-62.

[159] Thirone AC, Carvalho CR, Brenelli SL, Velloso LA, Saad MJ. Effect of chronic growth hormone treatment on insulin signal transduction in rat tissues. *Mol Cell Endocrinol* 1997; 130:33-42.

[160] Dominici FP, Cifone D, Bartke A, Turyn D. Alterations in the early steps of the insulin-signaling system in skeletal muscle of GH-transgenic mice. *Am J Physiol* 1999; 277:E447-54.

[161] Takano A, Haruta T, Iwata M, et al. Growth hormone induces cellular insulin resistance by uncoupling phosphatidylinositol 3-kinase and its downstream signals in 3T3-L1 adipocytes. *Diabetes* 2001; 50:1891-900.

[162] Weinstein SP, Wilson CM, Pritsker A, Cushman SW. Dexamethasone inhibits insulin-stimulated recruitment of GLUT4 to the cell surface in rat skeletal muscle. *Metabolism* 1998; 47:3-6.

[163] Sakoda H, Ogihara T, Anai M, et al. Dexamethasone-induced insulin resistance in 3T3-L1 adipocytes is due to inhibition of glucose transport rather than insulin signal transduction. *Diabetes* 2000; 49:1700-8.

[164] Khani S, Tayek JA. Cortisol increases gluconeogenesis in humans: its role in the metabolic syndrome. *Clin Sci (Lond)* 2001; 101:739-47.

[165] Bernal-Mizrachi C, Weng S, Feng C, et al. Dexamethasone induction of hypertension and diabetes is PPAR-alpha dependent in LDL receptor-null mice. *Nat Med* 2003; 9:1069-75.

[166] Berg AH, Combs TP, Scherer PE. ACRP30/adiponectin: an adipokine regulating glucose and lipid metabolism. *Trends Endocrinol Metab* 2002; 13:84-9.

[167] Scherer PE, Williams S, Fogliano M, Baldini G, Lodish HF. A novel serum protein similar to C1q, produced exclusively in adipocytes. *J Biol Chem* 1995; 270:26746-9.

[168] Arita Y, Kihara S, Ouchi N, et al. Paradoxical decrease of an adipose-specific protein, adiponectin, in obesity. *Biochem Biophys Res Commun* 1999; 257:79-83.

[169] Weyer C, Funahashi T, Tanaka S, et al. Hypoadiponectinemia in obesity and type 2 diabetes: close association with insulin resistance and hyperinsulinemia. *J Clin Endocrinol Metab* 2001; 86:1930-5.

[170] Hotta K, Funahashi T, Arita Y, et al. Plasma concentrations of a novel, adipose-specific protein, adiponectin, in type 2 diabetic patients. *Arterioscler Thromb Vasc Biol* 2000; 20:1595-9.

[171] Berg AH, Combs TP, Du X, Brownlee M, Scherer PE. The adipocyte-secreted protein Acrp30 enhances hepatic insulin action. *Nat Med* 2001; 7:947-53.

[172] Combs TP, Berg AH, Obici S, Scherer PE, Rossetti L. Endogenous glucose production is inhibited by the adipose-derived protein Acrp30. *J Clin Invest* 2001; 108:1875-81.

[173] Fruebis J, Tsao TS, Javorschi S, et al. Proteolytic cleavage product of 30-kDa adipocyte complement-related protein increases fatty acid oxidation in muscle and causes weight loss in mice. Proc Natl Acad Sci U S A 2001; 98:2005-10.

[174] Yamauchi T, Kamon J, Waki H, et al. The fat-derived hormone adiponectin reverses insulin resistance associated with both lipoatrophy and obesity. *Nat Med* 2001; 7:941-6.

[175] Maeda N, Shimomura I, Kishida K, et al. Diet-induced insulin resistance in mice lacking adiponectin/ACRP30. *Nat Med* 2002; 8:731-7.

[176] Kubota N, Terauchi Y, Yamauchi T, et al. Disruption of adiponectin causes insulin resistance and neointimal formation. *J Biol Chem* 2002; 277:25863-6.

[177] Yamauchi T, Kamon J, Minokoshi Y, et al. Adiponectin stimulates glucose utilization and fatty-acid oxidation by activating AMP-activated protein kinase. *Nat Med* 2002; 8:1288-95.

[178] Yamauchi T, Kamon J, Ito Y, et al. Cloning of adiponectin receptors that mediate antidiabetic metabolic effects. *Nature* 2003; 423:762-9.

[179] Tsuchida A, Yamauchi T, Ito Y, et al. Insulin/Foxo1 pathway regulates expression levels of adiponectin receptors and adiponectin sensitivity. *J Biol Chem* 2004.

[180] Vasseur F, Helbecque N, Dina C, et al. Single-nucleotide polymorphism haplotypes in the both proximal promoter and exon 3 of the APM1 gene modulate adipocyte-secreted adiponectin hormone levels and contribute to the genetic risk for type 2 diabetes in French Caucasians. *Hum Mol Genet* 2002; 11:2607-14.
[181] Hara K, Boutin P, Mori Y, et al. Genetic variation in the gene encoding adiponectin is associated with an increased risk of type 2 diabetes in the Japanese population. *Diabetes* 2002; 51:536-40.
[182] Pajvani UB, Scherer PE. Adiponectin: systemic contributor to insulin sensitivity. *Curr Diab Rep* 2003; 3:207-13.
[183] Fumeron F, Aubert R, Siddiq A, et al. Adiponectin gene polymorphisms and adiponectin levels are independently associated with the development of hyperglycaemia during a 3-year period: the epidemiologic data on the insulin resistance syndrome prospective study. *Diabetes* 2004; 53:1150-7.
[184] Menzaghi C, Ercolino T, Di Paola R, et al. A haplotype at the adiponectin locus is associated with obesity and other features of the insulin resistance syndrome. *Diabetes* 2002; 51:2306-12.
[185] Havel PJ. Update on adipocyte hormones: regulation of energy balance and carbohydrate/lipid metabolism. *Diabetes* 2004; 53 Suppl 1:S143-51.
[186] Ceddia RB, Koistinen HA, Zierath JR, Sweeney G. Analysis of paradoxical observations on the association between leptin and insulin resistance. *Faseb J* 2002; 16:1163-76.
[187] Ravussin E, Pratley RE, Maffei M, et al. Relatively low plasma leptin concentrations precede weight gain in Pima Indians. *Nat Med* 1997; 3:238-40.
[188] Considine RV, Sinha MK, Heiman ML, et al. Serum immunoreactive-leptin concentrations in normal-weight and obese humans. *N Engl J Med* 1996; 334:292-5.
[189] Zierath JR, Frevert EU, Ryder JW, Berggren PO, Kahn BB. Evidence against a direct effect of leptin on glucose transport in skeletal muscle and adipocytes. *Diabetes* 1998; 47:1-4.
[190] Kamohara S, Burcelin R, Halaas JL, Friedman JM, Charron MJ. Acute stimulation of glucose metabolism in mice by leptin treatment. *Nature* 1997; 389:374-7.
[191] Minokoshi Y, Alquier T, Furukawa N, et al. AMP-kinase regulates food intake by responding to hormonal and nutrient signals in the hypothalamus. *Nature* 2004; 428:569-74.
[192] Minokoshi Y, Kim YB, Peroni OD, et al. Leptin stimulates fatty-acid oxidation by activating AMP-activated protein kinase. *Nature* 2002; 415:339-43.
[193] Musi N, Goodyear LJ. AMP-activated protein kinase and muscle glucose uptake. *Acta Physiol Scand* 2003; 178:337-45.
[194] Kellerer M, Koch M, Metzinger E, Mushack J, Capp E, Haring HU. Leptin activates PI-3 kinase in C2C12 myotubes via janus kinase-2 (JAK-2) and insulin receptor substrate-2 (IRS-2) dependent pathways. *Diabetologia* 1997; 40:1358-62.
[195] Niswender KD, Morton GJ, Stearns WH, Rhodes CJ, Myers MG, Jr., Schwartz MW. Intracellular signalling. Key enzyme in leptin-induced anorexia. *Nature* 2001; 413:794-5.
[196] Szanto I, Kahn CR. Selective interaction between leptin and insulin signaling pathways in a hepatic cell line. *Proc Natl Acad Sci U S A* 2000; 97:2355-60.

[197] Cohen B, Novick D, Rubinstein M. Modulation of insulin activities by leptin. *Science* 1996; 274:1185-8.
[198] Sweeney G, Keen J, Somwar R, Konrad D, Garg R, Klip A. High leptin levels acutely inhibit insulin-stimulated glucose uptake without affecting glucose transporter 4 translocation in l6 rat skeletal muscle cells. *Endocrinology* 2001; 142:4806-12.
[199] Kellerer M, Lammers R, Fritsche A, et al. Insulin inhibits leptin receptor signalling in HEK293 cells at the level of janus kinase-2: a potential mechanism for hyperinsulinaemia-associated leptin resistance. *Diabetologia* 2001; 44:1125-32.

In: Insulin Resistance in Children and Adolescents ISBN 1-59454-215-5
Editors: D. Daneman and J. Hamilton, pp. 31-56 ©2005 Nova Science Publishers, Inc.

*Chapter 2*

# INSULIN RESISTANCE IN YOUTH: DEFINITION AND METHODS OF MEASUREMENT

***Silva A. Arslanian**, *Rola Saad and Fida Bacha***
Children's Hospital of Pittsburgh, Pennsylvania
Division of Pediatric Endocrinology,
Metabolism and Diabetes Mellitus

## ABSTRACT

As conditions associated with insulin resistance, including obesity, sedentary lifestyle, type 2 diabetes mellitus, polycystic ovary syndrome, continue to escalate among children and adolescents, the need to assess insulin sensitivity in this age group becomes more apparent. Even though insulin resistance plays an important role in disorders of glucose metabolism and other pathological conditions, both insulin sensitivity and insulin secretion should be determined for a comprehensive evaluation of various disorders. Insulin sensitivity and secretion are intricately related with a delicate feedback mechanism governing their relationship. In this chapter we will provide an overview of insulin resistance and discuss the various experimental methodologies for assessing both insulin sensitivity and secretion. We will specifically focus on techniques applied in children. Finally, we would like to provoke thought and challenge existing attitudes with respect to where the future should lead us.

## INTRODUCTION

As we start our journey in the new millennium, we find ourselves faced with socioeconomic advancements and civilization which are impacting children's health adversely. The increasingly prevalent trend of a sedentary lifestyle in the era of information

* Please address correspondence and reprint requests to: Silva A. Arslanian, M.D., Division of Endocrinology, Children's Hospital of Pittsburgh, 3705 Fifth Avenue at DeSoto Street, Pittsburgh, Pennsylvania 15213, U.S.A., Phone: (412) 692-6565, Fax: (412) 692-5834, Email: Silva.Arslanian@chp.edu

technology is keeping children glued to a screen for hours on end. This compounded with an environment of food abundance of calorically dense and nutritionally deplete choices has resulted in the emergence of diseases once considered unique to adults. Among these, obesity, insulin resistance, type 2 diabetes and dyslipidemia have taken the lead. Health care providers are confronted not only with the acute comorbidities of these conditions but the heightened risk for future atherosclerotic cardiovascular disease. This change of scenery in pediatric health care has created a new need to understand what insulin resistance is, how to measure it, and what to do about it. Accurate assessment of insulin sensitivity is crucial especially when evaluating the early markers/predictors of future morbidity and the success of various prevention or intervention strategies. In this chapter we will: 1) provide a definition of insulin resistance; 2) question why insulin resistance needs to be investigated in children, and 3) discuss the various experimental methods for assessing both insulin sensitivity and secretion. We will focus particularly on techniques that have been used in children highlighting advantages and limitations of the different methodologies. Finally, we would like to challenge existing attitudes with respect to future directions.

## What is Insulin Resistance?

The term insulin resistance is not easy to define. A frequently quoted definition of insulin resistance is one proposed by Berson and Yalow more than 30 years ago [1]. They defined insulin resistance as "a state in which greater than normal amounts of insulin are required to elicit a quantitatively normal response." In 1978, Kahn put forward the following definition "insulin resistance may be said to exist whenever normal concentrations of hormone produce a less than normal biologic response" [2]. This was an effort to make a distinction between states of decreased sensitivity to insulin, a decrease in the maximal response to insulin, and combinations of decreased sensitivity and decreased responsiveness. Usually, the sensitivity of a hormonal response is characterized by the dose-response curve considering the hormone concentration that produces half-maximal stimulation of response. The higher the concentration required, the lower the sensitivity, i.e. a shift in the dose-response curve to the right. Thus, greater than normal concentrations of hormone are required to elicit a quantitatively normal response. Decreased responsiveness is a situation in which the maximal response to a hormone is decreased. Another simplistic definition of insulin resistance is a physiological setting in which a normal response to insulin does not occur. In 1998, the American Diabetes Association consensus panel on insulin resistance defined insulin resistance as "an impaired biological response to either exogenous or endogenous insulin" [3]. However, none of these definitions are clinically useful because they do not indicate 1) what the normal response is; 2) what metabolic pathways regulated by insulin are abnormal (i.e., glucose, lipids or amino acids); 3) for what populations the normal values have been defined; and 4) what criteria to use, insulin concentration vs insulin action to define the resistance.

Normal glucose homeostasis is a function of the interplay between insulin sensitivity (liver, muscle and adipocytes) and insulin secretion from the β-cell. Insulin stimulates glucose uptake by muscle and adipose tissue and suppresses glucose production by the liver. While most discussions of insulin resistance center on glucose-insulin relationship because of its clinical relevance, insulin resistance is not confined to glucose metabolism only. Insulin resistance applies to any of its biological actions including suppression of lipolysis and proteolysis, stimulation of protein synthesis, vascular endothelial function and gene expression. However, the various metabolic pathways may have differential sensitivity to insulin's effect. One such example of insulin resistance involving glucose, lipid and protein metabolism in pediatrics is the insulin resistance of puberty. Our studies have demonstrated that insulin action in inhibiting proteolysis and suppressing lipid oxidation is decreased during puberty in addition to an approximately 25-30% decrease in insulin-stimulated glucose disposal [4,5]. Such an observation would suggest that the temporary evolution of insulin resistance and hyperinsulinemia during puberty may serve a teleological function conducive to mass accretion and accelerated growth.

Insulin sensitivity among healthy individuals spans a wide spectrum with significant variations that are determined both by genetics and environmental factors [6,7]. Bearing this in mind, there is no universally accepted, clinically useful, numeric expression that defines insulin resistance [3]. Moreover, there is no well-defined cut-point differentiating normal from abnormal.

## Why Does Insulin Resistance Matter?

A common misconception exists that all insulin resistance, per se, is harmful. However, insulin resistance plays an important role in several conditions including physiological, pathological, and drug-induced states. The physiological states are fasting, puberty, pregnancy, aging, physical inactivity, dietary habits and race. In some physiological states the presence of insulin resistance may be beneficial. For example, during fasting the biological innate drive to prevent hypoglycaemia is associated not only with a fall in circulating insulin concentrations, but also a decrease in insulin sensitivity [8,9,10]. This may be important teleologically because energy substrates must be mobilized from peripheral tissues to maintain metabolic functions. Resistance to insulin permits mobilization of free fatty acids from adipocytes, serving as a source for gluconeogenesis and energy in the fasting state.

Similarly, insulin resistance during puberty may have a beneficial effect. Compensatory hyperinsulinemia consequent to pubertal insulin resistance is associated with lower postabsorptive rates of proteolysis and protein oxidation in pubertal adolescents compared with prepubertal children. This translates to sparing of protein breakdown on average of 1g/day/kg fat free mass during puberty [5]. Because growth involves net deposition of protein, the rate of synthesis must be greater than that of breakdown. It is proposed that the most economical way of achieving this would be by a reduction in protein breakdown. Thus, protein accretion and acceleration of growth during puberty is achieved in an energy efficient manner mediated, at least in part, through hyperinsulinemia/insulin resistance.

The causes and mechanisms of physiological insulin resistance are not clear. A popular theory at the systemic or cellular level involves the Randle cycle, in which free fatty acids (FFA) inhibit glucose oxidation and utilization in heart and skeletal muscle [11,12]. The Randle theory has been investigated extensively in adults, but to our knowledge the only available data in pediatrics is a study by our group [13]. Infusion of intralipid in prepubertal and pubertal normal subjects demonstrated that the Randle cycle plays a role in pubertal insulin resistance. During puberty, decreased insulin action in suppressing fat oxidation, i.e. increased fat oxidation, results in decreased glucose oxidation and glucose storage during a hyperinsulinemic-euglycemic clamp [4]. Furthermore, it appears that developmental-maturational changes during childhood growth and puberty alter tissue sensitivity and/or specificity to the glucose-FFA interaction resulting in a differential response of FFA-glucose interaction in prepubertal and pubertal subjects. In the former group the interaction is conducive to fat accretion while in the latter group to insulin resistance [13].

Among the pathological states, obesity is the commonest and the most important condition associated with insulin resistance and hyperinsulinemia [14-17]. In our studies of normal children, adiposity accounts for 55% of the variance in insulin sensitivity [15]. Moreover, among obese youth those with higher visceral fat are more insulin resistant than those with lower visceral fat despite comparable BMI [16]. Not surprisingly therefore obesity is a major risk factor for type 2 diabetes in children in whom insulin resistance is present early in the natural course of the disease [18,19]. Other pathologic conditions associated with insulin resistance and well documented in pediatrics are polycystic ovary syndrome, premature adrenarche, and rare syndromes of severe insulin resistance [20,21,22]. Even though the association of insulin resistance with essential hypertension, dyslipidemia and atherosclerotic cardiovascular disease is well documented in adults [23], data are limited in pediatrics. We and others have shown that insulin resistance explains a significant portion of the variance in lipid levels [15,17,24]. Drugs that induce states of insulin resistance include corticosteroids, GH, some contraceptive pills, diuretics and some antipsychotic medications. With the introduction of the second generation antipsychotic drugs over the last decade, their use has soared. This has been associated with reports of dramatic weight gain, diabetes and an atherogenic lipid profile [25].

An important and primary role for insulin resistance in human disease was proposed by Reaven in 1988. He formulated that "syndrome X", which is a cluster of related metabolic abnormalities of hyperinsulinemia, glucose intolerance, increased triglycerides and very low density lipoproteins, decreased high density lipoprotein (HDL) and hypertension, determines to a large extent who will or who will not develop cardiovascular disease [26]. Since then, the concept has been popularized with different terminologies, such as the "metabolic syndrome" or the "insulin resistance syndrome" or the "dyslipidemic syndrome." Definitions of the metabolic syndrome in adults have been established by the WHO and the National Cholesterol Education Program [27,28]. To date, however, there are no established and accepted definitions of this syndrome in children despite the fact that interest in the field is increasing [29,30].

The ADA consensus panel stressed that the "fact that insulin resistance is associated with so much morbidity and mortality does not prove that it is the cause of these outcomes, or amelioration of insulin resistance will prevent them." Therefore, in the absence of outcome data, particularly in children, clinicians must exercise caution and not prescribe insulin sensitizers to youth for the treatment of obesity and insulin resistance whether it is for the primary prevention of diabetes or the secondary prevention of CVD [31,32]. Elimination of those components of the metabolic syndrome that are individually amenable to treatment should remain the top priority of management as recommended by the ADA panel [3]. The American Heart Association Scientific Statement recommends "on the basis of current knowledge and extrapolation from studies in adults, it is reasonable to suggest that lifestyle modification and weight control in childhood could reduce the risk of developing the insulin resistance syndrome, type 2 diabetes mellitus and cardiovascular disease [33].

## MEASUREMENT OF INSULIN SENSITIVITY

A comprehensive evaluation of the pathophysiological mechanisms responsible for disorders of glucose homeostasis requires the assessment of two important physiological components in glucose metabolism: 1) In vivo insulin action or the sensitivity of the body's tissues to insulin and 2) the pancreatic β-cell response to glucose. Even though traditionally the commonest glucose metabolic disorder in childhood has been type 1 diabetes, which is characterized with absolute insulin deficiency, conditions associated with insulin resistance have been on the rise in youth. It appears that the increasing rates of obesity in childhood have pulled the trigger for type 2 diabetes, the metabolic syndrome, and the polycystic ovary syndrome, all conditions associated with insulin resistance [18,20] (to be discussed in detail in the various chapters of this book). Despite the fact that investigations in the field of insulin resistance have been ongoing for several decades in adults, it is only recently that interest in this field in pediatrics has grown. As a result, there has been an escalating need for the development and application of methodologies to evaluate in vivo insulin action in children and adolescents.

Our objective in the present chapter is to describe the various approaches that have been used to evaluate insulin sensitivity in adults (Table 1). However, rather than reviewing the detailed methodologies of each test, we will highlight those techniques which have been applied to children and adolescents and their major contributions to our understanding of the physiology and the pathophysiology of glucose metabolism in youth.

**Table 1: Methods for Evaluation of In Vivo Insulin Sensitivity**

- Glucose clamp technique
- Intravenous glucose tolerance test and minimal model technique
- Oral glucose tolerance test
- Insulin tolerance test
- Insulin suppression test
- Forearm perfusion technique
- Surrogate estimates of insulin sensitivity

## Glucose Clamp Technique

This is universally accepted as the "gold standard" technique to determine insulin-stimulated whole body glucose disposal, insulin sensitivity, and pancreatic insulin secretion. It was initially introduced by Andres in 1966 [34] and developed to its present form by DeFronzo et al in 1979 [35]. The technique is based on the fact that in vivo there is a complex and highly integrated feedback loop governing the interplay between glucose and insulin on both the peripheral tissues and the β-cell. There are two variations of this technique, 1) the hyperinsulinemic-euglycemic clamp and 2) the hyperglycemic clamp both of which have been used in pediatrics by a limited number of investigators.

***Hyperinsulinemic-Euglycemic Clamp***

It is commonly accepted that the euglycemic insulin clamp technique allows the "purest" measure of tissue sensitivity to insulin overcoming the limitations of other techniques. The goal of the insulin clamp technique is to acutely raise and maintain the plasma insulin concentration at the desired experimental level while holding the plasma glucose concentration constant at the basal level. Thus, both insulin and glucose levels are "clamped" during the procedure.

For setting up a clamp study the following are needed: 1) vascular access: an antecubital catheter for infusions (insulin and glucose) and an "arterialized" heated-hand intravenous line for frequent sampling of blood. The latter permits the derivation of arterial equivalent of glucose from venous data [36,37]; 2) a bedside glucose analyzer for the measurement of plasma glucose obtained every 2.5-5 min; 3) 20% dextrose for intravenous infusion; and 4) regular crystalline insulin infusion: 5-120 mu/m$^2$/min depending on the desired steady-state plasma insulin concentration to be achieved. The typical rate however is 40 mu/m$^2$/min which raises the plasma insulin concentration by ~ 100 μu/ml above baseline. Some investigators use a 10-min priming infusion followed by a constant rate infusion in which case the priming dose results in a slight overshoot in the plasma insulin concentration during the first 20 min. We have always used a constant rate infusion of insulin which results in a gradual increase in plasma insulin concentration reaching a plateau at around 30 min (Figure 1) [38]. Hypoglycaemia is prevented by the application of the glucose clamp technique. Each subject's arterialized plasma glucose concentration is maintained at the basal level by a variable rate infusion of 20% dextrose. The glucose infusion is begun after 2-10 min of initiating the insulin infusion, and it is empirically set at 1-2 mg/kg/min. Thereafter, the glucose infusion rate is adjusted based on the negative feedback principle to maintain the plasma glucose level constant. To achieve this, the plasma glucose concentration is measured (glucose analyzer) every 5 min (more frequently if the rate of glucose metabolism is very fast) and the glucose infusion rate is adjusted appropriately. Thus, if the actual glucose concentration is lower than desired, the glucose infusion is increased and vice versa. Deciding how to alter the glucose infusion rate based on a given plasma glucose reading may seem like an impossible task for the novice who is performing a clamp experiment for the first time. Algorithms have been developed by several groups to facilitate setting the glucose infusion rate appropriate to the measured plasma glucose level and its rate of change [39]. The required calculations for most methods are quite simple and can be performed on a hand-held calculator. Within a 1-2 week period, anyone working with an established clamper can quickly become more proficient than the best computer algorithm. It must be stressed that the pumps used for insulin and dextrose infusion should be accurate and they should be recalibrated frequently to ensure their accuracy. In diabetic subjects with hyperglycaemia, after starting the insulin infusion, we let the plasma glucose concentration decline to euglycemic levels before beginning the glucose infusion (Figure 1).

Measurements obtained during a hyperinsulinemic-euglycemic clamp are; 1) insulin-stimulated glucose metabolism (M) and/or glucose disposal (Rd); 2) insulin sensitivity; and 3) the metabolic clearance rate of insulin (MCR). Under steady-state plasma glucose conditions, the amount of glucose infused is equal to the amount of glucose metabolized (mg/kg/min) by the total body, provided endogenous (hepatic) glucose production is completely suppressed. We routinely perform steady-state calculations over the last 30 min of a 3-hr clamp. We use [6,6-$^2H_2$]glucose stable isotope in combination with insulin clamp studies to quantitate hepatic glucose production [13]. It has to be cautioned to use the appropriate tracer methodology to obtain accurate and physiologically plausible estimates [40]. If endogenous glucose production is not suppressed, it is added to the exogenous glucose infusion rate to provide a measure of total-body glucose uptake [13]. The insulin clamp technique thus allows one to assess the individual contributions of both hepatic and peripheral tissues to the observed insulin resistance. Peripheral tissue insulin sensitivity is calculated by dividing insulin-stimulated glucose metabolism by the steady-state plasma insulin concentration (M/I) (mg/kg/min per μu/ml) [35]. This measurement is important when comparing two groups who have different steady-state insulin concentrations during the clamp in which case expressing only M is not sufficient [41]. An index of hepatic insulin sensitivity can be calculated as the inverse of the product of hepatic glucose production and the plasma insulin concentration [42,43]. The metabolic clearance rate of insulin (MCR) (ml/kg/min) can be computed by dividing insulin infusion rate by Δ increase in circulating insulin concentrations during the clamp [35,41,44]. We obtain plasma samples for insulin measurement at 15 min intervals throughout the clamp and at 10 min intervals during the baseline and the last 30 min of the steady state. In most investigations the duration of the clamp varies from 2-4 hours. However, when clamps are prolonged to 8 hours, there is a gradual increase in exogenous glucose infusion rate which reaches a plateau between 4 and 5 hours [45].

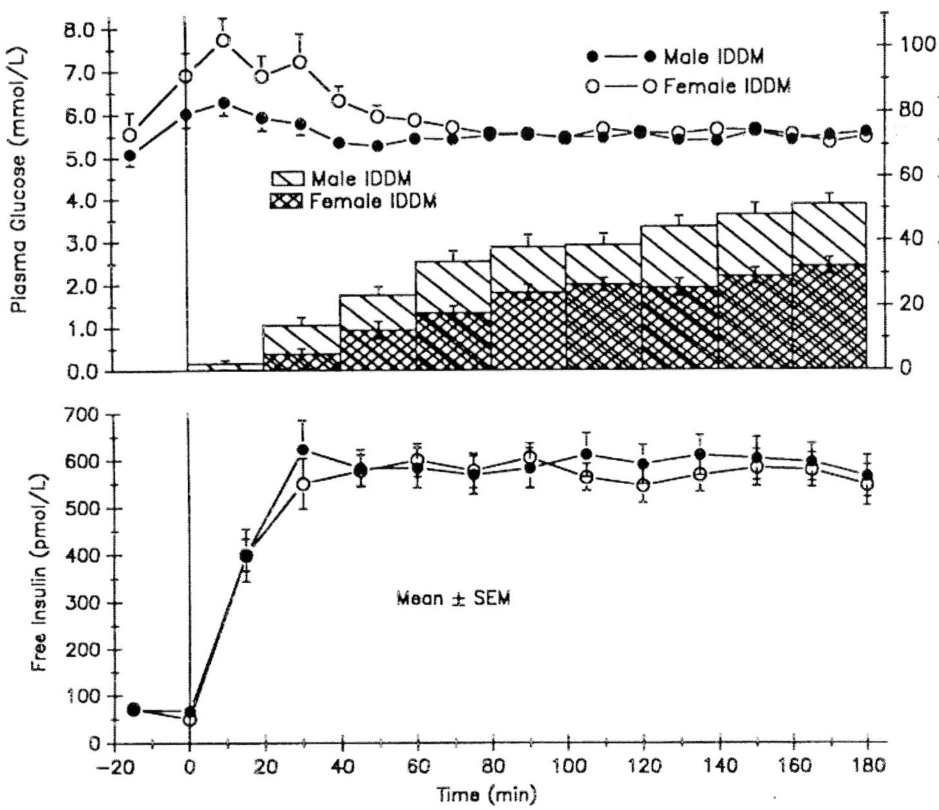


Figure 1: Plasma glucose, free insulin and exogenous glucose infusion rates during a 3-hour hyperinsulinemic-euglycemic clamp in male and female patients with type 1 diabetes (IDDM). (M: insulin-stimulated glucose metabolism). Reproduced with permission [35].

***Hyperglycemic Clamp***

This technique provides a method for assessing the response of the β-cell to glucose and for quantifying the amount of glucose metabolized during a controlled hyperglycemic condition [35,46-49]. During a hyperglycemic clamp the plasma glucose concentration is acutely increased and maintained at any given hyperglycaemia for the duration of the experiment. We typically raise the plasma glucose concentration and maintain it at 225 mg/dl ± 10% for 2 hours (Figure 2) [48]. This is achieved by a bolus infusion of 25-50% dextrose solution over a 2-min period followed by a variable rate infusion of 20% dextrose. During the first 15 min of the hyperglycemic clamp, very little of the infused glucose is metabolized; most goes to fill the glucose space. We have been successful in using the following formula for calculating the glucose priming bolus (mg) to raise the plasma glucose concentration to 225 mg/dl (225 – the mean of 3 baseline fasting plasma glucose) (mg/dl) x subject's weight (kg) x glucose distribution factor (dl/kg) (1.5 for normal weight children and 1.1 for overweight and obese children.) Occasionally, we have found that this may overshoot or undershoot the desired glucose plateau. However, since the plasma glucose concentration is measured at 0.5 min after the bolus infusion and thereafter every 2.5 min, rapid adjustments in the variable rate infusion of dextrose can be made to achieve the desired hyperglycaemia. During the first 15 min of the hyperglycemic clamp, we obtain plasma samples every 2.5 min for determination of glucose, insulin and C-peptide, and from 15-120 min every 5 min for glucose and every 15 min for insulin and C-peptide. Measurement of C-peptide is important especially if groups of experimental subjects differ in their insulin clearance rates.

Measurements obtained during a hyperglycemic clamp are: 1) the plasma insulin response to glucose and 2) whole body glucose metabolism. The plasma insulin response to glucose is biphasic with a rapid first phase in the first 10 min after the glucose bolus followed by a gradual increase of the second phase (Figure 2). We traditionally calculate the first-phase insulin concentration as the mean of five insulin determinations at times 2.5, 5, 7.5, 10.0, and 12.5 min of the clamp and the second phase as the mean of eight determinations from 15 to 120 min [48-50]. It is important that if the MCR of insulin is known, one can calculate the post-hepatic systemic delivery of insulin [46]. Because the portal insulin concentration cannot be measured in man, the true rate of insulin secretion can not be determined [47]. Alternate estimates have been proposed using C-peptide deconvolution methods in adults [51]. This technique has not been used in pediatrics because it is a two-day method which requires a separate assessment of C-peptide kinetics and infusion of human C-peptide. Even in adults an alternative has been proposed to minimize the complexity of the testing by using a population model of C-peptide kinetics [52]. Minimal modeling of C-peptide during the hyperglycemic clamp has also been used to overcome these difficulties [53].

During the hyperglycemic clamp, the rate of glucose metabolism (M) is calculated from the rate of exogenous glucose infusion minus urinary glucose loss since renal threshold is exceeded secondary to hyperglycaemia. We typically make the calculation of M (mg/kg/min) over the last 60 min of the hyperglycemic clamp. In healthy individuals under conditions of hyperglycaemia, hepatic glucose production is suppressed completely. However, this may not be the case in diabetic subjects. Therefore, in diabetic subjects, the concurrent use of isotopes will allow for the determination of hepatic glucose production. This should be added to the exogenous glucose infusion rate to calculate M. In addition to obtaining rates of glucose metabolism, one can derive an index of insulin sensitivity by dividing M with the plasma insulin concentration over the last 60 min of the clamp. This calculation assumes a linear relationship between the plasma insulin concentration and M which is a simplification of a more complex relationship. In our studies insulin sensitivity index calculated during the last 60 min of the hyperglycemic clamp and insulin sensitivity from the euglycemic clamp correlated strongly (r = 0.92, p <0.01), however, others have reported lower correlations ranging from 0.45-0.65 [54].

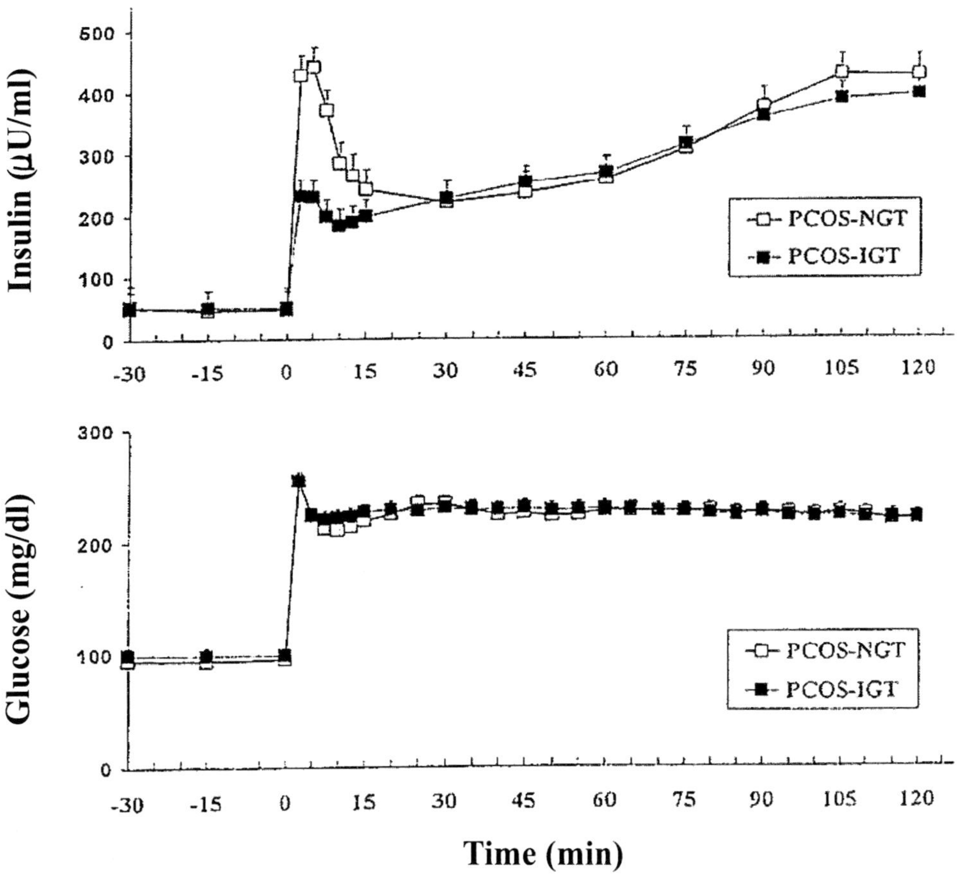


Figure 2: Insulin (upper panel) and glucose concentration (lower panel) during a hyperglycemic clamp in adolescents with polycystic ovary syndrome (PCOS) with normal vs impaired glucose tolerance (NGT vs IGT). Reproduced with permission [45].

The insulin-glucose clamp technique is accepted as the "gold standard" because of several advantages: 1) both glucose and insulin levels are controlled and "clamped" at the desired experimental level; 2) both hepatic and peripheral tissue insulin sensitivity can be measured; 3) when combined with indirect calorimetry, both glucose oxidation and glucose storage can be calculated; and 4) the test is highly reproducible with a coefficient of repeatability of 1.0 and low intra-individual coefficient of variation [37,45,55]. However, none of these reproducibility studies were performed in the pediatric age group.

*Use of Isotopes and Indirect Calorimetry*

Insulin clamp experiments can be performed with the concurrent use of isotopes to study substrate turnover and the effect of insulin on different metabolic pathways. In adults, radioactive isotopes are used (cheaper and easier to analyze) while in pediatrics safety concerns preclude the use of radioactive isotopes. Stable isotopes which are safe are expensive and require gas chromatography/mass spectroscopy techniques for analysis. We have used multiple stable isotopes simultaneously with clamp experiments to study glucose, protein and fat metabolism (Figure 3) at baseline and during hyperinsulinemia [44,56]. Readers interested in the field of isotopes are recommended to refer to Radioactive and Stable Isotope Tracers in Biomedicine [57] since a detailed discussion is beyond the scope of this chapter.

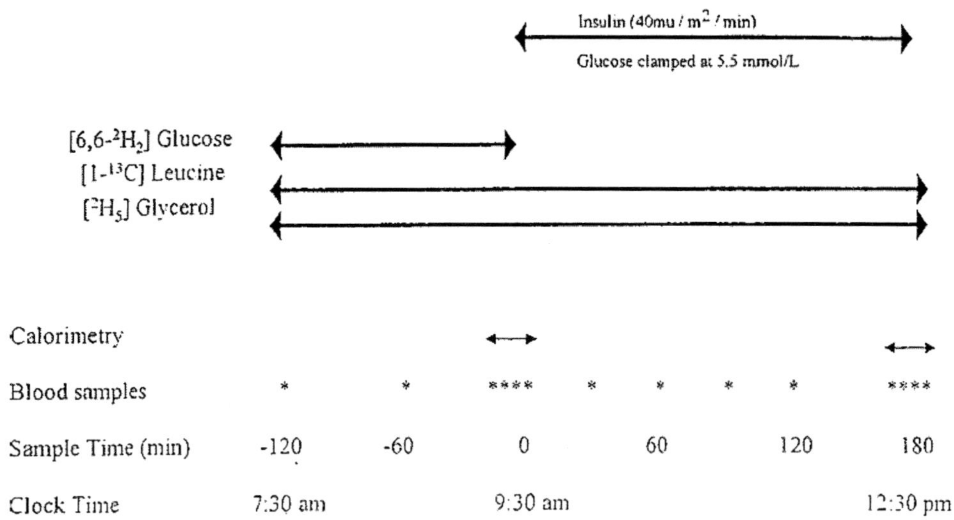


Figure 3: Study design to assess glucose, protein (leucine) and lipid (glycerol) metabolism and the effect of insulin during a hyperinsulinemic-euglycemic clamp combined with multiple stable isotope infusions. Reproduced with permission [53].

Indirect calorimetry can be used in conjunction with the glucose clamp to provide information on relative fuel oxidation (i.e. glucose vs fatty acids) and its modulation with insulin. Indirect calorimetry consists of the measurement of whole-body oxygen consumption ($VO_2$) and carbon dioxide production ($VCO_2$) and assessment of energy metabolism. The respiratory quotient (RQ) which is the ratio of $VCO_2/VO_2$ varies according to the fuel oxidized. RQ for carbohydrates is 1, for lipid 0.707 and for protein 0.835 [58]. Using equations based on $VCO_2$, $VO_2$ and urinary nitrogen excretion, rates of glucose, fat and protein oxidation and energy expenditure are computed [58-60]. A comprehensive review of indirect calorimetry is beyond the scope of this chapter and the reader is referred to other sources [58-60] Our use of indirect calorimetry combined with clamp experiments has enabled us to investigate the role of the Randle cycle, i.e. glucose-fatty acid competition in explaining pubertal insulin resistance [4,13]. Indirect calorimetry application to examine energy metabolism has demonstrated differences in resting energy expenditure between black and white children providing a potential explanation for the increased risk of obesity in black children [49].

***Relationship between Insulin Sensitivity and β-Cell Function***

Glucose homeostasis is maintained through a delicate balance between insulin secretion from the β-cells and insulin action in insulin-sensitive tissues. This relationship between insulin sensitivity and acute insulin release in response to glucose is best described by a hyperbolic function [41,61-65] suggesting that the β-cells and insulin-sensitive tissues interact in a tightly regulated manner governed by a negative feedback loop. The latter would require reciprocal changes in insulin sensitivity and secretion to maintain carbohydrate metabolism unchanged. Thus, for a given level of glucose tolerance, the product of insulin sensitivity and β-cell function, termed glucose disposition index, is a constant. When insulin sensitivity decreases, insulin secretion must increase for glucose tolerance to remain constant. If this compensatory increase in insulin secretion is incomplete deterioration in glucose tolerance will occur (Figure 4) [62,63,66]. Another implication of this hyperbolic relationship is that, although insulin responses may be identical in two groups of individuals, if insulin sensitivity is different, then glucose tolerance may differ between the groups. Thus, β-cell function should be assessed relative to insulin sensitivity. Individuals at risk of developing type 2 diabetes mellitus will have poorer β-cell function than controls with similar degrees of insulin resistance. In our studies evaluating the relationship of insulin sensitivity to insulin secretion, we demonstrated that: 1) black children have a limited β-cell capacity to increase insulin secretion in compensation to puberty – related insulin resistance [50]; 2) obese black adolescents have a more diabetogenic risk profile because of decreased glucose disposition index [16]; and 3) white youth with a family history of type 2 diabetes have impaired glucose disposition index compared with those without such a family history [67].

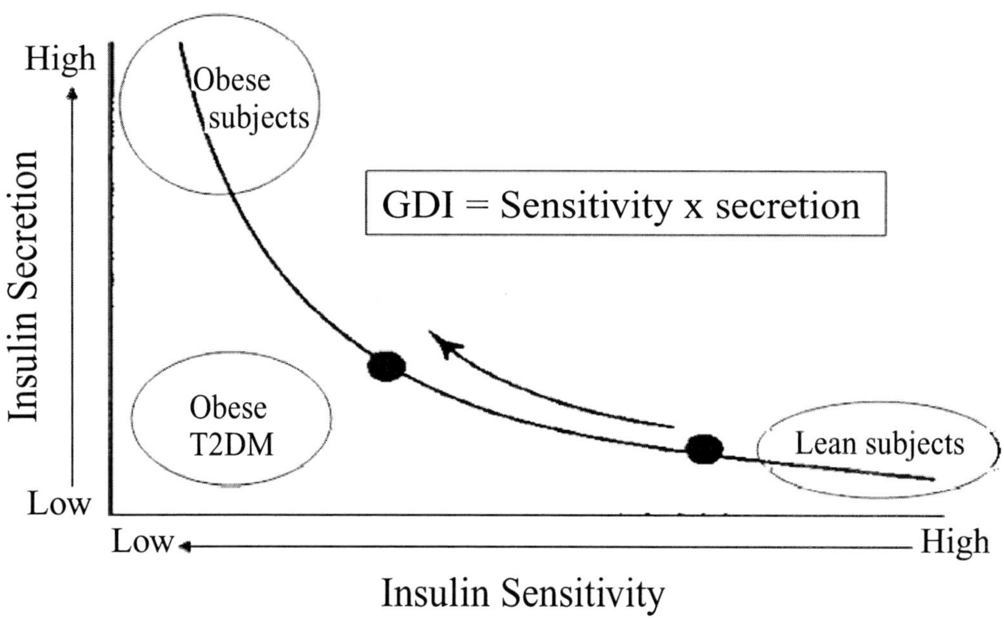


Figure 4: Hyperbolic relationship between insulin sensitivity and secretion. (GDI: glucose disposition index; T2DM: type 2 diabetes mellitus). Adapted with permission [60,63].

## The Frequently Sampled Intravenous Glucose Tolerance Test with Minimal Model Analysis

In an attempt to provide a simpler technique for in vivo assessment of metabolic function of islet cells and insulin sensitive tissues, the minimal model method was introduced by Bergman and colleagues in 1979 [68-71]. The model is based on the frequently sampled intravenous glucose tolerance test (FSIGTT). Computer mathematical minimal model (MINMOD) analysis of glucose utilization and insulin kinetics is applied to analyze plasma glucose and insulin dynamics following intravenous glucose injection [70]. In the fasted state the FSIGTT protocol involves injection of a bolus of 50% glucose solution (0.3g/kg body weight) over 0-1 min period. Basal samples are collected for 3 hours at -15, -10, -5 and -1 min and post injection samples are obtained at 2, 3, 4, 5, 6, 8, 10, 12, 14, 16, 19, 22, 24, 25, 27, 30, 40, 50, 60, 70, 80, 90, 100, 120, 140, 160 and 180 min [46]. Not infrequently, the sampling times have been altered in different publications [72].

Two modifications to the FSIGTT were introduced to ensure an endogenous insulin response of sufficient magnitude to enhance the ability of the computer to estimate the model parameters. The first was the tolbutamide enhanced FSIGTT [73]. The modification involves the intravenous injection of tolbutamide (300 mg in normal weight individuals, 500 mg in overweight or obese subjects) at 20 min. Additional blood sampling to the standard FSIGTT includes samples obtained at 23, 24 and 27 minutes. The insulin-modified FSIGTT was an attempt to use the FSIGTT model in patients with diabetes [74,75]. Insulin (0.03 units/kg) is administered as an IV bolus at 20 min of the FSIGTT with additional sampling similar to the tolbutamide protocol. Insulin sensitivity estimates from both protocols correlate with each other in the same individual, however, they are quantitatively discrepant [72]. Additional modifications of the minimal model have included radioactive or stable isotope labeling of the IVGTT [76,77]. The latter has been used in pediatrics [78,79]. This modification allows the separation of insulin and glucose effects on peripheral uptake from their effects on hepatic glucose production.

In order to simplify the actual performance of the FSIGTT with its relatively large number of samples (n=30) a modification was introduced to reduce the total number of blood samples to 12 [80]. It is well accepted that the full sample protocol is preferable for small studies designed to detect small changes in $S_I$, whereas the reduced sample protocol is appropriate for epidemiological studies with large numbers of subjects or large anticipated changes [81].

During the FSIGTT, in contrast to the euglycemic clamp, both insulin and glucose vary over a significant fraction of their respective physiological concentration ranges. In our unpublished experience some patients develop hypoglycaemia during the test necessitating discontinuation of the test. The computer MINMOD program assesses several estimates based on multiple assumptions [70]. The parameters derived from the MINMOD FSIGTT are: 1) insulin sensitivity index ($S_I$) which is the increase in fractional glucose disappearance per unit insulin increase, i.e. the ability of insulin to enhance glucose uptake and to inhibit hepatic glucose production; 2) insulin-independent fractional glucose disappearance ($S_G$) which is the increase in fractional disappearance of glucose per unit increase of glucose at basal insulin; 3) β-cell function with the most commonly used index being acute insulin release ($AIR_G$) which is an index of first-phase insulin secretion. Mathematical modeling of β-cell function yields two parameters describing the sensitivity to glucose of first and second-phase insulin secretion, respectively ($\phi_1$, $\phi_2$); 4) fractional insulin clearance [46].

Even though the minimal model FSIGTT has been used extensively in adults, it has received criticisms and suggestions for model improvement because of its limitations [82,83]. In repeated experiments in the same subject, the interday coefficients of variation were: for $S_I$ 20.2 ± 3.2% (range 6-44%); for $S_G$ 25.1 ± 8.8%, and for first-phase insulin secretion 20.1 ± 3.5% [81]. Though $S_I$ estimates from FSIGTT correlate with insulin sensitivity measured during the glucose clamp, the former is remarkably lower. $S_I$ from the tolbutamide FSIGTT was 13 ± 6% lower, and from insulin-FSIGTT was 44 ± 4% lower compared with clamp insulin sensitivity [72]. Studies have also demonstrated that the minimal-model results in overestimates of $S_G$ [84,85]. In adults, the stable-label IVGTT estimates of $S_I$ and $S_G$ have an average precision of ±5% compared to an average precision of ±74% for $S_G$ and ±22% for $S_I$ of non-tracer estimates [77]. A study in pediatrics reveals that the average precision from labeled vs unlabeled IVGTT is 22 and 47%, respectively for $S_I$, and 7 and 82% for $S_G$, respectively [78].

A careful review of the pediatric FSIGTT literature reveals several inconsistencies and wide deviations/variations from the protocol. In 1990 a modification of the model was proposed by shortening the FSIGTT to 90 min in children, with a tolbutamide dose of 5 mg/kg [86]. Even though the parameters derived from the abbreviated and the actual test correlated, the fractional standard deviation for $S_I$ from the former was significantly greater than that from the actual. Also, 5% of the subjects had insufficient insulin response during the FSIGTT for the minimal model program to calculate $S_I$. The authors appropriately pointed out "several shortcomings in the measurement of insulin sensitivity by the minimal model" [86]. It was their conclusion that extreme insulin resistance cannot be easily measured and conversely, insulin sensitivity is difficult to measure by the MINMOD when an inadequate amount of insulin is released. Despite this, assortments of the FSIGTT in pediatrics have included using highly variable sampling schedules during the test ranging from 11 [65] to 13 [87-89] to 18 [90,91] to 19 [92] to 22 [93] to 24 samples [94]. Glucose bolus dose has varied too from 0.3g/kg [88,92,94] to 11.4g/$m^2$ [90], to 100 gm without accounting for body weight [89], while the tolbutamide dose has differed from 5 mg/kg [86,92] to 125 mg/$m^2$ [90,91] to 300 mg/1.73$m^2$ [87-89]. The insulin dose has varied from 0.02 u/kg to 0.03 u/kg [65,95,96]. The smaller dose has even been used in obese insulin resistant children raising doubts about such a small dose producing a sufficient response in these insulin resistant subjects [65]. Moreover, almost all publications report that the glucose bolus is injected over 0.5-1 min. It remains unclear how feasible it is to infuse large volumes of 25% dextrose solutions in very obese children weighing more than 100 kg and sometimes reported to be as heavy as 139 kg who require large volumes exceeding 100cc [65,96]. Moreover, in obese children who had repeat FSIGTT on two or three occasions the $S_I$ varied by ~ 30-40% from the first to the other times [96]. Therefore, in the presence of such inconsistencies in the FSIGTT protocol in the pediatric age group and in the absence of its validation against the gold standard of the glucose clamp technique, the reliability of the data remains questionable. It is a reasonable expectation to have a standardized protocol in pediatrics that is applied across all centers in a uniform fashion following its careful and adequate validation.

## Oral Glucose Tolerance Test

One of the earliest attempts to assess insulin sensitivity in vivo employed the oral glucose tolerance test. A standard oral glucose load (1.75 g/kg body weight (max. 75 g)) is ingested over 5-10 min after an overnight fast. Blood is sampled every 15-30 min for 2-5 hrs for measurement of plasma glucose and insulin concentrations. Studies in the late sixties revealed the heterogeneity of response from mildly intolerant to severely diabetic states and formed the basis of modern diagnostic use of the OGTT [97]. While it is well accepted that the 2-hr glucose level determines glucose tolerance status (normal glucose tolerance vs impaired glucose tolerance vs diabetes) [98,99], the validity of the OGTT in deriving indices of insulin sensitivity and secretion indices has been questioned. Initially, the change in insulin/glucose ratio (Δinsulin/Δglucose) during the OGTT was used as an index of insulin sensitivity [100]. Later on several mathematical equations were proposed for the derivation of insulin sensitivity [101-103]. Common among all models is the use of fasting and post load glucose and insulin values as well as the applications of several assumptions. The overall concept is that the higher the rise in plasma glucose per unit of insulin the lower is insulin sensitivity. Even though the OGTT is a relatively simple test to perform, it has several drawbacks. The test is poorly reproducible, the rate of gastrointestinal absorption of glucose varies considerably from one person to another, glucose and insulin levels are constantly changing and are not "clamped", hepatic glucose production is unknown and lastly glucose uptake by the peripheral tissues is affected independently by hyperglycaemia and hyperinsulinemia [104-106]. OGTT data are also used to derive indices of β-cell function [101,103,107]. The most common empirical one is the insulinogenic index calculated as the ratio of $\Delta I_{30}/\Delta G_{30}$ (i.e. the difference in insulin and/or glucose level between 30 min and zero min). Other modifications have included the use of the 15 min data or the area under the OGTT curve [100]. Limited studies in pediatrics demonstrate that the composite whole body insulin sensitivity index (WBISI), calculated using the OGTT [102), correlate well with insulin sensitivity derived from the FSIGTT ($r = 0.67$) in overweight youth [108], and with the hyperinsulinemic-euglycemic clamp in obese children ($r = 0.78$) [109]. However, similar data are not available in normal weight youth or those with diabetes.

## Insulin Tolerance Test (ITT)

Insulin tolerance test is one of the earliest techniques used to evaluate insulin action in vivo [39,46]. During this technique, following a bolus of intravenous insulin, the rate at which serum glucose falls and the nadir it reaches are determined. After an overnight fast, and determination of the baseline plasma glucose, a bolus of fast acting insulin (0.1 unit/kg/day) is given intravenously. The plasma glucose concentration is determined every 5 minutes for 70-80 minutes. An index of insulin mediated glucose metabolism is then calculated expressed as glucose disappearance rate [$K_{ITT} = (0.693/t_{1/2})$ x100 percent/min] where $t_{1/2}$ is the half-life of plasma glucose decay. It is usually calculated by plotting plasma glucose concentration versus time (usually between 10-30 or 10-40 minutes time interval). Normal values of $K_{ITT}$ are greater than 2 percent/min. Values less than 1.5 are abnormal and between 1.5 and 2 are equivocal.

The disadvantages of the above test are: a) hypoglycaemia which is unpleasant and triggers a counterregulatory hormonal response that affects glucose decline by stimulating hepatic glucose production and impairing peripheral glucose uptake. Thus the test does not reflect pure insulin action; b) insulin level is supraphysiologic; c) the test does not allow one to derive a quantitative measure of insulin-mediated glucose metabolism; it only provides a relative ranking of insulin sensitivity; d) the test does not provide information about which tissues are responsible for impaired insulin action (liver versus periphery). The advantages are: a) The test is simple and rapid; b) it is reproducible and accurate. In fact a modified version of the ITT called short ITT (SITT) has been used and studied by many investigators. The SITT is terminated after 15-20 minutes to avoid hypoglycaemia and the subsequent counterregulatory response. Hirst et al and Akinmokun et al demonstrated that the SITT is reproducible in 18 healthy individuals (23-61 years) with within-subject coefficient of variation equal to 13% and 6%, respectively [110,111]. In addition the $K_{ITT}$ determined by the SITT correlated well with the glucose disposal rate determined by euglycemic clamps, the gold standard method of determining insulin sensitivity [111]. However, a study performed in adolescents with type 1 diabetes demonstrated that the SITT lacks validity because the insulin sensitivity derived from the SITT did not correlate with the sensitivity measured by the euglycemic clamp [112]. The ITT has not been popularized in pediatrics because of the risks consequent to hypoglycaemia.

## Insulin Suppression Test

This technique introduced in 1970 by Reaven and collegues[1] consists of quadruple infusion of epinephrine, propranolol, insulin and glucose [39,46]. Epinephrine suppresses insulin secretion and stimulates hepatic glucose production, while propranolol inhibits hepatic glucose production. The test allows one to evaluate disposal of a glucose load (given IV) by a constant and fixed level of hyperinsulinemia. After an overnight fast, a bolus of propranolol (5mg) is given IV, continuous infusions of epinephrine (6 mcg/min), propranolol (0.08 mg/min), regular insulin (80mU/min) and glucose (6 mg/kg/min) are started and given over 180 minutes. Steady state plasma glucose concentrations (SSPG) and insulin (SSPI) are achieved after 90 minutes. Blood samples are drawn every 5-10 minutes during the last hour of the test for determination of insulin and glucose levels. SSPI levels are approximately 100 μU/ml in most subjects. SSPG concentration reflects the insulin mediated glucose metabolism. The higher the SSPG, the higher is the insulin resistance. There is a high degree of correlation between assessment of insulin sensitivity by the insulin suppression test and the euglycemic clamp ($r=0.92$ $p<0.001$) [113]. Also the test is reproducible regardless of the degree of glucose intolerance.

The potential problems with the insulin suppression test are: a) propranolol may not be able to suppress hepatic glucose production completely especially in individuals with diabetes so one cannot infer with certainty that the sites of insulin resistance are the peripheral tissues; b) the SSPG reached is different between individuals and hyperglycaemia has its own effects on peripheral glucose uptake and suppression of hepatic glucose production. Therefore metabolic clearance rate was used to measure insulin action by some investigators; c) epinephrine may have different effects on peripheral tissue glucose uptake and blood flow in diabetic and normal individuals; d) epinephrine may cause arrhythmias in elderly and it is contraindicated in individuals with abnormal ECG or hypertension. Last, but not least, because of its complexity, this technique has not been used and in all likelihood will never be used in the pediatric age group.

A modification of the insulin suppression test was introduced in which somatostatin is infused instead of epinephrine and propranolol to inhibit both insulin and glucagon secretion. Suppression of glucagon and the infusion of insulin and glucose inhibit hepatic glucose production. After baseline blood samples are obtained, 125 mcg of somatostatin is given IV bolus then continuous infusions of somatostatin (250 mcg/hour), glucose (6 mg/kg.min) and insulin (0.77 mU/kg/min). Blood samples are drawn every 10-15 minutes throughout the study for determination of SSPG (reached during the last hour of the test) and SSPI (reached between 60-180 minutes). SSPG provides a measure of in vivo insulin sensitivity. Insulin sensitivity index can be calculated by dividing glucose infusion rate by the SSPG.

This modified test avoids the potential antagonistic effects of epinephrine on glucose metabolism and its side effects. However somatostatin inhibits some pituitary and gastrointestinal hormones (like growth hormone) which may affect glucose metabolism. In this test, one still cannot determine insulin mediated glucose disposal and cannot determine the site of insulin resistance and cannot overcome the effect of different SSPG levels. Because of the complexity of the test and some of its drawbacks, it was not adopted universally.

## Forearm Perfusion Technique

This technique quantitates glucose uptake directly by the muscles [39,46]. Because of its invasive nature it has not been widely used in children despite the robustness of the technique. A catheter is placed in an antecubital vein retrogradely and is advanced toward the wrist to sample the deep forearm tissues (mostly muscles). Another catheter is inserted also in a retrograde fashion in a superficial vein of the same forearm to get samples from skin and adipose tissue. A third catheter is inserted retrogradely in the brachial artery. Brachial plasma flow is determined by venous occlusion plethysmography, and the metabolism of forearm tissues is calculated according to the Fick principle.

Insulin can be infused in the brachial artery to determine the insulin mediated glucose disposal by the muscle directly. The latter is a major advantage of the described technique. The principal limitation of this technique is its invasive although relatively safe nature. Also this technique does not provide any information about hepatic response to insulin or whole body glucose uptake although the latter can be estimated. Another limitation of this technique is the inability to control glucose levels and the effect of hyperglycaemia in diabetic individuals. Also, since glucose is not produced by the muscle, the net balance reflects only uptake. However, a major advantage of this technique is that it can be used to study any substrate metabolism across any organ including the lower limbs, the kidney, the liver, the brain provided arterial and venous catheterization is performed [39]. Caution should be used, however, if other substrates (e.g. amino acids) are studied. The net balance of such a substrate is equal to uptake + production. Using Isotopes and specific formula the uptake of such a substrate can be determined.

## Surrogate Estimates of Insulin Sensitivity and Secretion

The above stated methods, particularly the clamp technique, of assessing in vivo insulin sensitivity and secretion are invasive, cost- and labor-intensive procedures that are not applicable to routine clinical practice or large-scale epidemiological studies. Therefore, simple but reliable surrogate estimates of insulin sensitivity and secretion have been developed. These include: (i) fasting insulin level ($I_F$), (ii) fasting glucose to insulin ratio ($G_F/I_F$) [114,115], (iii) the homeostasis model assessment (HOMA) [HOMA insulin sensitivity = $22.5/(I_F X G_F)$] [116], (iv) the quantitative insulin sensitivity check index (QUICKI = $1/[\text{Log}(I_F) + \text{Log}(G_F)]$) [117], and (v) insulin sensitivity indices derived from OGTT [101,107-109,118].

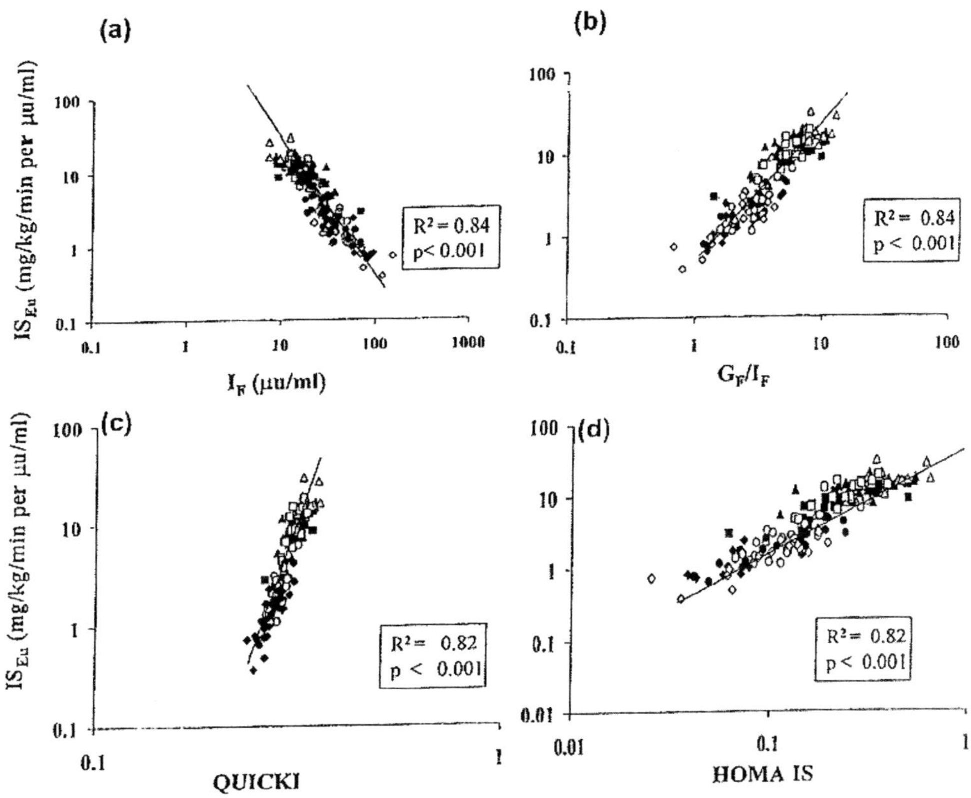


Figure 5: The correlations between in vivo insulin sensitivity measured by the hyperinsulinemic-euglycemic clamp and surrogate estimates. Reproduced with permission [117].

Despite a wealth of adult data showing a fairly good correlation between measured and estimated indices of insulin sensitivity, data are limited in pediatrics. A study in prepubertal girls with premature adrenarche showed a significant correlation ($r = 0.75$) between $G_F/I_F$ and insulin sensitivity index derived from FSIGTT [119]. Another study in white and black children (Tanner I and II) revealed that the predictive value of a modified HOMA equation was similar to fasting insulin alone in comparison with insulin sensitivity measured by FSIVGTT [120]. A study of children ages 6.2 – 11.3 years, Tanner stage I-III (81% obese) comparing estimates of insulin sensitivity with those derived from clamp identified QUICKI as the best estimate in comparison with HOMA and $G_F/I_F$ [121]. In a limited number of obese youth, insulin sensitivity from FSIGTT correlated with HOMA insulin resistance (r -0.81 to -0.90), and QUICKI (r 0.81 - 0.90) [96]. In a recent study of 156 black and white children and adolescents, we demonstrated that insulin sensitivity measured with the hyperinsulinemic-euglycemic clamp correlated significantly and strongly with $I_F$ (r = -0.92), $G_F/I_F$ (r = 0.92), HOMA IS (r = 0.91), QUICKI (r = 0.91) and insulin sensitivity index derived from the hyperglycemic clamp (Figure 5) [122]. Furthermore, the estimates reflected differences in insulin sensitivity related to race, puberty and obesity. On the other hand, the correlations between estimates of β-cell function and first- and second-phase insulin secretion measured during a hyperglycemic clamp were not as strong (Figure 6). Thus, fasting glucose and insulin derived estimates of insulin sensitivity may serve as valuable surrogate measures of insulin sensitivity and β-cell function in normal non-diabetic children. These estimates could be utilized in the longitudinal follow-up of large cohorts of normal children in intervention/prevention trials where more invasive methods of measurements are not feasible.

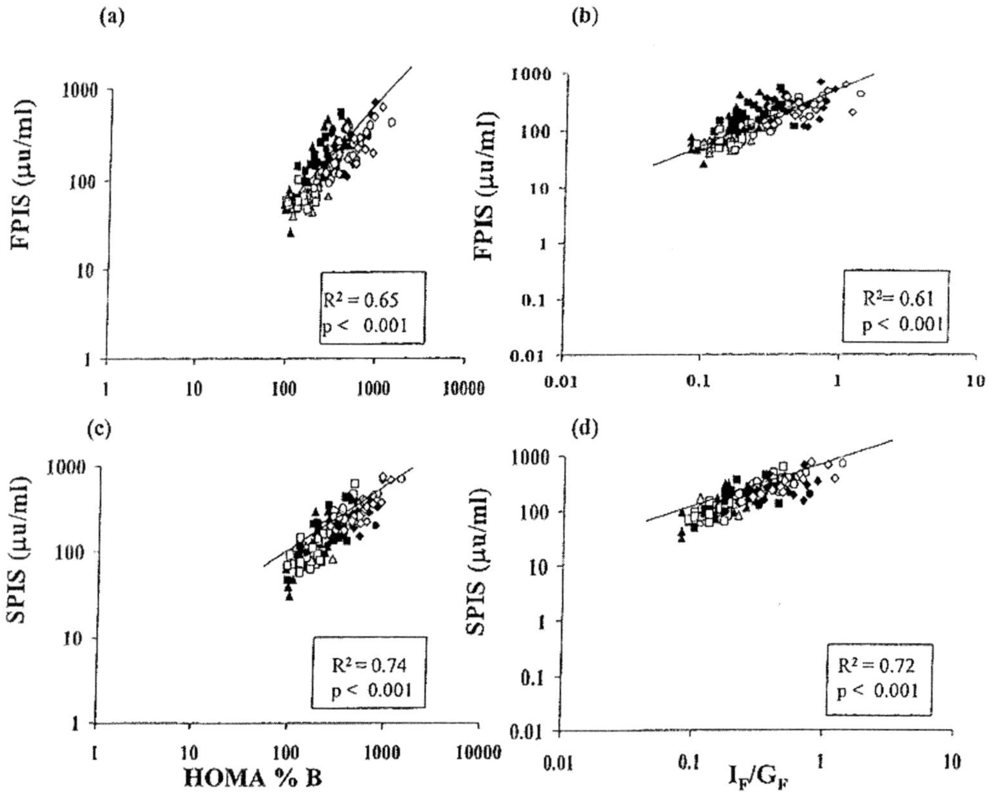


Figure 6: The correlations between in vivo insulin secretion measured by the hyperglycemic clamp and surrogate estimates of β-cell function. Reproduced with permission [117].

It cannot be stressed enough that there are limitations to using fasting glucose and insulin [123]. First, because of significant variability in insulin measurements across various laboratories, as demonstrated by the American Diabetes Association Task Force [124], there will be important differences in these estimates among different centers. Therefore, these estimates are center/laboratory specific and cannot be applied uniformly across centers.

Second, at the moment, these estimates are only validated in children with normal glucose homeostasis. Further studies are needed to assess the predictive value of these estimates for the full spectrum of glucose tolerance including impaired glucose tolerance and type 2 diabetes. In fact, while the $G_F/I_F$ ratio may be a good proxy of insulin sensitivity in non-diabetic children, this will not be the case when fasting glucose is elevated in the case of diabetes. This will result in a falsely elevated ratio which does not truly reflect increased insulin sensitivity. On the other hand, as fasting insulin declines due to a progressively failing pancreas, the increased $G_F/I_F$ ratio will give the false impression of improved insulin sensitivity. Furthermore, fasting estimates have no utility in children with type 1 diabetes and no endogenous insulin secretion. For all these reasons, readers are cautioned in their use of these estimates until further pediatric data are amassed.

## Summary and Future Directions

With the increasing rates of conditions associated with insulin resistance, the need for sensitive and specific methods for the evaluation of insulin sensitivity/resistance, especially in the research set up, will continue to escalate. Despite the multiplicity of methods available for adults, the techniques applicable to children and adolescents are limited. Some of the available methodologies, e.g. FSIGTT, need to be refined, standardized, and validated across the spectrum of glucose tolerance in children. The "gold standard" method of the clamp should be used by more investigators who have the research infrastructure and capabilities that would enable them to perform such experiments in a safe and reproducible fashion. Institutional Review Boards should have the foresight to realize that insulin resistance will continue to escalate as a pediatric problem and that the safe, careful and ethical conduct of such investigations should not be prohibited. Only with the proper experimental tools or assessment techniques will researchers be able not only to measure but also trust the outcome of prevention/intervention strategies.

## Acknowledgements

This work was supported by United States Public Health Service grant RO1 HD27503, K24 HD01357, MO1-RR00084 General Clinical Research, Eli Lilly and Company, Genentech Foundation for Growth and Development and Bristol-Myers Squibb Company.

## References

[1] Yalow RS, Berson SA. Immunoassay of endogenous plasma insulin in man. *J Clin Invest* 1960; 39:1157-75.
[2] Kahn CR. Insulin resistance, insulin insensitivity, and insulin unresponsiveness: A necessary distinction. *Metabolism* 1978;27:1893-1902.
[3] American Diabetes Association. Consensus development conference on insulin resistance. *Diabetes Care* 1998;21:310-14.

[4] Arslanian SA, Kalhan SC. Correlations between fatty acid and glucose metabolism. *Diabetes* 1994;43:908-914.
[5] Arslanian SA, Kalhan SC. Protein turnover during puberty in normal children. *Am J Physiol* 1996;270:E79-E84.
[6] Hollenbeck C, Reaven GM. Variations in insulin-stimulated glucose uptake in healthy individuals with normal glucose tolerance. *J Clin Endocrinol Metab* 1987;64:1169-1173.
[7] Matthaei S, Stumvoll M, Kellerer M, Häring H-U. Pathophysiology and pharmacological treatment of insulin resistance. *Endocrine Reviews* 2000;21:585-618.
[8] Norrelund H, Nielsen S, Christiansen J S, Jorgensen J O L and Moller N. Modulation of basal glucose metabolism and insulin sensitivity by growth hormone and free fatty acids during short term fasting. *European Journal of Endocrinology* 2004; 150:779-787.
[9] Svanfeldt M, Thorell A, Brismar K, Nygren J and Ljungqvist O. Effects of 3 days of postoperative low caloric feeding with or without bed rest on insulin sensitivity in healthy subjects. *Clinical Nutrition* 2003; 22(1):31-38.
[10] Stannard S R and Johnson N A. Insulin resistance and elevated triglyceride in muscle: more important for survival than thrifty genes ? *J Physiol* 2003;554.3:595-607.
[11] Randle PJ, Garland PB, Hales CN, Newsholme EA. The glucose fatty acid cycle. Its role in insulin sensitivity and the metabolic disturbances of diabetes mellitus. *Lancet* 1963;1:785-789.
[12] Randle PJ, Priestman DA, Mistry SC, Halsall A. Glucose fatty acid interactions and the regulation of glucose disposal. *J Cell Biochem* 1994;555:1-11.
[13] Arslanian S, Suprasongsin C. Glucose-fatty acid interactions in prepubertal and pubertal children: effects of lipid infusion. *Am J Physiol* 1997;272:E523-E529.
[14] Kahn BB, Flier JS. Obesity and insulin resistance. *J Clin Investigation* 2000;106-473-81.
[15] Arslanian S, Suprasongsin C. Insulin sensitivity, lipids, and body composition in childhood: Is "syndrome X" present? *J Clin Endocrinol Metab* 1996;81:1058-1062.
[16] Bacha F, Saad R, Gungor N, Janosky J, Arslanian SA. Obesity, regional fat distribution, and syndrome X in obese black versus white adolescents: Race differential in diabetogenic and atherogenic risk factors. *J Clin Endocrinol Metab* 2003;88:2534-2540.
[17] Caprio S, Tamborlane WV. Metabolic impact of obesity in childhood. *Endocrinol Metab Clin North Am* 1999;28:731-747.
[18] Arslanian S. Type 2 diabetes in children: Clinical aspects and risk factors. *Horm Res* 2002;57:19-28.
[19] Gungor N, Arslanian S. Pathophysiology of type 2 diabetes mellitus in children and adolescents. *Treat Endocrinol* 2002;1:359-371.
[20] Arslanian SA, Witchel SF. Polycystic ovary syndrome in adolescents: is there an epidemic? *Curr Opin Endocrinol Diabetes* 2002;9:32-42.
[21] Ibanez L, Dimartino-Nardi J, Potau N, et al. Premature adrenarche: normal variant or forerunner of adult disease? *Endocrine Rev* 2000;21:671-696.
[22] Flier JS. Lilly Lecture: Syndromes of insulin resistance. From patient to gene and back again. *Diabetes* 1992;41:1207-219.
[23] Reaven GM: Insulin resistance/compensatory hyperinsulinemia, essential hypertension, and cardiovascular disease. *J Clin Endocrinol Metab* 2003;88(6):2399-2403.

[24] Steinberger J, Moorehead C, Katch V, Rocchini AP. Relationship between insulin resistance and abnormal lipid profile in obese adolescents. *J Pediatr* 1995; 126:690-95.

[25] American Diabetes Association, American Psychiatric Association, American Association of Clinical Endocrinologists, North American Association for the Study of Obesity. Consensus development conference on antipsychotic drugs and obesity and diabetes. *Diabetes Care* 2004;27:596-601.

[26] Reaven GM. Role of insulin resistance in human disease. *Diabetes* 1988;37:1595-1607.

[27] Alberti KG, Zimmet PZ. Definition, diagnosis and classification of diabetes mellitus and its complications. Part 1. Diagnosis and classification of diabetes mellitus, provisional report of a WHO consultation. *Diabet Med* 1998;15:539-553.

[28] Expert Panel on Detection, Evaluation, and Treatment of High Blood Cholesterol in Adults. Executive summary of the third report of the National Cholesterol Education Program (NCEP) expert panel on detection, evaluation, and treatment of high blood cholesterol in adults (Adult Treatment Panel III). *JAMA* 2001;285-2486-97.

[29] Srinivasan SR, Frontini MG, Berenson GS. Longitudinal changes in risk variables of insulin resistance syndrome from childhood to young adulthood in offspring of parents with type 2 diabetes: The Bogalusa Heart Study. *Metabolism* 2003;52:443-450.

[30] Srinivasan SR, Myers L, Berenson GS. Predictability of childhood adiposity and insulin for developing insulin resistance syndrome (Syndrome X) in young adulthood: The Bogalusa Heart Study. *Diabetes* 2002;51:204-209.

[31] Hill JO. What to do about the metabolic syndrome? *Arch Intern Med* 2003;163:395-397.

[32] Davidson MB. Is treatment of insulin resistance beneficial independent of glycaemia? *Diabetes Care* 2003;26:3184-3186.

[33] Steinberger J, Daniels SR. Obesity, insulin resistance, diabetes, and cardiovascular risk in children. *Circulation* 2003; 107:1448-53.

[34] Andres R, Swerdloff R, Pozefsky T, Coleman D. Manual feedback technique for the control of blood glucose concentration. In: LT Skeggs, Jr, ed. *Automation in Analytical Chemistry,* New York: Mediad, 1966:486-491.

[35] DeFronzo RA, Tobin JD, Andres R. Glucose Clamp Technique: A Method for Quantifying Insulin Secretion and Resistance. *Am J Physiol* 1979;237(3):E214-E223.

[36] Abumrad NN, Rabin D, Diamond MP, Lacy WW. Use of a heated superficial hand vein as an alternative site for the measurement of amino acid concentrations and for the study of glucose and alanine kinetics in man. *Metabolism* 1981;30:936-940.

[37] Morris AD, Ueda S, Petrie JR, Connell JM, Elliott HL, Donnelly R. The euglycaemic hyperinsulinaemic clamp: an evaluation of current methodology. *Clin Exp Pharmacol Physiol* 1997;24:513-8.

[38] Arslanian SA, Heil BV, Becker DJ, Drash AL. Sexual dimorphism in insulin sensitivity in adolescents with insulin-dependent diabetes mellitus. *J Clin Endocrinol Metab* 1991;72:920-926.

[39] Scheen AJ, Paquot N, Castillo MJ, Lefebvre PJ. How to measure insulin action in vivo. *Diabetes/Metabolism Reviews* 1994;10:151-188.

[40] Finegood DT, Bergman RN, Vranic M. Estimation of endogenous glucose production during hyperinsulinemic-euglycemic glucose clamps. *Diabetes* 1987;36:914-24.

[41] Arslanian SA, Saad R, Lewy V, Danadian K, Janosky J. Hyperinsulinemia in African-American children. Decreased insulin clearance and increased insulin secretion and its relationship to insulin sensitivity. *Diabetes* 2002;51:3014-3019.

[42] Bacha F, Saad R, Gungor N, Arslanian SA. Adiponectin in youth. *Diabetes Care* 2004; 27:547-552.

[43] Miyazaki Y, Glass L, Triplitt C, Wajcberg E, Mandarino LJ, DeFronzo RA. Abdominal fat distribution and peripheral and hepatic insulin resistance in type 2 diabetes mellitus. *Am J Physiol Endocrinol Metab* 2002;283:E1135-E1143.

[44] Arslanian S, Suprasongsin C. Testosterone treatment in adolescents with delayed puberty: Changes in body composition, protein, fat, and glucose metabolism. *J Clin Endocrinol Metab* 1997;82:3213-3220.

[45] Soop M, Nygren J, Brismar K, Thorell A, Ljungqvist O. The hyperinsulinaemic-euglycemic glucose clamp: reproducibility and metabolic effects of prolonged insulin infusion in healthy subjects. *Clin Sci* 2000;98:367-74.

[46] Del Prato S, Ferrannini E, Defronzo RA. Evaluation of Insulin Sensitivity in Man. In: Clarke WL, Larner J, Pohl SL eds. *Methods in Diabetes Research.* New York:John Wiley & Sons, Inc. 1986:36-76.

[47] Hovorka R, Jones RH. How to measure insulin secretion. *Diabetes/Metabolism Reviews* 1994; 10(2):91-117.

[48] Arslanian SA, Lewy VD, Danadian K. Glucose intolerance in obese adolescents with polycystic ovary syndrome: Role of insulin resistance and β-cell dysfunction and risk of cardiovascular disease. *J Clin Endocrinol Metab* 2001;86:66-71.

[49] Arslanian S, Suprasongsin C, Janosky JE. Insulin secretion and sensitivity in black versus white prepubertal healthy children. *J Clin Endocrinol Metab* 1997;82:1923-1927.

[50] Saad RJ, Danadian K, Lewy V, Arslanian SA. Insulin resistance of puberty in African-American children: lack of a compensatory increase in insulin secretion. *Pediatric Diabetes* 2002;3:4-9.

[51] Polonsky KS. The β-cell in diabetes: From molecular genetics to clinical research. *Diabetes* 1995;44:705-717.

[52] Hovorka R, Koukkou E, Southerden D, Powrie JK, Young MA. Measuring prehepatic insulin secretion using a population model of C-peptide kinetics: accuracy and required sampling schedule. *Diabetologia* 1998;41:548-554.

[53] Bonadonna RC, Stumvoll M, Fritsche A, Muggeo M, Häring H, Bonora E, et al. Altered homeostatic adaptation of first- and second-phase β-cell secretion in the offspring of patients with type 2 diabetes. *Diabetes* 2003;52:470-480.

[54] Uwaifo GI, Parikh SJ, Elberg KJ, Chin J, Yanovski JA. Comparison of insulin sensitivity, clearance, and secretion estimates using euglycemic and hyperglycemic clamps in children. *J Clin Endocrinol Metab* 2002; 87:2899-2905.

[55] Bokemark L, Froden A, Attvall S, Wikstrand J, Fagerberg B. The euglycemic hyperinsulinemic clamp examination: variability and reproducibility. *Scand J Clin Lab Invest* 2000;60:27-36.

[56] Saad RJ, Keenan BS, Danadian K, Lewy VD, Arslanian SA. Dihydrotestosterone treatment in adolescents with delayed puberty: Does it explain insulin resistance of puberty? *J Clin Endocrinol Metab* 2001;86:4881-86.

[57] Wolfe RR. *Radioactive and stable isotope tracers in biomedicine. Principles and Practice of Kinetic Analysis,* New York, 1992; Wiley-Liss, Inc.

[58] Schultz Y. The Basis of Direct and Indirect Calorimetry and their Potentials. *Diabetes/Metabolism Reviews* 1995;11(4):383-408.

[59] Ferrannini E. Calorimetry. *Research Methodologies in Human Diabetes Part 2. Walter de Gruyter*. Berlin. New York 1995:97-112.

[60] Bursztein S, Elwyn DH, Askanazi J, Kinney JM. *Energy metabolism, indirect calorimetry, and nutrition*. Grayson TH, ed: Baltimore;Williams & Wilkins, 1989.

[61] Kahn SE, Prigeon RL, McCulloch DK, Boyko EJ, Bergman RN, Schwartz MW, et al. Quantification of the relationship between insulin sensitivity and β-cell function in human subjects. *Diabetes* 1993;42:1663-72.

[62] Kahn SE. The importance of β-cell failure in the development and progression of type 2 diabetes. *J Clin Endocrinol & Metab* 2001;86:4047-58.

[63] Bergman RN, Ader M, Huecking K, VanCitters G. Accurate assessment of β-cell function: The hyperbolic correction. *Diabetes* 2002;51:S212-S220.

[64] Arslanian S: Insulin resistance and insulin secretion in childhood and adolescence: their role in type 2 diabetes in youth. In: Silink M, Kida K, Rosenbloom AL eds. *Type 2 Diabetes in Childhood and Adolescence*, London and New York: Martin Dunitz, 2003:93-116.

[65] Goran MI, Bergman RN, Avila Q, Watkins M, Ball GDC, Shaibi GQ, et al. Impaired glucose tolerance and reduced β-cell function in overweight Latino children with a positive family history for type 2 diabetes. *J Clin Endocrinol Metab* 2004;89:207-212.

[66] Weyer C, Bogardus C, Mott DM, Pratley RE. The natural history of insulin secretory dysfunction and insulin resistance in the pathogenesis of type 2 diabetes mellitus. *J Clin Invest* 1999; 104:787-794.

[67] Bacha F, Saad R, Arslanian S. Family history of type 2 diabetes (T2DM) is associated with an impaired balance between insulin secretion and insulin sensitivity in white children. *Diabetes* 2003;52:A69.

[68] Bergman RN, Ider YZ, Bowden CR, Cobelli C. Quantitative estimation of insulin sensitivity. *Am J Physiol* 1979;236-E667-77.

[69] Bergman RN, Beard JC, Chen M. The minimal modeling method: Assessment of insulin sensitivity and β-cell function in vivo. In: Clarke WL, Larner J, Pohl SL eds. *Methods in Diabetes Research*. New York:John Wiley and Sons, Inc. 1986:15-34.

[70] Bergman RN. Toward physiological understanding of glucose tolerance: Minimal-model approach. *Diabetes* 1989;38:1512-1527.

[71] Bergman RN, Hope ID, Yang YJ, Watanabe RM, Meador MA, Youn JH, et al. Assessment of insulin sensitivity in vivo: a critical review. *Diabetes/Metab Rev* 1989;5:411-429.

[72] Saad MF, Steil GM, Kades WW, Ayad MF, Elsewafy WA, Boyadjian R. Differences between the tolbutamide-boosted and the insulin-modified minimal model protocols. *Diabetes* 1997;46:1167-71.

[73] Yang YJ, Youn JH, Bergman RN. Modified protocols improve insulin sensitivity estimation using the minimal model. *Am J Physiol* 1987; 253:E595-602.

[74] Finegood DT, Hramiak IM, Dupre J. A modified protocol for estimation of insulin sensitivity with the minimal model of glucose kinetics in patients with insulin-dependent diabetes. *J Clin Endocrinol Metab* 1990;70:1538-1549.

[75] Welch S, Gebhart SS, Bergman RN, Phillips LS. Minimal model analysis of intravenous glucose tolerance test-derived insulin sensitivity in diabetic subjects. *J Clin Endocrinol Metab* 1990; 71:1508-18.

[76] Cobelli C, Pacini G, Toffolo G, Sacca L. Estimation of insulin sensitivity and glucose clearance from minimal model: new insights from labeled IVGTT. *Am J Physiol* 250 (*Endocrinol Metab* 13) 1986;E591-E598.

[77] Avogaro A, Bristow JD, Bier DM, Cobelli C, Toffolo G: Stable-label intravenous glucose tolerance test minimal model. *Diabetes* 1989;38:1048-55.

[78] Sunehag AL, Treuth MS, Toffolo G, Butte NF, Cobelli C, Bier DM, et al. Glucose production, gluconeogenesis, and insulin sensitivity in children and adolescents: An evaluation of their reproducibility. *Pediatr Res* 2001; 50:115-123.

[79] Hoffman RP, Armstrong PT. Glucose effectiveness, peripheral and hepatic insulin sensitivity, in obese and lean pre-pubertal children. *Int J Obes Relat Metab Disord* 1996;20:521-525.

[80] Steil GM, Volund A, Kahn SE, Bergman RN. Reduced sample number for calculation of insulin sensitivity and glucose effectiveness from the minimal model. Suitability for use in population studies. *Diabetes* 1993; 42:250-56.

[81] Steil GM, Murray J, Bergman RN, Buchanan TA. Repeatability of insulin sensitivity and glucose effectiveness from the minimal model. Implications for study design. *Diabetes* 1994;43:1365-71.

[82] Ferrannini E and Mari A. How to measure insulin sensitivity. *J Hypertension* 1998;16:895-906.

[83] Mari A. Mathematical modeling in glucose metabolism and insulin secretion. *Current Opinion in Clinical Nutrition and Metabolic Care* 2002;5:495-501.

[84] Quon MJ, Cochran C, Taylor SI, Eastman RC. Non-insulin-mediated glucose disappearance in subjects with IDDM. Discordance between experimental results and minimal model analysis. *Diabetes* 1994;43:890-896.

[85] Finegood DT, Tzur D. Reduced glucose effectiveness associated with reduced insulin release: an artifact of the minimal-model method. *Am J Physiol* 1996;271:E485-E495.

[86] Cutfield WS, Bergman RN, Menon RK, Sperling MA. The modified minimal model: Application to measurement of insulin sensitivity in children. *J Clin Endocrinol Metab* 1990;70:1644-1650.

[87] Travers SH, Jeffers BW, Bloch CA, Hill JO, Eckel RH. Gender and Tanner stage differences in body composition and insulin sensitivity in early pubertal children. *J Clin Endocrinol Metab* 1995; 80:172-178.

[88] Travers SH, Jeffers BW, Eckel RH. Insulin resistance during puberty and future fat accumulation. *J Clin Endocrinol Metab* 2002; 87:3814-18.

[89] Freemark M, Bursey D. The effects of metformin on body mass index and glucose tolerance in obese adolescents with fasting hyperinsulinemia and a family history of type 2 diabetes. *Pediatrics* 2001; 107:1-7.

[90] Lindquist CH, Gower BA, Goran MI. Role of dietary factors in ethnic differences in early risk of cardiovascular disease and type 2 diabetes. *Am J Clin Nutr* 2000;71:725-32.

[91] Goran MI, Bergman RN, Gower BA. Influence of total vs visceral fat on insulin action and secretion in African American and white children. *Obes Res* 2001;9:423-431.

[92] Cook JS, Hoffman RP, Stene MA, Hansen JR. Effects of maturational stage on insulin sensitivity during puberty. *J Clin Endocrinol Metab* 1993;77:725-730.
[93] Hoffman RP, Vicini P, Sivitz WI, Cobelli C. Pubertal adolescent male-female differences in insulin sensitivity and glucose effectiveness determined by the one compartment minimal model. *Pediatr Res* 2000;48:384-388.
[94] Hofman PL, Cutfield WS, Robinson EM, Bergman RN, Menon RK, Sperling MA, et al. Insulin resistance in short children with intrauterine growth retardation. *J Clin Endocrinol Metab* 1997; 82:402-406.
[95] Hamilton J, Cummings E, Zdravkovic V, Finegood D, Daneman D. Metformin as an adjunct therapy in adolescents with type 1 diabetes and insulin resistance. *Diabetes Care* 2003; 26:138-143.
[96] Conwell LS, Trost SG, Brown WJ, Batch JA. Indexes of insulin resistance and secretion in obese children and adolescents. *Diabetes Care* 2004;27:314-319.
[97] Reaven G, Miller R. Study of the relationship between glucose and insulin responses to an oral glucose load in man. *Diabetes* 1968;17:560-69.
[98] World Health Organization: Definition, diagnosis and classification of diabetes mellitus and its complications: Report of a WHO Consultation. *Part 1: Diagnosis and Classification of Diabetes Mellitus*, Geneva, 1999; World Health Org.
[99] The Expert Committee on the Diagnosis and Classification of Diabetes Mellitus. Follow-up report on the diagnosis of diabetes mellitus. *Diabetes Care* 2003; 26(11):3160-67.
[100] Pacini G, Mari A. Methods for clinical assessment of insulin sensitivity and β-cell function. *Best Pract Res Clin Endocrinol & Metab* 2003;17:305-322.
[101] Cederholm J, Wibell L. Insulin release and peripheral sensitivity at the oral glucose tolerance test. *Diabetes Res and Clin Practice* 1990;10:167-75.
[102] Matsuda A, DeFronzo R. Insulin sensitivity indices obtained from oral glucose tolerance testing. *Diabetes Care* 1999;22:1462-70.
[103] Breda E, Cavaghan MK, Toffolo G, Polonsky KS, Cobelli C. Oral glucose tolerance test minimal model indexes of β-cell function and insulin sensitivity. *Diabetes* 2001;50:150-158.
[104] Mooy JM, Grootenhuis PA, de Vries H, Kostene PJ, Popp-Snijders C, Bouter LM, et al. Intra individual variation of glucose, specific insulin and proinsulin concentrations measured by two oral glucose tolerance tests in a general Caucasian population: The Hoorn Study. *Diabetologia* 1996;39:298-305.
[105] Barrett-Connor E. The oral glucose tolerance test revisited. *European Heart Journal* 2002;23(16):1229-1231.
[106] Davidson MB. Counterpoint: The oral glucose tolerance test is superfluous. *Diabetes Care* 2002;25(10):1883-85.
[107] Stumvoll M, Mitrakou A, Pimenta W, Jenssen T, Yki-Jarvinen H, Haeften TV, et al. Use of the Oral Glucose Tolerance Test to Assess Insulin Release and Insulin Sensitivity. *Diabetes Care* 2000; 23:295-301.
[108] Weigensberg M J. Cruz M L and Goran M I. Association between insulin sensitivity and Post-glucose challenge plasma insulin values in overweight Latino youth. *Diabetes Care* 2003; 26: 2094-2099.
[109] Yeckel C W. Weiss R. Dziura J. Taksali S E. Dufour S. Burgert T S. Tamborlane W V and Caprio S. Validation of insulin sensitivity indices from oral glucose tolerance test

parameters in obese children and adolescents. *J Clin endocrinol Metab* 2004; 89: 1096-1101.

[110] Hirst S, Phillips DJW, Vines SK, Clark PM, Hales CN. Reproducibility of the Short Insulin Tolerance Test. *Diabetic Medicine* 1993;10:839-842.

[111] Akinmokun A, Selby PL, Ramaiya K, Alberti KGMM. The Short Insulin Tolerance Test for Determination of Insulin Sensitivity: A Comparison with the Euglycemic Clamp. *Diabetic Medicine* 1993;9:432-437.

[112] Sarnblad S, Kroon M, Aman J. The short insulin tolerance test lacks validity in adolescents with type 1 diabetes. *Diab Med* 2002;19:51-6.

[113] Greenfield MS, Doberne L, Kraemer F, Tobey T, Reaven G. Assessment of Insulin Resistance with the Insulin Suppression Test and the Euglycemic Clamp. *Diabetes* 1981;30:387-392.

[114] Legro RS, Finegold D, Dunalf A. A fasting Glucose to Insulin Ratio is a useful Measure of Insulin Sensitivity in Women with Polycystic Ovary Syndrome. *J Clin Endocrinol Metab* 1998; 83:2964-68.

[115] Silfen ME, Manibo AM, McMahon DJ, Levine LS, Murphy AR, Oberfield SE. Comparison of simple measures of insulin sensitivity in young girls with premature adrenarche: The fasting glucose to insulin ratio may be a simple and useful measure. *J Clin Endocrinol Metab* 2001;86: 2863-68.

[116] Matthews DR, Hosker JP, Rudenski AS, Naylor BA, Treacher DF, Turner RC. Homeostasis model assessment: insulin resistance and beta cell function from fasting plasma glucose and insulin concentrations in man. *Diabetologia* 1985;28:412-419.

[117] Katz A, Nambi SS, Mather K, Baron AD, Follmann DA, Sullivan G, et al. Quantitative Insulin Sensitivity Check Index: A Simple, Accurate Method for Assessing Insulin Sensitivity in Humans. *J Clin endocrinl Metab* 2000;85:2402-10.

[118] Gutt M, Davis CL, Spitzer SB, Llabre MM, Kumar M, Czarnecki EM, et al. Validation of the insulin sensitivity index (ISI(0,120)): comparison with other measures. *Diabetes Res Clin Pract* 2000; 47:177-184.

[119] Vuguin P, Saenger P, DiMartino-Nardi J. Fasting Glucose Insulin Ratio: A Useful Measure of Insulin Resistance in Girls with Premature Adrenarche. *J Clin Endocrinol Metab* 2001; 86:4612-21.

[120] Huang TK, Johnson MS, Goran MI. Devlopment of a Prediction Equation for Insulin Sensitivity From anthropometry and Fasting Insulin in Prepubertal and Early Pubertal children. *Diabetes Care* 2002;25:1203-1210.

[121] Uwaifo GI, Fallon EM, Chin J, Eberg J, Parikh SJ, Yanovski JA. Indices of insulin action, disposal, and secretion derived from fasting samples and clamps in normal glucose-tolerant black and white children. *Diabetes Care* 2002; 25:2081-87.

[122] Gungor N, Saad R, Janosky J, Arslanian S. Validation of surrogate estimates of insulin sensitivity and insulin secretion in children and adolescents. *J Pediatr* 2004;144:47-55.

[123] Quon MJ. Editorial: Limitations of the fasting glucose to insulin ratio as an index of insulin sensitivity. *J Clin Endocrinol Metab* 2001;86(10):4615-17.

[124] Robbins DC, Anderson L, Bowsher R, Chance R, Dinesen B, Frank B, et al. Task Force Report. Report of the American Diabetes Association's Task Force on standardization of the insulin assay. *Diabetes* 1996;45:242-256.

In: Insulin Resistance in Children and Adolescents
Editors: D. Daneman and J. Hamilton, pp. 57-86
ISBN 1-59454-215-5


*Chapter 3*

# FETAL INFLUENCES ON INSULIN RESISTANCE

***Craig Jefferies, Paul Hofman and Wayne S. Cutfield***
Starship Children's Hospital, New Zealand

## ABSTRACT

Epidemiological studies have repeatedly demonstrated an association between fetal growth retardation and the adult onset of hypertension, ischaemic heart disease, and type 2 diabetes mellitus (DM). Insulin resistance is a common metabolic abnormality underlying all of these conditions. It has been hypothesized that glucose homeostasis is fundamentally altered as a consequence of an intra-uterine adaptation to reduced fetal nutrition. This adaptation is then thought to permanently reset crucial endocrine functioning and is mainly reflected in associated reduced fetal growth.
There is also now general agreement that type 2 DM results from a combination of ß-cell failure and the presence of pre-existing insulin resistance. The majority of cases of type 2 DM can be directly linked to secondary effects of obesity and inactivity. However, there are marked individual variations in insulin resistance prior to the onset or effect of obesity. Certain ethnic groups in particular need to gain only a disproportionately small amount of weight to markedly increase their risk of type 2 DM. Fetal influences that permanently increase insulin resistance from birth would result in an increased susceptibility to type 2 DM. Identification of intra-uterine influences on insulin resistance has particular relevance to the third world; where both fetal malnutrition and type 2 DM are rife and occurring within the same generation. The most studied area to date is the small-for-gestational-age (SGA) infant. New research also suggests that prematurely born and twin children are also insulin resistant, although this is not necessarily reflected in reduced birth weight. In this chapter we will review fetal influences on insulin resistance, in particular studies that relate to detecting insulin resistance in children.

## INTRODUCTION

Insulin resistance is the most common metabolic abnormality detected prior to the development of type 2 DM [1]. There is general agreement that type 2 DM results from a combination of insulin resistance and progressive ß-cell failure. Although the majority of cases of type 2 DM can be directly linked to the adverse effects of obesity, what modulates one's susceptibility to the effects of obesity is the subject of much research.

To the dismay of many health experts and planners, type 2 DM is both a current and future global problem of major proportions. The annual cost of diabetes related care in the U.S. alone is predicted to be nearly $US 200 billion by the year 2020 [2]. Interestingly, the majority of those predicted to need diabetes care are in high risk ethnic groups such as African American, Hispanic, American Indian and Asian. Even more alarming is the escalating incidence of type 2 DM in the more populous developing world. For example, India has an estimated 33 million cases and China is not far behind with 23 million cases. Paradoxically, in Western countries marked obesity is associated with the development of type 2 DM, whereas in developing countries a lesser degree of obesity is associated with type 2 DM. Therefore, although genetic and lifestyle risk factors are important in the development of type 2 DM, the identification of pre and postnatal influences are of particular importance to the developing world.

The metabolic syndrome has been coined to describe the clustering of impaired glucose tolerance, dyslipidemia and hypertension. In 1988 Reaven proposed that insulin resistance was the key common underlying abnormality resulting in these metabolic diseases and the metabolic syndrome [3]. This chapter will explore the role of the fetal and early post-natal environment on programmed changes in glucose regulation.

## The Fetal Origins of Adult Disease

In the late 1980s and early 1990s, Barker and colleagues at the Southampton Epidemiology Unit made a number of landmark epidemiological observations linking reduced size at birth with a range of diseases later in adult life: type 2 DM, "Syndrome X" (metabolic syndrome), hypertension, cerebrovascular disease, coronary heart disease and chronic bronchitis [4-9]. These observations were possible due to the meticulous neonatal and infancy records kept across several counties in England, including Hertfordshire and Preston from 1911 onwards. Based upon these earliest studies it was argued that adult stroke was related to the intrauterine environment, chronic bronchitis was due to adverse early postnatal influences, and coronary heart disease had its origins in fetal and early postnatal life [5-7, 9]. These initial studies led Barker to propose the *fetal origins of adult disease* hypothesis: that the origins of common adult diseases begins in-utero. Subsequent studies by the Southampton Epidemiology Unit examined the relationship between birth weight and both hypertension and type 2 DM. These studies provided precise endpoints to more closely examine the relationship between actual birth weight and systolic blood pressure or plasma glucose values during a 2 hour glucose tolerance test [10, 11]. In 1228 adult men and women from Hertfordshire, there was a trend of progressive increase in systolic blood pressure with progressive reduction in birth weight from >8.5 lb to ≤5.5 lb [12]. The same trends were observed in studies of 59 to 70 years old men from Hertfordshire and Preston between birth weight and 2 hour plasma glucose during an oral glucose tolerance test [10, 13]. Higher 2-hour plasma glucose values were seen with a progressive fall in birth weight from >9.5 lb to ≤5.5 lb [13]. Only 6% of those with the heaviest birth weight compared to 30% of those with a birth weight ≤5.5 lb were classified as Syndrome X [7].

Criticisms of this hypothesis have focused mainly on two areas: The first is an initial lack of correction for important social factors such as social class and lifestyle [14, 15]. These original observations were only made in a few counties in England where unrecognised confounding factors could be present. Secondly, studies in relatively small numbers of non-identical twins showed a lack of difference in blood pressure between the larger and smaller born twins [16]. Differences in blood pressure would have been expected, with the smaller twin exhibiting higher blood pressure in adult life.

The observations linking birth weight and later disordered glucose metabolism have now been made by many research groups across different ethnicities and countries, negating the contention that the original observations were distorted by unmeasured confounding variables [17]. One of the most important of these studies was conducted on survivors of the 1944-5 Dutch famine, a period of well documented famine exposure in recent history. Of the 702 50-year old men and women studied, 2 hour plasma glucose values following an oral glucose tolerance test were higher in those born during, than those born before or conceived after, the famine [18]. Furthermore, late gestation famine exposure was associated with the highest 2 hour plasma glucose values [18]. This was the one of the first human studies to link fetal undernutrition to long term abnormalities in glucose regulation.

Subsequently a study in San Antonio, Texas, USA, also demonstrated an association between lower birth weight and Syndrome X; those at greatest risk having had the lowest birth weight along with the highest current BMI [19]. In this bi-ethnic population of 30-year old Mexican Americans and non-Hispanic Whites, the odds of developing Syndrome X increased 1.72 fold for each tertile decrease in birth weight. In Upsala, Sweden, Lithell and colleagues have also demonstrated in a study of 971 men aged 60 years [20], that not just birth weight, but thinness at birth, was important in later development of type 2 DM. Those with the lowest ponderal index quintile had an odds ratio of 4.4 for developing type 2 DM. Other studies in the USA that have confirmed the association between lower birth weight and increased type 2 DM risk include the Health Professionals Study, and that conducted in Pima Indians [21, 22]. Further associations were also made by the original Southampton Epidemiology Unit between lower birth weight and death from coronary heart disease [23]. The lowest tertile of birth weight was associated with a two- to three-fold increased risk of death from heart disease. This association between lower birth weight and coronary heart disease has subsequently been made by others [24-26]. The link made by the Southampton Epidemiology Unit between lower birth weight and hypertension in adults is supported by higher blood pressure found in Swedish adolescents with progressive reduction in birth weight [27]. Furthermore, a trend towards a greater increase in blood pressure has been found in infants and children of lower birth weight [28].

With regard to the question of twins and the fetal origins hypothesis, we have recently shown that prepubertal twin children have an abnormal blood pressure profile and are insulin resistant when compared to normal singleton children [29]. These findings were independent of birth weight or gestation, and suggested that there are potentially unrecognised in-utero effects independent of nutrition that may influence blood pressure and glucose regulation in twins. Therefore, we believe that twins are not a valid model to use in the study of the fetal origins hypothesis and that twin studies cannot be used as criticism of this hypothesis.

More detailed evidence of reprogramming of specific organ functions continues to be shown, which include immune system (thyroid autoantibodies) [30], large vessel compliance [31], endothelial function [32], vital capacity [33], hypothalamic-pituitary-adrenal axis [34], skeletal muscle insulin resistance [35], growth hormone-IGF-I axis [36], menarche [37], polycystic ovarian syndrome [38], schizophrenia [39], renin-angiotensin regulation [31], and cholesterol metabolism [40]. However, specific mechanisms linking perinatal events, presumed nutritional, to these organ changes or disorders have not been identified.

## Thrifty Phenotype Hypothesis

Epidemiological studies linking reduced birth weight and type 2 diabetes mellitus led Hales to propose the *thrifty phenotype hypothesis* [41]. Accordingly, insulin resistance and deficiency are the outcome of the undernourished fetus having to be nutritionally thrifty. If the individual remains undernourished during post-natal life, glucose and insulin regulation is adequate. However, a change to adequate or over-nutrition, exposes deficiencies in β-cell function and tissue sensitivity to insulin, ultimately leading to type 2 diabetes [41]. Similarly, lower renin levels reported in adults of lower birth weight has led to the speculation that fetal undernutrition leads to a reduction in nephron number which may cause nephrosclerosis and hypertension [42, 43]. This concept of undernutrition leading to organ hypoplasia has been incorporated within the thrifty phenotype hypothesis to explain the development of type 2 DM.

## The Fetal Insulin Hypothesis (Thrifty Genotype)

According to the *thrifty-genotype* hypothesis proposed by Neel, diseases such as type 2 DM results from discordance between certain features of our present-day environment and our genetic make-up which evolved to fit the life of Paleolithic humans. This concept implies that while affected individuals harbour the ancestral version of the relevant genes, healthy unaffected individuals have acquired recent mutations leading to a loss of thriftiness of these genes [44]. Subsequently, Hattersley and Tooke coined the *fetal insulin hypothesis* to relate reduced birthweight with later type 2 DM [45]. They proposed that genetically determined insulin resistance results in impaired insulin-mediated growth in the fetus as well as insulin resistance in adult life. Low birthweight, measures of insulin resistance in life, and ultimately glucose intolerance, diabetes, and hypertension could all be phenotypes of the same insulin-resistant genotype. Insulin is an important growth factor in fetal life. The presence of mutations in diabetes susceptibility genes would potentially result in fetal growth retardation. Hattersley and colleagues showed that in sib-pairs discordant for a glucokinase mutation, the child with the mutation had a lower birth weight with a mean difference of 521gm [46]. However, mutations in MODY genes are rare, and would not account for more than a very small percentage of SGA infants. Polymorphisms in MODY genes including hepatic nuclear factor (HNF)-1α, HNF-4 α and HNF-6 were not shown to have a major influence on birth size in a Danish cohort [47]. Interestingly maternal hyperglycaemia (due to MODY2) during fetal life had no effect on metabolic phenotypes of the adult offspring with or without MODY2 (glucokinase mutations). In a study of 447 family members from 37 MODY2 kindreds, regardless of the MODY2 status of the mothers, offspring without the mutation were similar for insulin secretion, insulin sensitivity, blood pressure and lipid profile in adulthood [48]. Therefore, in this model, although maternal environment and fetal genotypes could alter growth in utero by changing fetal insulin secretion, these effects do not result in a persistent programming in later life.

It is likely that that both the thrifty genotype and thrifty phenotype contribute to the association between reduced birth weight and later type 2 DM. Genetic and early environmental abnormalities could be additive in determining the risk of later type 2 DM, as a "double hit" phenomenon for the development of clinical disease, further amplified by adverse lifestyle changes such as inactivity, diet and smoking. In addition, the early fetal environment may influence expression of genes (epigenetics), involved in glucose regulation through altered methylation patterns of imprinted genes [49].

## Animal Models of Fetal Programming

Human studies are valuable to more precisely demonstrate the metabolic and endocrine consequences of lower birth weight. However, it is inevitable that identification of the mechanisms leading to these changes can only be explored in animal studies. The environment can be manipulated and tissues examined from animal studies, which is not possible with human studies. A number of rodent models have been developed to explore the effects of placental dysfunction on reduced birth size and later disease which are summarised in Table 1.

Unfortunately, none of these models replicates the human fetal environment that leads to a reduction in birth weight. In developed countries in humans, placental dysfunction leading to the combination of a reduction in oxygen and all nutrients is likely to be the principal cause of restricted fetal weight gain. Despite these limitations, some valuable insights into the effects of fetal restriction have been obtained from these animal models. In late gestation, bilateral uterine artery ligation model of growth restriction in rats, Simmons and colleagues showed that insulin-mediated glucose uptake and glucose transporter (GLUT-1) protein levels are reduced in skeletal muscle of weight restricted fetuses [50]. However, no changes were seen in glucose transport or GLUT-1 protein levels in the fetal brain. These observations support the notion that fetal nutrient restriction leads to diversion of glucose from skeletal muscle to the brain to ensure survival of the fetus. In the rat, total calorie undernutrition during pregnancy and a high calorie diet postnatally leads to hyperphagia and obesity when compared to control rats with normal nutrition during pregnancy and the same high calorie diet postnatally [51]. This suggests that hyperphagia may be a factor in the abdominal obesity seen in human adults born of lower birth weight. Key hepatic enzymes of glucose homeostasis programmed in offspring of protein restricted dams retain the ability to respond to over nutrition during adult life [52]. This study suggests that protein restriction in utero leads to changes in hepatic enzyme function involved in glucose regulation.

It must be noted that there is a sexual dimorphism, and almost always it appears that only the male offspring are able to be programmed [51, 53].

**Table 1. Animal Models of Fetal Programming**

| Author | Model | Outcome in growth retarded offspring. |
|---|---|---|
| Woodall et al, (1996).<br>Vickers et al, (2000).<br>Garofano, (1997). | Maternal total calorie undernutrition (30% of *ad libitum* intake) | Postnatal growth failure & abnormal somatotrophic axis [54].<br>Hyperphagia, obesity, hyperinsulinaemia, hyperleptinaemia & hypertension [51].<br>Impairment of β-cell development [55]. |
| Langley, (1994).<br>Desai, (1997).<br>Ozanne, (2001).<br>Petry, (2001). | Protein undernutrition (~8% vs. 20% diet composition) | Increased systolic blood pressure [53].<br>Key changes in hepatic enzymes of glucose homeostasis [52].<br>Age-related loss of glucose tolerance, adipocyte insulin resistance [56].<br>Insulin resistance & diabetes [57]. |
| Simmons, (1992). | Uterine artery ligation | Reduced insulin-mediated glucose uptake & GLUT-1 protein in skeletal muscle [58]. |
| Cleasby, (2003).<br>Benediktsson, (1993).<br>Lindsay, (1996). | Fetal glucocorticoid overexposure | Attenuated fatty acid uptake specifically in visceral fat [59].<br>Hypertension [60].<br>Raised blood glucoses in adulthood [61]. |

Protein under nutrition rat models suggest that reduced β-cell development is the early feature of later development of diabetes mellitus. However this is in contrast to the literature in human studies where there is stronger evidence for reduced insulin sensitivity than a primary defect in β-cell function [62-64]. The literature has long been swayed toward fetal pancreas underdevelopment by an anatomical report in severe growth retarded fetuses 25 years ago [65]. However, subsequent and more recent evaluation utilising sophisticated and standardised techniques of islet number has shown that being SGA does not alter fetal pancreas development [66]. Mean beta-cell fraction was 2.53% in the growth retarded fetuses and 2.86% in the control fetuses (P = 0.47) [66].

# Insulin Resistance in Small for Gestational Age (SGA) Children

## Defining SGA

The term SGA is descriptive and denotes babies born either short or low birth weight for a given gestational age. In some countries where accurate birth length is possible the SGA definition has been further refined to include $SGA_W$ (low birth weight), $SGA_L$ (low birth length), or $SGA_{WL}$ (low birth weight and length) [67]. Although this more refined definition appears to be predictive for late growth and metabolic abnormalities, birth length is generally measured unreliably and inaccurately. Because of this inaccuracy, SGA most commonly refers only to low birth weight and will be used in this context throughout the rest of this chapter.

SGA is used as a marker for intrauterine growth restriction. In the past the term intra uterine growth retardation (IUGR) frequently has been used interchangeably with SGA. However IUGR suggests there has been pathological growth restriction whereas this may not always be the case. The term SGA therefore is now preferred, although most SGA probably is the result of an adverse in utero environment.

The definition of SGA has varied among studies including a birth weight <$10^{th}$ percentile for gestational age, <$3^{rd}$ percentile for gestational age and <-2 standard deviations [62, 68, 69]. Recently an expert working group defined SGA as "a birth weight [ ]and/or length that is at least 2 SD below the mean ($\leq$-2 SD) for gestational age (approximately the $3^{rd}$ percentile)" [67]. Whatever definition is employed it is important to recognize that SGA has been arbitrarily set. Clearly the more stringent the SGA definition, the more likely all subjects will have intrauterine growth retardation, while the less stringent definition will be more inclusive of all growth retarded subjects but also include more subjects with normal growth who were destined to be small. In our experience defining SGA as being a birth weight < $10^{th}$ percentile (or -1.7 SD score) accurately separates the metabolic abnormalities in the SGA group from normal birth weight controls.

## Insulin Resistance in SGA Children

The fetal origins hypothesis was derived from the neonatal and infant growth data on older adults. Survival from infancy dictated these adults were born either at or near term as survival of premature infants was uncommon. Thus most low birth weight infants documented at this time were term and SGA and most subsequent studies in both animal and human, examining the fetal origins hypothesis, have involved normal gestation, SGA subjects.

It has been postulated that fetal adaptation to an adverse intrauterine environment involves altered programming of endocrine pathways, leading to permanent metabolic changes, including insulin resistance [62]. Many of the later adult sequelae therefore, could be explained as a consequence of this insulin resistance and secondary hyperinsulinism, especially considering the central role of insulin resistance in the development of the adult diseases comprising syndrome X [1, 3, 70-72]. Insulin resistance has been demonstrated in low birth weight, older adults, supporting this probable link [73].

If adverse perinatal events cause programming and an alteration in insulin sensitivity, these changes should be present from birth. Using oral glucose tolerance tests (OGTT), insulin resistance has been demonstrated in young adults (20 year olds) in SGA compared to age-matched case controls [74]. Insulin resistance was further identified in a similar aged group of young adults by the more sophisticated euglycaemic hyperinsulinaemic clamp [64]. This defect in insulin resistance appears to be due to a reduction in peripheral glucose uptake [64]. It also appears that hyperinsulinaemia is the only overt feature of syndrome X present in young adults with SGA, although subtle differences in lipid parameters and adiposity have been documented by some [64, 74]. However if more sophisticated measures are used, such as ambulatory blood pressure monitoring of blood pressure, subtle abnormalities in blood pressure profiles can also be detected in insulin resistant populations [29].

We have further extended the observation of isolated insulin resistance into the prepubertal years in SGA subjects. By using Bergman's minimal model in 4-10 year old currently healthy SGA children, we were able to demonstrate that they were markedly insulin resistant compared to an age, height and weight matched group of normal children [62], see Figures: 1 A & B.

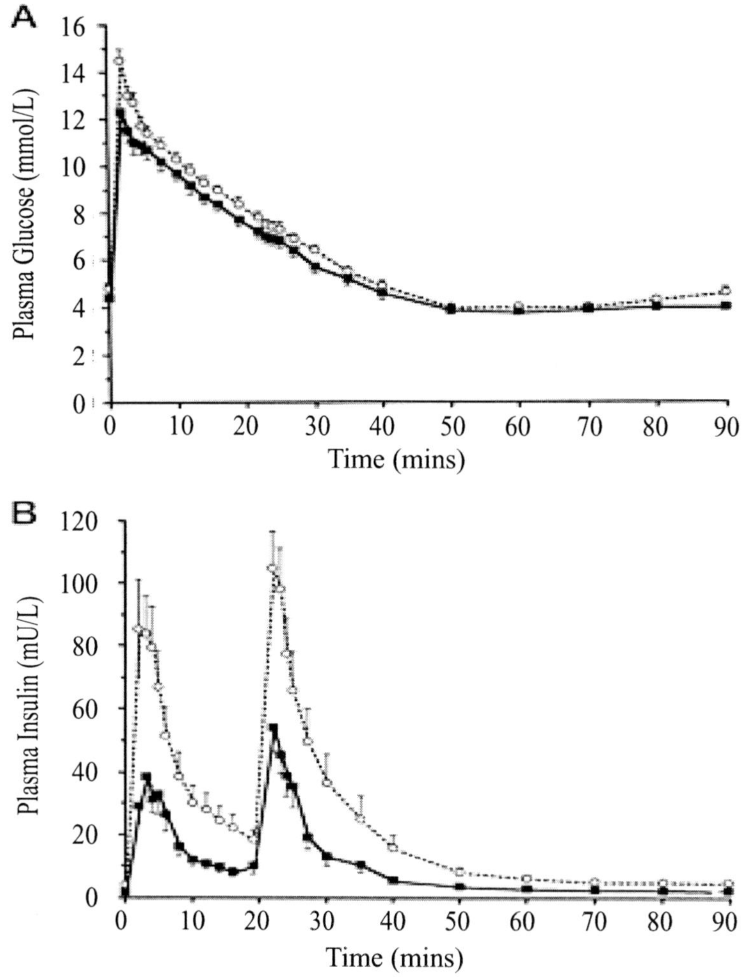


Figure 1 A). Glucose excursions during frequently sampled IV glucose test (FSIGT) in small-for-gestational, (open circles) and control (closed circles) subjects.
Figure 1 B). Insulin excursions in small-for-gestational (open circle) subjects and control (closed circle) subjects during FSIGT, (from Hofman [62]). The time zero minutes is the insulin response to IV dextrose, time 20 minutes is the response to IV tolbutamide, $p < 0.01$ between groups.

In our study the relationship between birth weight SD score and insulin resistance was not linear. Further studies, though using less sensitive techniques, have confirmed insulin resistance is present down to at least 12 months of age; suggesting this effect is an early abnormality and probably present from birth. The degree of insulin resistance that results in later adult disease is likely determined by unfolding of secondary genetic predisposition and life style choices. The latter mainly include sedentary life style and obesity that exaggerate any underlying degree of insulin resistance. The genetic influences that have been identified include polymorphisms of IGF-1, angiotensin converting enzyme 1, and β-3 adrenoreceptor and PPARγ [75-77].

Other studies have confirmed that isolated abnormalities in insulin sensitivity do increase the later risk of type 2 DM. In asymptomatic first degree adult children of patients with type 2 DM, their risk of similarly developing DM could be accurately predicted by assessment of insulin sensitivity and glucose effectiveness [1]. Over the next 25 years, those with normal insulin sensitivity and glucose effectiveness did not develop type 2 DM, while those with an isolated defect in insulin sensitivity had the cumulative risk for developing diabetes of 40% [1]. The current data also suggests that SGA subjects have a high risk of developing type 2 DM late in adult life. The risk likely increases into adulthood as insulin resistance increases with the cumulative effect of puberty, sedentary life style and obesity. Most children studied have been very slim, with relative adiposity being the most important factor influencing insulin sensitivity in childhood [78]. There is adult evidence to suggest these children born SGA have an increased risk of adult obesity and this may be the added metabolic burden that eventually leads to the β-cell failure and type 2 DM [79-81].

## Insulin Resistance in Premature Children

The majority of the studies to date have focused on SGA adults and children. If the fetal salvage hypothesis is correct and the metabolic abnormalities observed in later life reflect programming from an early adverse environment, then groups other than those born SGA may also be at risk. Prematurely born children and adults also suffer an adverse early environment. The early neonatal life of premature babies, especially those very premature (<32 weeks) is often turbulent. They are not physiologically mature enough to cope and have a range of problems from nutrient access and growth to respiratory, CNS and immunological immaturity. While SGA usually reflects utero-placental insufficiency and an adverse in utero environment, prematurity reflects predominantly an early postnatal adverse environment. Some have discounted prematurity as a factor associated with insulin resistance, due to the independent association with thinness at birth, though this was mainly based on the early studies by Barker and colleagues where prematurity as known now was not common [4, 22]. The postnatal environment occurs during the equivalent of third trimester of pregnancy and therefore is similar to the adverse late in-utero environment resulting in SGA babies.

The few studies published to date support the hypothesis that prematurity may also result in metabolic programming. Irving et al studied 34 premature young adults with birth weight <2000g and 27 controls [82]. Although they weren't very premature (mean gestation 34 weeks) they had an elevated BMI and systolic blood pressure compared to the controls. Baseline fasting insulin, an indirect marker of insulin resistance, was also significantly raised in the premature group. Fewtrell and colleagues recently studied 200 premature 12 year olds using a 30 minute glucose and insulin following a standard oral glucose load [83]. They found an association with birth weight and glucose level but not insulin when adjusted for current weight. However this study had the major flaw of the subjects being at various stages of puberty which markedly alters insulin resistance. Nonetheless these studies both suggested a possible effect of prematurity on insulin sensitivity.

We have recently completed a more sophisticated assessment of insulin sensitivity using the FSIGT and Bergman's minimal model in 47 premature (11 SGA and 36 AGA, gestational age 24-32 weeks), and 20 control prepubertal children aged 4 to 10 years. The results confirm that these children have a reduction in insulin sensitivity similar to that observed in term SGA subjects (see Figure: 2). Unlike term SGA children they also have a reduction in glucose effectiveness which reflects glucose's ability to increase its own uptake and suppress its own production. It has been demonstrated that defects in both insulin sensitivity and glucose effectiveness are additive and greatly increase the risk of later metabolic complications such as type 2 DM [84]. There was no association between insulin sensitivity and either birth weight or prematurity. We also did not see any difference in any metabolic parameters between premature AGA and SGA subjects. The effect of prematurity alone seemed to predominate suggesting that the postnatal environment was more important in metabolic programming in prematurely born subjects. If this is a postnatal effect then these metabolic abnormalities could be potentially modified thus improving adult morbidity.

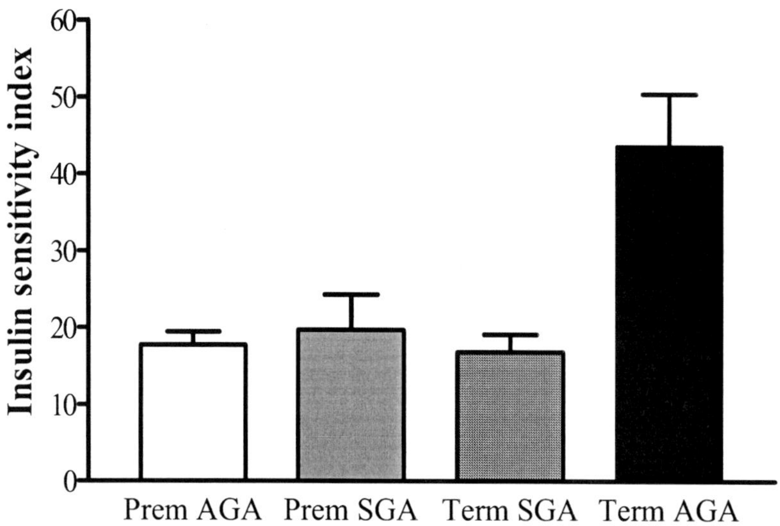


Figure 2. Insulin resistance in premature and term prepubertal children. Terms: appropriate-for-gestational-age (AGA), small-for-gestational-age (SGA). ($p<0.001$ Premature AGA and SGA compared to Term AGA).

To identify the possible postnatal events associated with these metabolic changes we have subsequently analysed the neonatal records of these children. Although we found no effect of chronic illness and pre- or post-natal glucocorticoid therapy it was clear that all the premature children were protein malnourished, with none receiving the recommended adequate protein intake in the first month and the majority being below this in the following 2 months (unpublished data). Rodent models of maternal protein malnutrition result in a metabolic syndrome phenotype in the offspring, raising the interesting possibility that the metabolic changes we have observed may be in part related to macronutrient intake [54].

We also noted that premature infants delivered to mothers with gestational proteinuric hypertension (GPH) were more insulin sensitive than other prematurely born children (although still less than the control children) despite this group being more growth retarded.

The protective factor(s) that GPH provide remain to be elucidated but one possibility may be the well documented hyper-leptinemia in these pregnancies [85, 86]. Leptin increases placental amino acid transport and may therefore ameliorate protein deficiency prior to delivery [87]. The studies to date indicate that prematurity especially with a gestation <32 weeks is associated with metabolic abnormalities, similar to those observed in term, SGA subjects. However unlike the SGA group, the timing of the insult to the post natal period suggests there may well be option of therapeutic interventions that can be implemented to reduce or prevent these metabolic sequelae. Studies are required to further define the metabolic profile in prematurely born subjects and define the postnatal causes of the insulin resistance that is observed in later life.

## INSULIN RESISTANCE IN TWINS

In human reproduction twins are a unique natural event and account for a small but significant proportion of society. Approximately 2% of the general population are estimated to be either twins or of multiple birth [88]. The "twin study" is the study of a disease in twin subjects, and has a specific "twin" design and evaluation. The underlying premise is that genetic influences are more common in monozygotic (MZ) than in dizygotic (DZ) twins. MZ twins are genetically 100% similar, whereas DZ twins are as genetically similar as siblings (i.e.: <50%). The important principles that underlie a twin study [89] are: (1) The trait being studied is not fundamentally influenced by being a twin, (2) Equal numbers of male and female subjects are included. Studies are often biased by over-representation of females. (3) Equal numbers of MZ and DZ twins are studied. MZ twins tend to want to join studies together unlike DZ twins [89]. As will be explained in more detail in this section, insulin resistance and therefore glucose homeostasis may be fundamentally influenced by being a twin which would invalidate the first principle of twin studies.

### Twins and Type 2 Diabetes Mellitus

The majority of studies of DM in adult twins have examined concordance rates between monozygotic and dizygotic twins for type 1 and type 2 DM, in an attempt to tease out the impact of genetic as compared to environmental influences [90-92]. Early twin studies reported very high concordance rates of 69 to 90% for type 2 DM in MZ twins, and have been used to justify the current intense search for genes associated with type 2 DM [93, 94]. These studies often do not use objective criteria in the diagnosis of type 2 DM (verbal reporting of DM status, or requirement for medications), were either volunteer or data-based, and suffered from recruitment bias. Two more recent, large, cross-sectional twin studies from the USA and Finland have reported much lower concordance rates of type 2 DM in MZ twins in the order of 17 to 20%, DZ twins had a concordance of 8 to 9% for type 2 DM [92, 95]. The weakness of a cross-sectional study design in determining concordance in a disease that increases in incidence with age was shown by Newman et al, whereby the concordance rate for type 2 DM in MZ twins increased from 17 to 42% over a 10 year follow-up period [95]. Recently, in the only prospective study of type 2 DM in twins, Medici et al reported a concordance rate in MZ twins of 76% over a 15 year follow-up period [94]. Furthermore, when Type 2 DM and impaired glucose tolerance were combined, the concordance rate in MZ twins was very high at 96% at 15 years of follow-up [94]. Unfortunately these authors did not determine the concordance rate of type 2 DM in DZ twins to more precisely determine the magnitude of the genetic effect on disease risk.

The strong genetic influence in determination of type 2 DM is more impressively evident when more detailed analysis of glucose homeostasis parameters for the development of type 2 DM is evaluated in MZ twin studies. In five unaffected MZ adult twins discordant for type 2 DM, reduced insulin secretion and increased glucose levels during an OGTT were observed [96]. Similarly, in 12 MZ adult twin pairs discordant for type 2 DM, only 7/12 had impaired glucose tolerance; however all 12 had diminished first phase insulin release, insulin resistance and a reduced insulin response during the hyperglycemic clamp [97].

Environmental factors appear also to have a role in the development of type 2 DM, as concordance of the disease even in MZ twins is less than 100%. Most unaffected MZ twins discordant for type 2 DM, (that is one twin has type 2 DM, the other is "normal), exhibit insulin resistance and or impaired insulin secretion, and are therefore at high risk of developing type 2 DM [1]. Adverse environmental factors such as obesity, lower birth weight and physical inactivity are likely to further enhance insulin resistance and diminish insulin secretion drawing them closer to clinical disease. In MZ twins discordant for type 2 DM, the index twin was obese when compared to the unaffected twin [90, 96, 98].

To date, no studies have examined the incidence of type 2 DM in adult twins to determine whether the twinning process is a risk factor in itself for the development of type 2 DM. Poulsen and colleagues found that 34% of 303 adult twin pairs had at least one member of the pair with either type 2 DM or impaired glucose tolerance [99]. This is a considerably higher incidence than that observed in the general adult Danish population of approximately ~10%. A study by Bo and colleagues in 30 year-old Italian twins was conducted in a select population with either diabetes or a family history of type 2 DM, the rate of type 2 DM overall in such a young population was much higher than expected [100]. The possible increased incidence of abnormal glucose regulation in twins suggests that some aspect of the twinning process itself may increase their type 2 DM risk. The in utero environment during fetal life and/or genes associated with enhanced twin survival may play a role in the development of insulin resistance and type 2 DM.

## Twins and the Fetal Origins Hypothesis

Commonly there is considerable disparity between the birth weights of twin pairs, thus this group has been selected as an obvious population to test the fetal origins of adult disease hypothesis [101, 102]. As twins have increased rates of low birth weight and prematurity, most have postulated then that type 2 DM and the rest of the metabolic syndrome may be expected to occur much more commonly in the twin with lower birth weight. There are only a small number of twin studies that have examined the fetal origins hypothesis in relation to type 2 DM in adulthood [4, 16, 103, 104]. These studies have not consistently demonstrated a relationship between reduced birth weight and disordered glucose regulation or hypertension [4, 16, 103, 104]. By using original midwife birthweight records in DZ and MZ twins, Poulsen and colleagues examined 303 twins aged 55 to 74 years from the Danish twin registry [101]. They showed that birthweight was lower in the MZ and DZ twins with type 2

DM twins than in the non-diabetic co-twins. The twin with the lower birth weight had the highest two hour plasma glucose concentrations during an OGTT [101]. In a population-based Danish twin study, Poulsen demonstrated a genetic influence for glucose intolerance, obesity, blood pressure and low HDL-cholesterol levels, however environmental influence for abdominal obesity, insulin resistance and hypertriglyceridaemia [105]. Furthermore they demonstrated a sexual discordance amongst male and female twins for components in the metabolic syndrome. They question the validity of conclusions drawn from classical twin studies due to a potentially more adverse intrauterine environment among MZ compared to DZ twins though provide further evidence for a prenatal component in the etiology of the components included in the metabolic syndrome [105]. In contrast, the Birmingham twin study which evaluated a younger population of adult twins failed to show an association between birthweight and glucose intolerance despite substantial within pair differences in birth weight [102]. The Birmingham study twins were born in a much later period of the last century, were examined several decades earlier in life, and were from a non-diabetes biased cohort when compared to the Danish registry. Therefore, whether or not twins conform to the model proposed by Barker and the fetal origins hypothesis remains unclear [99, 101, 102]. Conflicting results are seen with a lack of clear association between reduced birth weight and elevated blood pressure in twins [4, 16, 103, 104].

## Twins and Insulin Resistance

Poulsen and colleagues examined insulin sensitivity with the euglycaemic clamp in MZ and DZ twins in two age groups (25-34 and 57-66 years). Interestingly, in the young group MZ twins were found to be more insulin sensitive than younger DZ twins. Conversely, in the older group the MZ twins were more insulin resistant than the DZ twins. In contrast to the fetal origins hypothesis, they did not find birth weight to be associated with insulin secretion or action in the younger adult twins. However, there appeared to be an association between low birth weight and reduced insulin sensitivity and low insulin secretion in elderly MZ twins [105]. These authors postulated that ageing could unmask the influence of an adverse intrauterine environment that leads to insulin resistance and low insulin secretion in twins [105]. Vaag et al. found no difference in insulin sensitivity as assessed by OGTT insulin values in adult MZ twins discordant for type 2 DM. Not surprisingly, β-cell function was reduced in the diabetic twin, consistent with the progressive nature of β-cell decline in the development of type 2 DM [97, 106, 107].

There are clearly conflicting results from studies that have examined the relationship between birth weight and insulin sensitivity or overt type 2 DM in adults. Lifestyle influences such as obesity, activity levels, smoking, sex hormone use etc were not usually considered in these adult twin studies and may have served to increase variability in the assessment of insulin sensitivity consequently.

We examined insulin sensitivity in prepubertal twin children to minimize many of these lifestyle effects. Using a validated modification of the minimal model for use in children we found there was no difference ($p = 0.7$) in insulin sensitivity or insulin secretion between MZ and DZ twins [108]. This observation argues against a genetic influence on insulin sensitivity during the prepubertal years in twins. There was concordance for insulin sensitivity within twin pairs, that was predictably higher in MZ twins, ($r^2 = 0.84$, $p = 0.004$) than within DZ twin pairs, ($r^2 = 0.32$, $p = 0.03$).

However, the prepubertal twins we studied demonstrated considerably lower insulin sensitivity values than age and BMI matched control subjects ($p < 0.01$). To compensate for insulin resistance the twins displayed compensatory hyperinsulinism when compared to control subjects as illustrated in Figure 3.

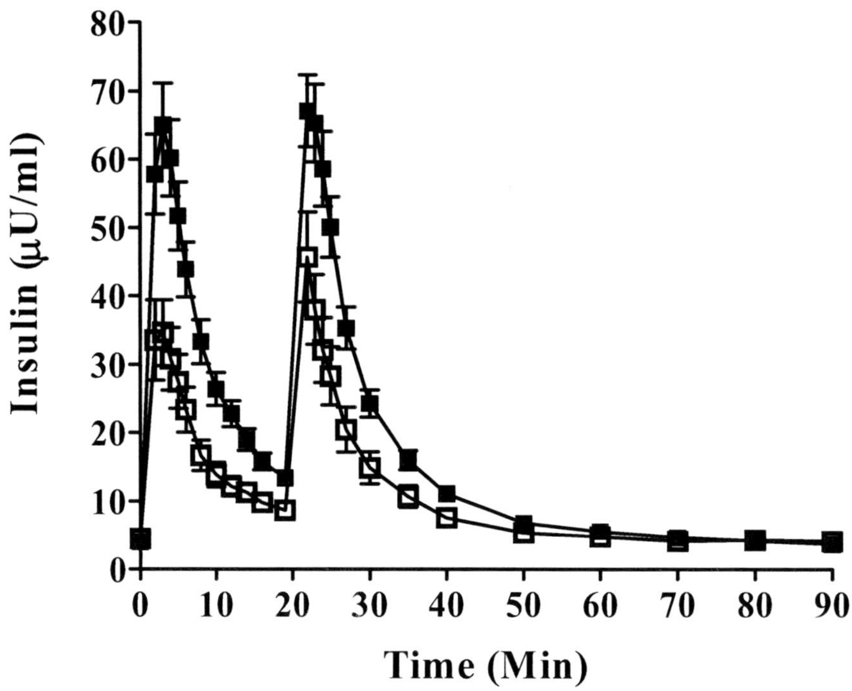


Figure 3. Insulin excursions in twins (MZ and DZ) and singleton controls during FSIGT: twins (solid squares, n =50) and singleton controls (open squares, n =19).

The insulin resistance in twins compared to singletons was independent of gestational age, birth weight, zygosity, age, sex, and BMI ($p < 0.001$). In twins, insulin sensitivity was only weakly associated with birthweight SD score ($p = 0.14$) and gestation ($p = 0.09$). Interestingly, there was no difference in insulin sensitivity when the heavier born twins were compared to the lighter born twins in MZ or DZ pair ($p = 0.6$), therefore all twins regardless of birth weight had lower insulin sensitivity than control subjects.

Glucose regulation appears to be fundamentally different in twins regardless of birth weight, suggesting that fetal undernutrition is unlikely to be a major factor in the development of insulin resistance in twins as has been proposed for SGA children [62]. Other potential candidates that lead to insulin resistance in twins include placental factors or genetic polymorphisms that enhance twin survival. As twins, irrespective of birth size, are insulin resistant they can longer be considered a valid group to test the fetal origins hypothesis linking birth size and latter adult disease.

## INSULIN RESISTANCE OR REDUCED BETA CELL FUNCTION

Insulin resistance refers primarily to the effect of insulin on glucose homeostasis. Thus, in non-diabetic subjects reduction in insulin sensitivity should result in a compensatory and appropriate hyperbolic increase in insulin secretion to maintain euglycaemia [109]. The evaluation of older adults with the euglycaemic hyperinsulinaemic clamp method has demonstrated that type 2 DM associated with a low birth weight is preceded by marked insulin resistance [73]. This insulin resistance coupled with the eventual loss or failure of appropriate beta cell function results in the typical picture of obesity induced type 2 DM [107]. Hyperinsulinaemia as determined by OGTT, has been demonstrated in young adults born SGA compared to age-matched subjects [63]. In addition, insulin resistance has also been shown in young adults born SGA by both minimal model and clamp techniques [64, 74]. This human data are in contrast to the reduced β-cell mass and reduced insulin secretion that predominate the animal models outlined earlier. In Figure 4, insulin sensitivity is compared to insulin secretory capacity (the acute insulin response) in SGA, twins premature and control subjects. The relationship between insulin resistance and the acute insulin response follows the expected hyperbolic relationship [110]. Collectively the data for SGA, twin and prematurely born children and SGA young adults indicate that insulin resistance rather than impaired β-cell function is likely to be the earliest defect in glucose regulation that precedes later development of type 2 DM in these groups.

Secondary baseline or stimulated hyperinsulinaemia may result in alterations to axes other than glucose regulation, such as increased sympathetic nervous system activation and sodium retention leading to an increased risk of elevated blood pressure, dyslipidemia and abnormalities in coagulation factors [70]. Insulin also stimulates hepatic release of IGF-I through actions on the GH receptor and at the IGF-I mRNA transcriptional level [111-114]. Insulin increases circulating IGF binding protein (BP)-3 levels by reducing IGFBP-3 degradation, suppressing circulating IGFBP-1, and allowing free IGF-I to contribute to post-prandial glucose disposal [115-117].

In two separate studies of SGA and prematurely born children we have demonstrated effects of hyperinsulinaemia on the IGF-I/ IGF BP-3 axis [118] [*GH IFGI Res* 2004 Jun 14 Suppl A 130-5] These children displayed strong correlations between fasting plasma insulin and IGF-I levels. In addition, fasting plasma insulin was correlated with IGF-I in prematurely born children. Both circulating insulin and glucose suppress IGFBP-I levels, supporting a role for IGFBP-I in glucose regulation. In control children IGFBP-I levels predictably fell following an IV glucose bolus during the FSIGT as shown in Figure: 5. However in SGA children there was no relationship between the level of acute insulin response and fall in IGFBP-I. Although the acute insulin response was twice as great in the SGA children the IGFBP-I levels only differed from control children at a single time point (see Figure: 5). These observations raise the possibility that SGA children exhibit insulin resistance to IGFBP-I regulation as well as to glucose regulation. The concept of insulin resistance to substrates other than glucose has not been well studied and could include, amino acids, free fatty acids, cation transport, IGF-I, IGFBP-I and IGFBP-3 levels.

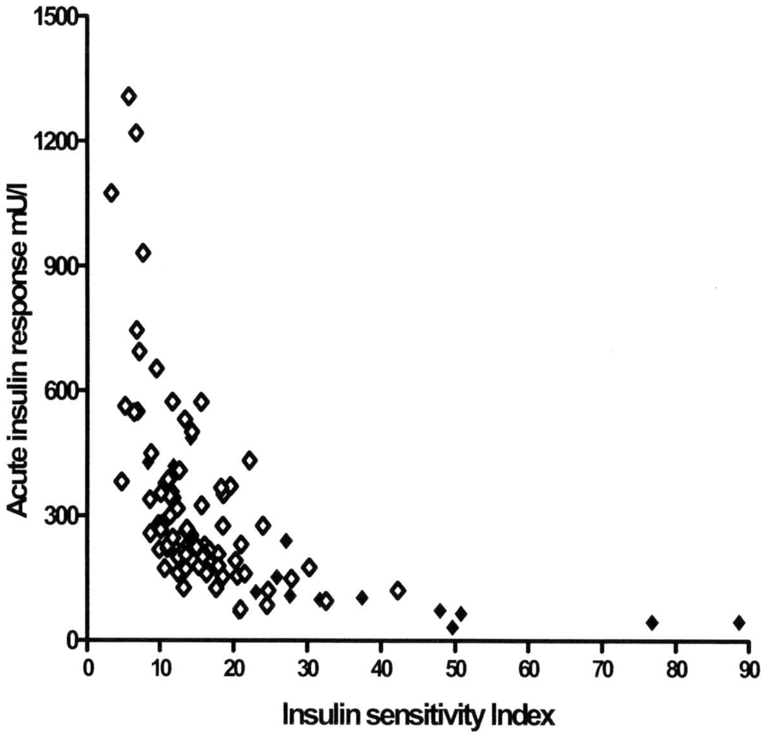


Figure 4. The hyperbolic relationship between insulin sensitivity and insulin response in prepubertal twin, SGA and prematurely born children (open diamond), and normal prepubertal children (closed diamond).

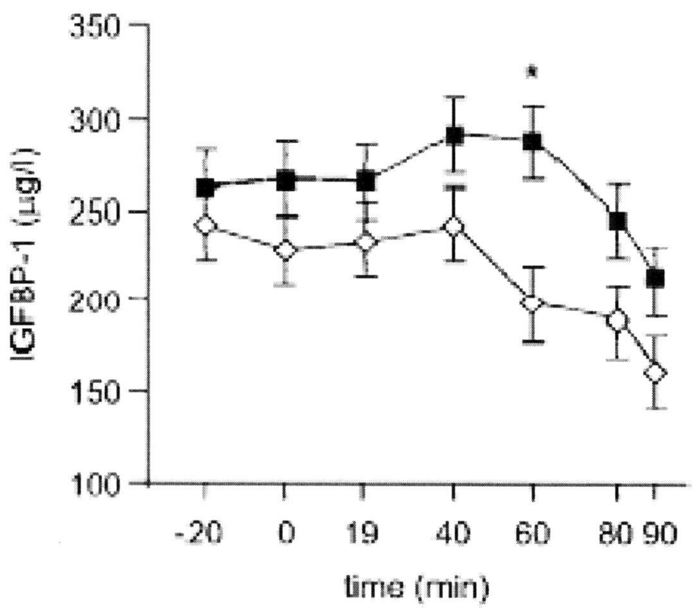


Figure 5. Plasma IGFBP-1 levels during a FSIGT (open diamond) and short normal (filled square) prepubertal subjects, *P = 0.016. From Cutfield (2002) [118].

# Infants of Diabetic Mothers, Later Obesity & Cortisol Metabolism

## Infants of Diabetic Mothers

To date we have examined the growth retarded or nutritionally constrained infant. At the other end of the nutritional spectrum is the over-nourished infant of the diabetic mother, the large-for-gestation infant (LGA). These infants represent the upper end of a "U" shaped curve for birthweight and risk of type 2 DM. Gestational DM is common and affects at least 130,000 women per year in the USA, with a prevalence rate that has increased from 2.9 to 8.8% over 20 years. A link between the fetal environment of a diabetic pregnancy and the later development of type 2 DM was first suggested by Freinkel approximately 20 years ago [119]. Early studies of glucose regulation in offspring of diabetic women have provided conflicting results: Silverman did not find an increased incidence of impaired glucose tolerance during childhood in offspring of diabetic women, whereas Plagemann suggested that impaired glucose tolerance was higher than expected for this age group [120, 121]. Both studies however compared the incidence of impaired glucose tolerance in their subjects to literature reports. With the recent increase in childhood obesity and the association between insulin resistance and obesity, conclusions based on comparisons with historical controls may be inaccurate. Using the minimal model, a more precise technique to measure insulin sensitivity, we found similar insulin sensitivity values in the prepubertal offspring of women with type 2 DM to offspring of women with type 1 DM and control subjects. Interestingly, larger maternal insulin doses were associated with lower insulin sensitivity values in offspring, raising the possibility that either maternal insulin had a programming effect on the glucose regulation of offspring or more severe maternal insulin resistance is associated with a stronger genetic risk of insulin resistance in the offspring. Therefore it appears that excessive glucose exposure to the fetus does not lead to a defect in glucose regulation during childhood. However, what is evident from serial evaluations of glucose homeostasis in a defined cohort of diabetic offspring is an increased incidence of impaired glucose tolerance after puberty [122].

Offspring of mothers with type 2 DM will have both a strong genetic predisposition to develop insulin resistance and obesity coupled with the potentially adverse environmental effects of fetal exposure to hyperglycaemia and or hyperinsulinaemia. However the genetic influence of type 2 DM is complex as only maternal family history of type 2 DM increases diabetes 2.5 fold, with paternal family history not reaching significance [123]. In offspring of diabetic women, Silverman and colleagues found that childhood obesity preceded a demonstrable impairment of glucose tolerance [122]. Similarly, we found that the offspring of women with type 2 DM were heavier than those offspring from normal or women with type 1 DM [124].

The impact of maternal glucose regulation on fetal events is also seen in non-diabetic women. Caruso and colleagues have shown increased insulin sensitivity in women with unexplained low birth weight infants compared to a control group of women with normal birth weight infants [125]. It is likely that the mother's enhanced insulin sensitivity and greater uptake of nutrients diminished available supply to the placenta and fetus.

In summary, offspring of diabetic mothers (particularly those with type 2 DM), are more likely to develop obesity during childhood, insulin resistance after puberty with an increased risk of type 2 DM during adult life. The prenatal events initiating and post-natal events accelerating these changes are likely to be multi-factorial and include genetic susceptibility, exposure to increased glucose and insulin levels during fetal life and post-natal nutrition.

## Low Birth Weight and Later Obesity

There is growing evidence linking lower birth weight with a greater risk of obesity in UK, Dutch and Indian adult populations [28, 52]. The Dutch famine study of 300,000 19-year-old males found a relationship between maternal undernutrition in the first half of pregnancy and the development of obesity [126]. Surprisingly, no relationship was found between maternal undernutrition in late pregnancy or early infancy and later obesity. The distribution of increased body fat in those of lower birth weight is principally truncal, which enhances the risks of metabolic disease. In men from Hertfordshire, lower birth weight and weight at 1 year were associated with greater waist to hip circumference ratios [17]. In those of lower birth weight, the greater likelihood of developing truncal obesity, which is usually visceral in males, will add further to the risk of cardiovascular disease and type 2 DM. Poor post-natal weight gain in men was associated with greater risks of disease in late adult life. In Hertfordshire, men with lower weights at 1 year had greater risks of impaired glucose tolerance, type 2 DM and ischaemic heart disease; suggesting that those who did not exhibit catch-up growth may be at greater risk of later adult disease [10, 11]. The same relationship between weight at 1 year and these adult diseases was not seen in women from Hertfordshire, suggesting either that a sex difference exists in fetal programming, or that there is uncertainty over these epidemiological observations [10, 11].

In a study performed on 1492 adults aged 26-32 years in South Delhi, thinness until the age of two years and then an acceleration in BMI demonstrated the greatest risk of impaired glucose tolerance or diabetes mellitus [127]. This observation reinforces the link between early poor nutrition and later metabolic disease with accelerated weight gain. In general accelerated childhood growth and increased physical size have been shown to be strongly associated with insulin resistance [128]. Studies on a large Finnish cohort with detailed birth and school health records for 7,086 have added to this and revealed interesting effects of post-natal weight gain and growth [129]. The cumulative incidence of type 2 DM was 7.9%, the odds ratio for type 2 DM was 1.38 for each 1-kg decrease in birthweight. Interestingly the odds ratio for type 2 DM was 1.39 for each standard deviation increase in weight between 7 and 15 years of age, and increased to 1.83 in an analysis restricted to those with birth weights below 3.0 kg. Maternal BMI in pregnancy was an added risk factor for rapid growth during childhood as well as an increased incidence of type 2 DM [129].

The exact impact of post-natal growth and "catch-up" growth is still being evaluated and even in normal and LGA infants abnormal postnatal growth patterns with rapid gain in BMI after age 2 years being associated with increased the risk of later disease in both normal, SGA and LGA infants [130]. Although maternal size (BMI) influences birthweight, paternal size has been shown to be associated with childhood growth velocity, at least in Indian populations [128]. What determines the accelerated growth is most likely a complex mix of food availability, genetics, maternal and paternal influence coupled with cultural and social beliefs. In animal models, if the undernourished rat is cross-fostered to a normal lactating dam, the animal will reach normal body and organ weights by weaning, though its subsequent longevity is reduced [131].

### Hypothalamic-Pituitary-Adrenal (HPA) Axis Abnormalities and Insulin Resistance

It has been hypothesised that stress to the fetus leads to irreversible increase in hypothalamic-pituitary-adrenal (HPA) axis activity that is pivotal in initiating fetal and post-natal insulin resistance. There is evidence that programming of the HPA axis occurs in animal models, however the data in humans is a little less convincing [132, 133]. Reduction in birth weight has been shown to be associated with increased early morning plasma cortisol levels in several different adult populations [134]. However, evidence in children appears less convincing. Clark and colleagues only showed a weak U-shaped relationship between birthweight and urinary glucocorticoids in prepubertal children [34]. In contrast to these adult studies we found lower early morning cortisol levels in SGA, premature and twin children when compared to control children [135]. Our own data in prepubertal children (SGA, premature and twin) does not support any increase in fasting cortisol and insulin resistance, and there was a significant reduction in insulin resistant subjects compared to controls (Unpublished data). In another study of SGA children extensive HPA axis evaluation (fasting plasma cortisol, adrenocorticotroph response, circadian rhythm and cortisol area under the curve) did not reveal any differences between control and SGA children [133]. The lack of a clear association, particularly in children, between cortisol overproduction and insulin resistance suggests that it is unlikely that HPA axis activation directly leads to programmed insulin resistance. At best the studies in adults may reflect common pathways of disease rather than a direct causative mechanism.

## The Relevance of Fetal Influences on Type 2 Diabetes Mellitus

Recent attempts to quantify the relative importance of impaired fetal growth and the overall incidence of 2 DM have down-played the importance of the fetal origins of insulin resistance [136]. In a review of six published studies Boyko concluded that impaired fetal growth accounted for only a minority of diabetes cases in adult life [136]. In his analysis up to 35% of cases of diabetes were attributable to reduced birth weight. Although not as strong a predictor as obesity, it would appear that birth weight is a meaningful risk factor for type 2 DM. Furthermore, these studies were performed in developed countries. It is very likely that there are different risk associations between low birth weight and later diabetes mellitus in large developing countries such as India. Low birth weight is common in India. Two thirds of middle aged non-obese Indian males are insulin resistant [137]. Over the past 30 years with the advent of better post-natal nutrition in India there has been a 500% increase in the incidence of impaired glucose tolerance and type 2 DM combined. Type 2 DM is now more common in India than in any other country in the world [138]. We speculate that post-natal over-nutrition of undernourished fetuses in developing countries is becoming a major factor in the worldwide epidemic of type 2 DM.

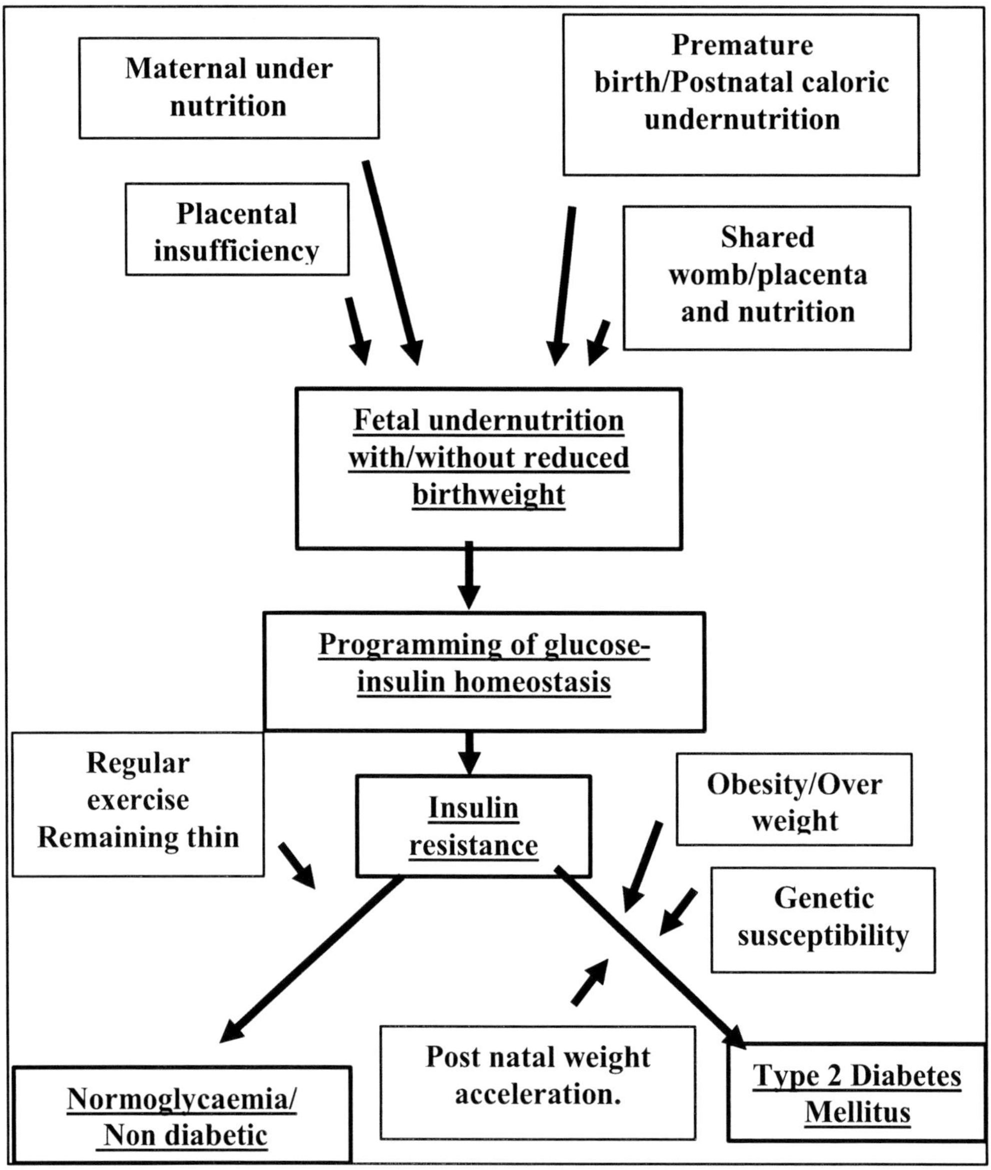


Figure 6. Fetal programming of glucose and insulin homeostasis.

The study of the fetal origins of disease provides two important roles: firstly to identify those at risk in the current generation, and secondly, to prevent subsequent disease in future generations [4, 139]. The continued development and popularity of assisted reproductive techniques, improvements in survival of very low birth weight infants due to the success of modern neonatal intensive care and the continued delivery of undernourished and idiopathic SGA infants, suggests that the impact of fetal programming of later adult metabolic disease will continue to be important for many decades. It will be equally important to ascertain which associated genetic traits or lifestyle and dietary factors enhance the risk of diabetes mellitus in these groups of individuals. Figure 6 outlines our current understanding of the fetal origins of insulin resistance. The emphasis on the fetal origins of adult disease is evolving from epidemiological associations to understanding the underlying cellular and physiological processes that lead to metabolic disease in adult life.

## CONCLUSIONS

Epidemiological studies have repeatedly demonstrated an association between reduced birth weight and the adult onset of hypertension, ischaemic heart disease, and type 2 diabetes mellitus (DM). Insulin resistance is a common metabolic abnormality underlying all of these conditions. It has been hypothesized that glucose homeostasis is fundamentally altered as a consequence of an intra-uterine adaptation to reduced fetal nutrition. This adaptation is then thought to permanently reset crucial endocrine and metabolic axes and is initially reflected in reduced fetal growth and small size at birth.

Studies in childhood indicate an early reduction in insulin sensitivity in SGA offspring, with growing evidence for a similar reduction in insulin sensitivity in twin and prematurely born populations. These studies suggest that reduced insulin sensitivity is an early marker for the later development of type 2 DM.

## REFERENCES


[1] Martin BC, Warram JH, Krolewski AS, Bergman RN, Soeldner JS, Kahn CR. Role of glucose and insulin resistance in development of type 2 diabetes mellitus: results of a 25-year follow-up study [comment]. *Lancet.* 1992; 340:925-9.

[2] Gorman C. Why so many are getting diabetes. *Time*, 2003:37-47.

[3] Reaven GM. Banting lecture 1988. Role of insulin resistance in human disease. *Diabetes* 1988; 37:1595-607.

[4] Barker DJ. The fetal and infant origins of adult disease. *BMJ.* 1990; 301:1111.

[5] Barker DJ, Winter PD, Osmond C, Margetts B, Simmonds SJ. Weight in infancy and death from ischaemic heart disease [comment]. *Lancet.* 1989; 2:577-80.

[6] Barker DJ, Osmond C, Golding J, Kuh D, Wadsworth ME. Growth in utero, blood pressure in childhood and adult life, and mortality from cardiovascular disease. *BMJ.* 1989; 298:564-7.

[7] Barker DJ, Fall CH. Fetal and infant origins of cardiovascular disease. *Archives of Disease in Childhood.* 1993; 68:797-9.

[8] Robinson S, Walton RJ, Clark PM, Barker DJP, Hales CN, Osmond C. The relation of fetal growth to insulin secretion in young men. *Diabetologia* 1992; 35:444-6.

[9] Martyn CN, Barker DJP, Osmond C. Mother's pelvic size, fetal growth, and death from stroke and coronary heart disease in men in the UK. *Lancet* 1996; 348:1264-8.

[10] Hales CN, Barker DJ, Clark PM, et al. Fetal and infant growth and impaired glucose tolerance at age 64 [comment]. *BMJ.* 1991; 303:1019-22.

[11] Barker DJ, Hales CN, Fall CH, Osmond C, Phipps K, Clark PM. Type 2 (non-insulin-dependent) diabetes mellitus, hypertension and hyperlipidaemia (syndrome X): relation to reduced fetal growth. *Diabetologia*. 1993; 36:62-7.

[12] Law CM, de Swiet M, Osmond C, Fayers PM, Barker DJ, Cruddas AM, Fall CH. Initiation of hypertension in utero and its amplification throughout life. *BMJ*. 1993 Jan 2;306(6869):24-7.

[13] Barker DJ. The intrauterine origins of cardiovascular disease. *Acta Paediatrica. Supplement*. 1993; 82:93-9; Discussion 100.

[14] Paneth N, Ahmed F, Stein AD. Early nutritional origins of hypertension- a hypothesis still lacking support. *J Hypertension* 1996; 14:S121-9.

[15] Susser M, Levine B. Ordeals for the fetal programming hypothesis. *BMJ* 1999; 318:885-6.

[16] Williams S, Poulton R. Twins and maternal smoking: ordeals for the fetal origins hypothesis. *BMJ* 1999; 318:897-900.

[17] Law CM, Barker DJP, Osmond C, Fall CHD, Simmonds SJ. Early growth and abdominal fatness in adult life. *J Epidemiol Community Health* 1992; 46:184-6.

[18] Ravelli AC, van der Meulen JH, Michels RP, et al. Glucose tolerance in adults after prenatal exposure to famine [comment]. *Lancet*. 1998; 351:173-7.

[19] Valdez R, Athens MA, Thompson GH, Bradshaw BS, Stern MP. Birthweight and adult health outcomes in a biethnic population in the USA. *Diabetologia* 1994; 37:624-31.

[20] Lithell HO, McKeigue PM, Berglund L, Mohsen R, Lithell UB, Leon DA. Relation of size at birth to non-insulin dependent diabetes and insulin concentrations in men aged 50-60 years. *BMJ* 1996; 312:406-10.

[21] Curhan GC, Willet WC, Rimm EB, Stampfer MJ. Birth weight and adult hypertension and diabetes mellitus in US men. *Am J Hypertens* 1996; 9:Abstract.

[22] McCance DR, Pettitt DJ, Hanson RL, Jacobsson LTH, Knowler WC, Bennett PH. Birth weight and non-insulin dependent diabetes: thrifty genotype, thrifty phenotype or surviving small baby genotype? *BMJ* 1996; 308:942-5.

[23] Osmond C, Barker DJP, Winter PD, Fall CH, Simmonds SJ. Early growth and death from cardiovascular disease in women. *BMJ* 1993; 307:1519-24.

[24] Leon DA, Lithell HO, Vagero D, al. e. Reduced fetal growth rate and increased risk of death from ischaemic heart disease: cohort study of 15 000 men and women born 1915-29. *BMJ* 1998; 317:241-5.

[25] Frankel S, Elwood P, Sweetnam P, Yarnell J, Smith GD. Birthweight, body mass index in middle age, and incident coronary heart disease. *Lancet* 1996; 348:1478-80.

[26] Rich-Edwards JW, Stampfer MJ, Manson J, al. e. Birth weight and risk of cardiovascular disease in a cohort of women followed up since 1976. *BMJ* 1997; 315:396-400.

[27] Nilsson PM, Ostergren PO, Nyberg P, Soderstrom M, Allebeck P. Low birth weight is associated with elevated systolic blood pressure in adolescence: a prospective study of a birth cohort of 149 378 Swedish boys. *J Hypertension* 1997; 15:1627-31.

[28] Launer LJ, Hofman A, Grobbee DE. Relation between birth weight and blood pressure: longitudinal study of infants and children. *BMJ* 1993; 307:1451-4.

[29] Jefferies CA, Hofman PL, Wong W, Robinson EM, Cutfield WS. Increased nocturnal blood pressure in healthy prepubertal twins. *J Hypertension* 2003; 21:1319-24.

[30] Phillips DI, Cooper C, Fall C, Prentice L, Osmond C, Barker DJ, Rees Smith B. Fetal growth and autoimmune thyroid disease. *Quart J Med* 1993; 86:247-53.
[31] Martyn CN, Barker DJ, Jespersen S, Greenwald S, Osmond C, Berry C. Growth in utero, adult blood pressure, and arterial compliance. *British Heart Journal.* 1995; 73:116-21.
[32] Lesson CP, Whincup PH, Cook DG. Flow mediated dilation in 9- to 11-year-old children: the influence of intrauterine and childhood factors. *Circulation.* 1997; 96:2233-8.
[33] Shaheen S, Barker DJ. Early lung growth and chronic airflow obstruction. *Thorax* 1994; 49:533-6.
[34] Clark PM, Hinmarsh PC, Shiell AW, Law CM, Honour JW, Barker DJ. Size at birth and adrenocortical function in childhood. *Clin Endocrinol* 1996; 45:721-6.
[35] Phillips DI. Insulin resistance as a programmed response to fetal undernutrition. *Diabetologia* 1996; 39:1119-22.
[36] Fall CH, Pandit AN, Law CM, et al. Size at birth and insulin-like growth factor-1 concentrations. *Archives of Disease in Childhood.* 1995; 73:287-93.
[37] Cooper C, Kuh D, Egger P, Wadsworth M, Barker D. Childhood growth and age at menarche. *Br J Obstet Gynae* 1996; 103:814-7.
[38] Cresswell JL, Barker DJ, Osmond C, Egger P, Phillips DI, Fraser RB. Fetal growth, length of gestation, and polycystic ovaries in adult life. *Lancet* 1997; 350:1131-5.
[39] Susser E, Neugebauer R, Hoek HW, et al. Schizophrenia after prenatal famine. Further evidence. *Arch Gen Psych* 1996; 53:25-31.
[40] Barker DJ, Martyn CN, Osmond C, Hales CN, Fall CH. Growth in utero and serum cholesterol concentrations in adult life. *BMJ* 1993; 307:1524-7.
[41] Hales CN, Barker DJP. Type 2 (non-insulin-dependent) diabetes mellitus: the thrifty phenotype hypothesis. *Diabetologia* 1992; 35:595-601.
[42] Martyn CN, Lever AF, Morton JJ. Plasma concentrations of inactive rennin in adult life are related to indicators of foetal growth. *J Hypertension* 1996; 14:881-8.
[43] MacKenzie HS, Brenner BN. Fewer nephrons at birth: a missing link in the aetiology of essential hypertension? *Am J Kidney Dis* 1995; 26:91-8.
[44] Sharma AM. The thrifty-genotype hypothesis and its implications for the study of complex genetic disorders in man. *J Mol Med* 1998; 76:568-71.
[45] Hattersley AT, Tooke JE. The fetal insulin hypothesis: an alternative explanation of the association of low birthweight with diabetes and vascular disease. *Lancet* 1999; 353:1789-92.
[46] Hattersley AT, Beards F, Ballantyne E, Appleton M, Harvey R, Ellard S. Mutations in the glucokinase gene of the fetus result in reduced birth weight. *Nat Genet* 1998; 19:268-70.
[47] Rasmussen SK, Urhammer SA, Hansen T, et al. Variability of the insulin receptor substrate-1, hepatocyte nuclear factor-1alpha (HNF-1alpha), HNF-4alpha, and HNF-6 genes and size at birth in a population-based sample of young Danish subjects. J *Clin Endocrinol Metab.* 2000; 85:2951-3.
[48] Velho G, Hattersley AT, Froguel P. Maternal diabetes alters birth weight in glucokinase-deficient (MODY2) kindred but has no influence on adult weight, height, insulin secretion or insulin sensitivity. *Diabetologia* 2000; 43:1060-3.

[49] Jaenisch R, Bird A. Epigenetic regulation of gene expression: how the genome integrates intrinsic and environmental signals. *Nat Genet* 2003; 33 Suppl:245-54.
[50] Simmons RA, Flozak AS, Ogata ES. The effect of insulin, and insulin-like growth factor 1 on glucose transport in normal and small for gestational age fetal rats. *Endocrinology* 1993; 133:1361-1368.
[51] Vickers MH, Breier BH, Cutfield WS, Hofman PL, Gluckman PD. Fetal origins of hyperphagia, obesity, and hypertension and postnatal amplification by hypercaloric nutrition. *American Journal of Physiology - Endocrinology & Metabolism.* 2000; 279:E83-7.
[52] Desai M, Hales CN. Role of fetal and infant growth in programming metabolism in later life. *Biol Rev Camb Phil Soc* 1997; 72:329-48.
[53] Langley SC, Jackson AA. Increased systolic blood pressure in adult rats induced by fetal exposure to low protein diets. *Clin Sci* 1994; 86:217-22.
[54] Woodall SM, Breier BH, Johnson BM, Gluckman PD. *A model of intrauterine growth retardation caused by chronic maternal undernutrition in the rat: Effects on the somatotropic axis and postnatal growth.* 1996; 150:231-42.
[55] Garofano A, Czernichow P, Breant B. In utero undernutrition impairs rat beta-cell development. *Diabetologia* 1997; 40:1231-4.
[56] Ozanne SE, Dorling MW, Wang CL, Nave BT. Impaired PI 3-kinase activation in adipocytes from early growth-restricted male rats. *Am J Physiol Endocrinol Metab.* 2001; 280:E534-9.
[57] Petry CJ, Dorling MW, Pawlak DB, Ozanne SE, Hales CN. Diabetes in old male offspring of rat dams fed a reduced protein diet. *Int J Exp Diabetes Res.* 2001; 2:139-43.
[58] Simmons RA, Gounis AS, Bangalore SA, Ogata ES. Intrauterine growth retardation: fetal glucose transport is diminished in lung but spared in brain. *Pediatric Research.* 1992; 31:59-63.
[59] Cleasby ME, Kelly PA, Walker BR, Seckl JR. Programming of rat muscle and fat metabolism by in utero overexposure to glucocorticoids. *Endocrinology* 2003; 144:999-1007.
[60] Benediktsson R, Lindsay RS, Noble J, Seckl JR, Edwards CR. Glucocorticoid exposure in utero: new model for adult hypertension. *Lancet.* 1993; 341:339-41.
[61] Lindsay RS, Lindsay RM, Waddell BJ, Seckl JR. Prenatal glucocorticoid exposure leads to offspring hyperglycaemia in the rat: studies with the 11 beta-hydroxysteroid dehydrogenase inhibitor carbenoxolone. *Diabetologia* 1996; 39:1299-305.
[62] Hofman PL, Cutfield WS, Robinson EM, et al. Insulin resistance in short children with intrauterine growth retardation. *Journal Clin Endocrinol & Metab.* 1997; 82:402-6.
[63] Flanagan DE MV, Godsland IF, Cockington RA, Robinson JS, Phillips DI. Fetal growth and the physiological control of glucose tolerance in adults: a minimal model analysis. *Am J Physiol Endocrinol Metab.* 2000; 2000:4.
[64] Jaquet D, Gaboriau A, Czernichow P, Levy-Marchal C. Insulin resistance early in adulthood in subjects born with intrauterine growth retardation. *J Clin Endocrinol Metab* 2000; 85:1401-6.
[65] Van Assche FA, De Prins F, Aerts L, Verjans M. The endocrine pancreas in small-for-dates infants. *Br J Obstet Gynaecol.* 1977; 84:751-3.

[66] Beringue F, Blondeau B, Castellotti MC, Breant B, Czernichow P, Polak M. Endocrine pancreas development in growth-retarded human fetuses. *Diabetes* 2002; 51:385-91.
[67] Lee PA, Chernausek SD, Hokken-Koelega AC, Czernichow P. International Small for Gestational Age Advisory Board International Small for Gestational Age Advisory Board consensus development conference statement: management of short children born small for gestational age, April 24-October 1, 2001. *Pediatrics* 2003; 111:1253-61.
[68] Leger J, Limoni C, Collin D, Czernichow P. Prediction factors in the determination of final height in subjects born small for gestational age. *Pediatric Research.* 1998; 43:808-12.
[69] Chatelain P, Peretti N, Lapillonne A, et al. New insights into the postnatal growth of infants born 'idiopathic' small for gestational age. *Journal of Pediatric Endocrinology & Metabolism.* 2001; 14:1515-9.
[70] Reaven GM, Lithell H, Landsberg L. Hypertension and associated metabolic abnormalities--the role of insulin resistance and the sympathoadrenal system. *NEJM.* 1996; 334:374-81.
[71] Frontoni S, Bracaglia D, Baroni A, et al. Early autonomic dysfunction in glucose-tolerant but insulin-resistant offspring of type 2 diabetic patients. *Hypertension.* 2003; 41:1223-7.
[72] Chen HS, Hwu CM, Kwok CF, et al. Insulin sensitivity in normotensive offspring of hypertensive parents. *Hormone & Metabolic Research.* 2000; 32:110-4.
[73] McKeigue PM, Lithell HO, Leon DA. Glucose tolerance and resistance to insulin-stimulated glucose uptake in men aged 70 years in relation to size at birth. *Diabetologia* 1998; 41:1133-8.
[74] Leger J, Levy-Marchal C, Bloch J, et al. Reduced final height and indications for insulin resistance in 20 year olds born small for gestational age: regional cohort study. *BMJ* 1997; 315:341-7.
[75] Arends N, Johnston L, Hokken-Koelega A, et al. Polymorphism in the IGF-I gene: clinical relevance for short children born small for gestational age (SGA). *J Clin Endocrinol Metab.* 2002; 87:2720.
[76] Cambien F, Leger J, Mallet C, Levy-Marchal C, Collin D, Czernichow P. Angiotensin I-converting enzyme gene polymorphism modulates the consequences of in utero growth retardation on plasma insulin in young adults. *Diabetes.* 1998; 47:470-5.
[77] Jaquet D, Czernichow P. Born small for gestational age: increased risk of type 2 diabetes, hypertension and hyperlipidaemia in adulthood. *Hormone Research.* 2003; 59:131-7.
[78] Cutfield WS, Bergman RN, Menon RK, Sperling MA. The modified minimal model: application to measurement of insulin sensitivity in children. *J Clin Endocrinol Metab.* 1990; 70:1644-50.
[79] Ong KK, Dunger DB. Perinatal growth failure: the road to obesity, insulin resistance and cardiovascular disease in adults. Best Practice & Research *Clinical Endocrinology & Metabolism.* 2002; 16:191-207.
[80] Roseboom TJ, van der Meulen JH, Ravelli AC, Osmond C, Barker DJ, Bleker OP. Effects of prenatal exposure to the Dutch famine on adult disease in later life: an overview. *Mol & Cell Endocrinology.* 2001; 185:93-8.
[81] Byberg L, McKeigue PM, Zethelius B, Lithell HO. Birth weight and the insulin resistance syndrome: association of low birth weight with truncal obesity and raised

plasminogen activator inhibitor-1 but not with abdominal obesity or plasma lipid disturbances. *Diabetologia*. 2000; 43:54-60.

[82] Irving RJ, Belton NR, Elton RA, Walker BR. Adult cardiovascular risk factors in premature babies.[comment][erratum appears in Lancet 2000 Aug 5;356(9228):514]. *Lancet*. 2000; 355:2135-6.

[83] Fewtrell MS, Doherty C, Cole TJ, Stafford M, Hales CN, Lucas A. Effects of size at birth, gestational age and early growth in preterm infants on glucose and insulin concentrations at 9-12 years. *Diabetologia*. 2000; 43:714-7.

[84] Bergman RN. Lilly lecture 1989. Toward physiological understanding of glucose tolerance. Minimal-model approach. *Diabetes*. 1989; 38:1512-27.

[85] McCarthy JF, Misra DN, Roberts JM. Maternal plasma leptin is increased in preeclampsia and positively correlates with fetal cord concentration. *American Journal of Obstetrics & Gynecology*. 1999; 180:731-6.

[86] Fernandez-Twinn DS, Ozanne SE, Ekizoglou S, et al. The maternal endocrine environment in the low-protein model of intra-uterine growth restriction. *British J Nutrition*. 2003; 90:815-22.

[87] Jansson N, Greenwood SL, Johansson BR, Powell TL, Jansson T. Leptin stimulates the activity of the system A amino acid transporter in human placental villous fragments. *J Clin Endocrinol Metab*. 2003; 88:1205-11.

[88] Gosdon R, Trasler J, Lucifero D, M. F. Rare congenital disorders, imprinted genes and reproductive technology. *Lancet* 2003; 361:1975-77.

[89] Kyvik KO. Twin research: nature versus nurture in common diseases. In: Day INM, Humphries SE, eds. Genetics of common diseases. Oxford: BIOS *Scientific Publishers LTD*, 1997.

[90] Barnett AH, Eff C, Leslie RDG, Pyke DA. Diabetes in identical twins. *Diabetologia* 1981; 20:87-93.

[91] Gottlieb MS, Root HF. Diabetes Mellitus in Twins. *Diabetes* 1968; 17:693-704.

[92] Kaprio J, Tuomilehto J, Koskenvuo M, et al. Concordance for type-1 and Type-2 diabetes mellitus in a population based cohort of twins in Finland. *Diabetologia* 1992; 35:1060-1067.

[93] Lo SSS, Tun RYM, Hawa M, Leslie RDG. Studies of diabetic twins. *Diabetes/Metab Rev* 1991; 7:223-228.

[94] Medici F, Hawa M, Ianari A, Pyke DA, Leslie RDG. Concordance rate for type 2 diabetes mellitus in monozygotic twins: actuarial analysis. *Diabetologia* 1999; 42:146-50.

[95] Newman B, Selby JV, King MC, Slemenda C, Fabsitz R, Friedman GD. Concordance for Type 2 (non-insulin dependent) diabetes mellitus in male twins. *Diabetologia* 1987; 30:763-8.

[96] Barnett AH, Spiliopoulos AJ, Pyke DA, Stubbs WA, Burrin J, Alberti KGMM. Metabolic studies in unaffected co-twins of non insulin dependent diabetics. *BMJ* 1981; 282:1656-8.

[97] Vaag A, Henriksen JE, Madsbad S, Holm N, Beck-Nielsen H. Insulin secretion, insulin action, and hepatic glucose production in identical twins discordant for non insulin dependent diabetes mellitus. *J Clin Invest* 1995; 95:690-98.

[98] Matsuda A, Uzuya T. Relationship between obesity and concordance rate for type 2 diabetes mellitus among twins. *Diabetes Research and Clinical practice* 1994; 26:137-143.

[99] Poulsen P, Vaag A, Beck-Nielsen H. Does zygosity influence the metabolic profile of twins? A population based cross sectional study. *BMJ* 1999; 319:151-4.

[100] Bo S, Cavallo-Perin P, Ciccone G, Scaglione L, Pagano G. The metabolic syndrome in twins: a consequence of low birth weight or of being a twin? *Exp Clin Endocrinol Diabetes*. 2001; 109:135-40.

[101] Poulsen P, Vaag A, kyvik K, Jensen D, Beck-Nielsen H. Low birth weight is associated with NIDDM in discordant monozygotic and dizygotic twin pairs. *Diabetologia* 1997; 40:439-446.

[102] Baird J, Osmond C, MacGregor A, Sneider H, Hales CN, Phillips DIW. Testing the fetal origins hypothesis in twins: the Birmingham twin study. *Diabetologia* 2001; 44:33-39.

[103] Zhang J, Brenner RA, Klebanoff MA. Differences in birthweight and blood pressure at age 7 years among twins. *Am Journal of Epidemiology*. 2001; 153:779-82.

[104] Dwyer T, Blizzard L, Morley R, Ponsonby A-L. Within pair association between birthweight and blood pressure at age 8 in twins from a cohort study. *BMJ* 1999; 319:1325-9.

[105] Poulsen P, Levin K, Beck-Nielsen H, Vaag A. Age-dependent impact of zygosity and birth weight on insulin secretion and insulin action in twins. *Diabetologia* 2002; 45:1649-57.

[106] Gerich JE. The genetic basis of type 2 diabetes mellitus: Impaired insulin secretion versus impaired insulin sensitivity. *Endocrine Rev* 1998; 19:491-503.

[107] Kahn SE. The Importance of β-Cell Failure in the Development and Progression of Type 2 Diabetes. *J Clin Endocrinol Metab*. 2001; 86:4047-4058.

[108] Jefferies C, Hofman PL, Robinson EM, Cutfield WS. Twin children are insulin resistant. *J Peds In Press*.

[109] Bergman RN, Ader M, Huecking K, Van Citters G. Accurate Assessment of beta-Cell Function: The Hyperbolic Correction. *Diabetes* 2002; 51:S212-220.

[110] Khan N, Couper JJ. Low-birth-weight infants show earlier onset of IDDM. *Diabetes Care*. 1994; 17:653-6.

[111] Boni-Schnetzler M, Binz K, Mary JL, Schmid C, Schwander J, Froesch ER. Regulation of hepatic expression of IGF I and fetal IGF binding protein mRNA in streptozotocin-diabetic rats. *FEBS Letters*. 1989; 251:253-6.

[112] Boni-Schnetzler M, Schmid C, Mary JL, et al. Insulin regulates the expression of the insulin-like growth factor binding protein 2 mRNA in rat hepatocytes. *Mol Endocrinology*. 1990; 4:1320-6.

[113] Boni-Schnetzler M, Schmid C, Meier PJ, Froesch ER. Insulin regulates insulin-like growth factor I mRNA in rat hepatocytes. *Am J Physiology*. 1991; 260:E846-51.

[114] O'Brien RM, Granner DK. Regulation of gene expression by insulin. *Biochemical Journal*. 1991; 278:609-19.

[115] Bereket A, Lang CH, Blethen SL, Fan J, Frost RA, Wilson TA. Insulin-like growth factor binding protein-3 proteolysis in children with insulin-dependent diabetes mellitus: a possible role for insulin in the regulation of IGFBP-3 protease activity [comment]. *J Clin Endocrinol Metab*. 1995; 80:2282-8.

[116] Baxter RC, Martin JL. Radioimmunoassay of growth hormone-dependent insulin like growth factor binding protein in human plasma. *Journal Clin Invest.* 1986; 78:1504-12.
[117] Yeoh SI, Baxter RC. Metabolic regulation of the growth hormone independent insulin-like growth factor binding protein in human plasma. *Acta Endocrinologica.* 1988; 119:465-73.
[118] Cutfield WS, Hofman PL, Vickers M, Breier B, Blum WF, Robinson EM. IGFs and binding proteins in short children with intrauterine growth retardation. *J Clin Endocrinol Metab.* 2002; 87:235-9.
[119] Freinkel N. Banting Lecture 1980. Of pregnancy and progeny. *Diabetes* 1980; 29:1023-35.
[120] Silverman BL, Metzger BE, Cho NH, Loeb CA. Impaired glucose tolerance in adolescent offspring of diabetic mothers. Relationship to fetal hyperinsulinism. *Diabetes Care* 1995; 18:611-7.
[121] Plagemann A, Harder T, Kohlhoff R, Rohde W, Dorner G. Glucose tolerance and insulin secretion in children of mothers with pregestational IDDM or gestational diabetes. *Diabetologia* 1997; 40:1094-100.
[122] Silverman BL, Rizzo TA, Cho NH, Metzger BE. Long-term effects of the intrauterine environment. The Northwestern University Diabetes in Pregnancy Center. *Diabetes Care* 1998; 21 Suppl 2:B142-9.
[123] Bjornholt JV, Erikssen G, Liestol K, Jervell J, Thaulow E, Erikssen J. Type 2 diabetes and maternal family history: an impact beyond slow glucose removal rate and fasting hyperglycaemia in low-risk individuals? Results from 22.5 years of follow-up of healthy nondiabetic men. *Diabetes Care* 2000; 23:1255-9.
[124] Hunter WA, Cundy T, Rabone D, et al. Insulin sensitivity in the offspring of women with type 1 and type 2 diabetes mellitus. *Diabetes Care* 2004 In press.
[125] Caruso A, Paradisi G, Ferrazzani S, Lucchese A, Moretti S, Fulghesu AM. Effect of maternal carbohydrate metabolism on fetal growth. *Obstet Gynecol* 1998; 92:8-12.
[126] Ravelli AC, van der Meulen JH, Osmond C, Barker DJ, Bleker OP. Obesity at the age of 50 years in men and women exposed to famine prenatally. *Am J Clin Nutr* 1999; 70:811-6.
[127] Bhargava SK, Sachdev HS, Fall CH, et al. Relation of serial changes in childhood body-mass index to impaired glucose tolerance in young adulthood. *NEJM* 2004; 350:865-75.
[128] Yajnik CS. Interactions of perturbations in intrauterine growth and growth during childhood and the risk of adult-onset disease. *Proceedings of the Nutrition Society.* 2000; 59:257-65.
[129] Forsen T, Eriksson J, Tuomilehto J, Reunanen A, Osmond, C, Barker D. The fetal and childhood growth of persons who develop type 2 diabetes. Ann Internal Med 2000; 133:176-82.
[130] Eriksson JG FT, Osmond C, Barker DJ. Pathways of infant and childhood growth that lead to type 2 diabetes. *Diabetes Care* 2003; 26:3006-10.
[131] Hales CN, Ozanne SE. The dangerous road to catch-up growth. Journal of physiology 2003; 547:5-10.
[132] Matthews SG. Early programming of the hypothalamic-pituitary-adrenal axis. *Trends in Endocrinology & Metab.* 2002; 13:373-380.

[133] Dahlgren J, Boguszewski M, Rosberg S, Albertsson-Wikland K. Adrenal steroid hormones in short children born small for gestational age. *Clin Endocrinol* 1998; 49:353-61.

[134] Phillips DI, Walker BR, Reynolds RM, et al. Low birth weight predicts elevated plasma cortisol concentrations in adults from 3 populations. *Hypertension*. 2000; 35:1301-6.

[135] Jefferies C, Keelan J, Robinson EM, Hofman P, Cutfield WS. Circulating tumour necrosis factor alpha (TNF-a) levels are reduced in healthy non-obese insulin resistant children. *Ped Diabetes* 2004 In press.

[136] Boyko EJ. Proportion of type 2 diabetes cases resulting from impaired fetal growth. *Diabetes Care* 2000; 23:1260-4.

[137] Banerji MA, Faridi N, Atluri R, Chaiken RL, Lebovitz HE. Body composition, visceral fat, leptin, and insulin resistance in Asian Indian men. *J Clin Endocrinol Metab* 1999; 84:137-44.

[138] Pradeepa R, Mohan V. The changing scenario of the diabetes epidemic: implications for India. *Indian J Med Res* 2002; 116:121-32.

[139] Barker DJ. In utero programming of chronic disease. *Clinical Science*. 1998; 95:115-28.

In: Insulin Resistance in Children and Adolescents ISBN 1-59454-215-5
Editors: D. Daneman and J. Hamilton, pp. 87-101 

*Chapter 4*

# PUBERTY AND INSULIN RESISTANCE

***Antoinette M. Moran and Betsy L. Rosenberg***
University of Minnesota

## ABSTRACT

A transient insulin resistant state occurs during puberty and is part of normal human development. Insulin resistance increases immediately at the beginning of puberty, peaks at mid-puberty, and then declines to nearly prepubertal levels by early adulthood. Girls are more insulin resistant than boys during puberty which is related in part to differences in adiposity between the sexes. Glucose homeostasis is maintained during puberty through compensatory hyperinsulinemia. While resistance to insulin's effect on glucose metabolism is present, insulin-stimulated protein metabolism is normal. Therefore, a physiologic consequence of insulin resistance during puberty may be augmentation of rapid growth by promotion of protein anabolism.

The causes of physiological insulin resistance during puberty have not been definitively established. Gonadal sex steroids do not appear to play a central role. There is strong evidence, however, that GH/IGF-I activity contributes to pubertal insulin resistance. GH and IGF-I levels increase and then decrease during puberty, following a pattern similar to that of insulin resistance. A significant association between IGF-I levels and pubertal insulin resistance has been demonstrated in many studies. Some studies find that African Americans are more insulin resistant during puberty than their white counterparts, although this was not found to be the case in a study where the black youth were lean and physically active.

## THE PATTERN OF PHYSIOLOGICAL INSULIN RESISTANCE DURING PUBERTY

During puberty children undergo dramatic changes in growth, sexual maturation, and emotional functioning. It is well known that a transient insulin resistant state is also part of normal pubertal development. This phenomenon was first described in a euglycemic insulin clamp study which showed that insulin-stimulated glucose uptake is significantly reduced in non-diabetic pubertal children compared to non-diabetic prepubertal children and adults [1].

Several other studies have confirmed that while prepubertal children and postpubertal young adults are equally sensitive to insulin, adolescents are insulin resistant compared to either of these groups [1-10].

A cross-sectional study evaluated insulin resistance in 357 healthy children and adolescents using the euglycemic insulin clamp technique. This large cohort allowed characterization of insulin resistance at each of the five Tanner stages of puberty. In both boys and girls, insulin resistance was found to increase immediately at the beginning of puberty (Tanner stage II), peak at mid-puberty (Tanner stage III), and then return to nearly prepubertal levels by the end of puberty (Tanner stage V) [2]. Insulin sensitivity decreased by about 20% in both boys and girls between Tanner stage I and Tanner stage III. At all Tanner stages, the girls in this study were significantly more insulin resistant than the boys (Figures 1 and 2).

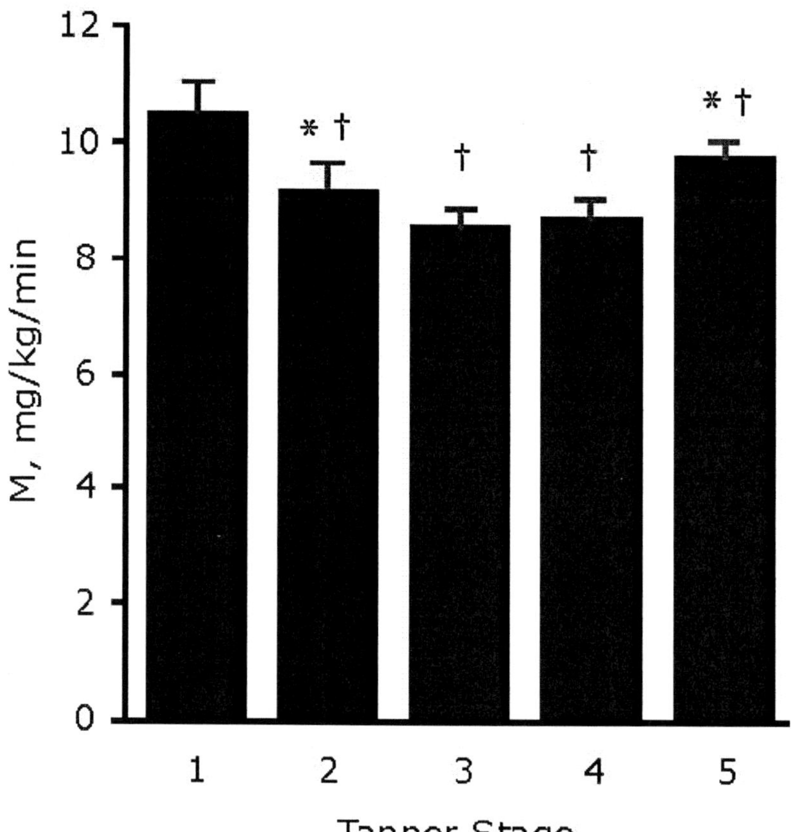


Figure 1. Insulin resistance (M) by Tanner stage, adjusted for sex and BMI. A lower M value represents greater insulin resistance. Data are expressed as means ± SE. *P < 0.05 compared with preceding Tanner stage, †P < 0.05 compared with T!.

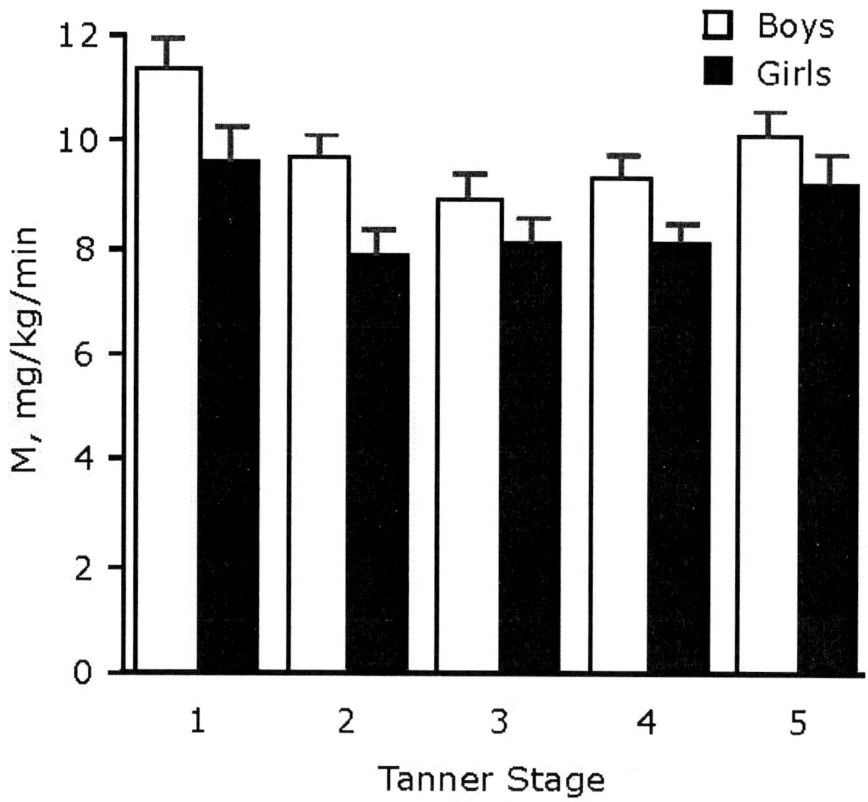


Figure 2. Insulin resistance (M) by Tanner stage and sex, adjusted for BMI. The cohort of 159 girls was more insulin resistant than the cohort of 198 boys ($P < 0.0001$). Girls appeared to be more insulin resistant than boys at each Tanner stage, but statistical significance was only achieved for T4 ($P < 0.01$).

In another cross-sectional study, Bergman's minimal model was used to compare two stages of puberty (Tanner stages II and III) in 96 children [3]. For a given BMI, insulin resistance was greater in Tanner stage III than Tanner stage II and greater in girls compared to boys. The minimal model was also used in a mixed-sex group of 58 girls and boys [4]; a sharp increase in insulin resistance was noted from Tanner stage II to V. A longitudinal study used the tolbutamide-modified intravenous glucose tolerance test to measure insulin sensitivity in 60 boys and girls at Tanner stage I, and then again two years later after about half of the subjects were at Tanner stages III and IV. It was shown that insulin sensitivity fell by 32% in children who had progressed to Tanner stage III [5].

## COMPENSATORY HYPERINSULINEMIA DURING PUBERTY

Insulin resistance during puberty is associated with elevated insulin levels [1, 4-7, 9, 10]. The fasting insulin level is sometimes used as an index of insulin resistance, since there is a close correlation between it and insulin resistance as measured by the euglycemic clamp. Fasting insulin and insulin resistance are not exactly the same measures, however, and cannot be directly compared. Determination of insulin resistance with the insulin clamp is an experimentally controlled model which isolates insulin resistance, whereas fasting insulin represents an active, integrated biological system of which insulin sensitivity is only one variable.

Hyperinsulinemia appears to be a successful compensatory response to insulin resistance since fasting glucose levels have not been shown to change during puberty [1, 4-9]. To study the nature of insulin secretion during puberty, hyperglycemic clamp studies were performed in 14 healthy adolescent children, 9 preadolescent children, and 14 adult controls [6]. During an identical hyperglycemic stimulus, insulin secretion was two to three times greater in adolescents than in either adults or prepubertal children. The rate of glucose infusion necessary to maintain a specific hyperglycemic plateau was similar in all three groups, again indicating that the exaggerated insulin response in puberty serves to compensate for increased insulin resistance and to maintain glucose homeostasis. Both first- and second-phase insulin responses were elevated in the adolescent subjects, demonstrating that beta cell function is preserved. Insulin and C-peptide levels were similarly elevated during the hyperglycemic clamp, which suggests that the hyperinsulinemia is due to augmented beta cell secretion rather than reduced hepatic degradation, since insulin but not C-peptide is extracted by the liver (Figure 3) [11].

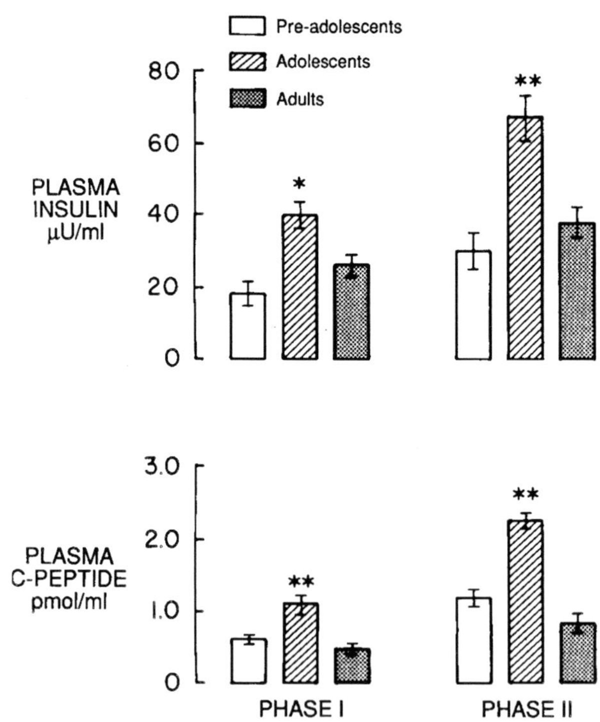


Figure 3. Mean (± SEM) first-phase (0 to 10 minutes) and second-phase (10 to 20 minutes) plasma insulin and C-peptide responses during glucose clamp procedure. Responses were significantly greater in adolescents (*p < 0.02 and ** p < 0.01) than in the other two groups. To convert plasma insulin values to picomoles per liter, multiply by 6.0. This figure is from "Increased insulin secretion in puberty: a compensatory response to reductions in insulin sensitivity for *J of Pediatrics*, Vol. 114 pg. 965-967, 1989, with permission.

# METABOLIC EFFECTS OF INSULIN RESISTANCE DURING PUBERTY

The physiologic significance of an insulin resistant state during puberty is not completely understood. Insulin is known to be an anabolic hormone that promotes the storage of glucose, fat, and protein primarily through the inhibition of their breakdown. Insulin's growth enhancing ability is illustrated by the improvement in growth in children with poorly controlled type 1 diabetes (T1D) after intensive insulin treatment [12]. Many believe that, given the anabolic properties of insulin, high insulin levels during puberty may serve to augment rapid growth.

## Glucose Metabolism

Insulin promotes blood glucose normalization and storage of carbohydrate by stimulating peripheral glucose uptake by skeletal muscle and other cells. In the liver, insulin inhibits hepatic glucose production and increases glycogen stores [13]. During normal puberty, carbohydrate metabolism becomes resistant to the effects of insulin, and a compensatory increase in insulin secretion occurs to maintain glucose homeostasis.

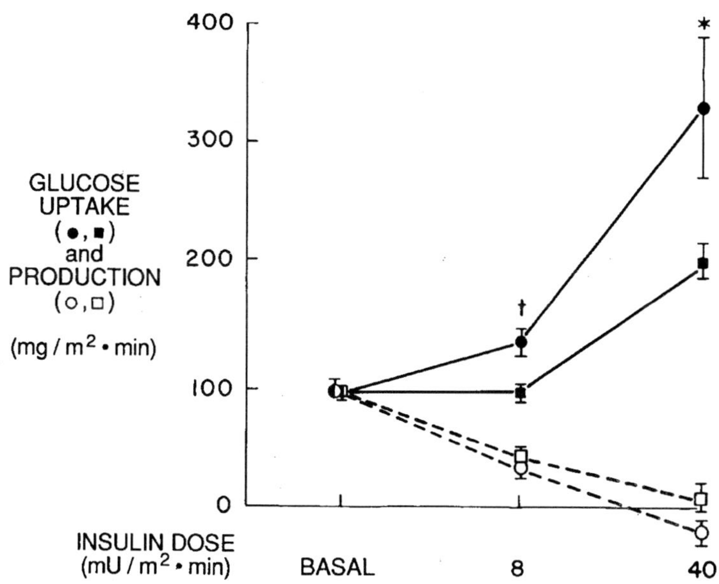


Figure 4. Effect of puberty on rates of glucose uptake and production in the basal state and at the end of the 8 and 40 mU/m$^2$/min insulin infusions; data are presented as means ± SE. Basal glucose turnover was nearly identical in prepubertal (circles, n = 6) and pubertal (squares, n = 7) subjects. Glucose uptake (closed symbols) increased onlu in prepubertal subjects during low-dose insulin (p < 0.05 versus baseline) and was markedly greater in prepubertal than in pubertal subjects (+p, 0.05) during the high-dose infusion. On the other hand, endogenous glucose production (open symbols) showed similar degrees of suppression during the insulin infusions in both groups. This figure is from "Insulin resistance of puberty: a defect restricted to peripheral glucose metabolism," *J Clin Endocrinol Metab* Vol. 2, pg. 277-282, 1991, with permission.

The defect in insulin-stimulated glucose metabolism during puberty appears to be restricted to the peripheral tissues. Euglycemic insulin clamp studies using tracer methodology have shown that hepatic glucose production is similar between prepubertal and pubertal subjects during both high and low dose insulin infusion, indicating that insulin's ability to suppress hepatic gluconeogenesis is normal during puberty [7]. Peripheral glucose uptake, however, was impaired in response to insulin infusion in pubertal children in these clamp studies (Figure 4).

To further assess this peripheral defect indirect calorimetry was used to measure glucose oxidation during euglycemic insulin clamp studies in eight healthy adolescents and six healthy young adult control subjects [8]. While the adolescents had a 40% reduction in insulin-stimulated glucose uptake compared to the adults, glucose oxidation rates increased to a similar degree in both groups during insulin infusion suggesting a defect in non-oxidative glucose metabolism. Non-oxidative glucose metabolism has been found to correlate with muscle glycogen synthesis [14] and, therefore, a defect in this process may be involved in altered glucose metabolism during puberty.

## Protein Metabolism

In contrast to carbohydrate metabolism, it appears that insulin's effect on the metabolism of protein is not affected by puberty. Fasting concentrations of branch-chain amino acids do not differ significantly between prepubertal and pubertal subjects, and amino acid concentrations suppress similarly in both groups of children in response to insulin infusion. [7] [$^{13}$C]leucine tracer studies and indirect calorimetry during the euglycemic insulin clamp have shown that leucine flux (an index of protein breakdown) and leucine oxidation are comparable in healthy adolescent and adult subjects in the basal state and during insulin infusion [8].

These studies suggest that, unlike glucose metabolism, protein metabolism is not impaired during the insulin resistant state of puberty. Insulin promotes protein storage primarily by inhibiting proteolysis. Since circulating levels of insulin are elevated during puberty, protein anabolism is likely magnified. Therefore, it is possible that a physiologic benefit of insulin resistance to carbohydrate metabolism during puberty is amplification of the protein anabolic effects of insulin at this time of rapid growth.

## Fat Metabolism

There is conflicting evidence regarding the effect of insulin on lipid metabolism during puberty. Rates of lipolysis and fat oxidation during the euglycemic insulin clamp were compared in nine prepubertal, nine pubertal, and five young adult healthy subjects [15]. Lipolysis was calculated by measuring rates of endogenous glycerol appearance and fat oxidation was measured with indirect calorimetry. Lipolysis was highest in the pubertal group, and insulin did not appropriately suppress lipid oxidation in these subjects. Lipolysis involves the release of fatty acids and glycerol from triglyceride stores in adipose tissue. An increase in lipolysis during puberty would lead to higher concentrations of free fatty acids and increased rates of fatty acid oxidation. Increased fatty acid oxidation may impair glucose uptake because of substrate competition with glucose oxidation [16]. These investigators, therefore, concluded that increased lipid oxidation during puberty may contribute to pubertal insulin resistance by reducing glucose uptake [15].

Other studies have not shown a difference in insulin-stimulated fatty acid oxidation between pubertal subjects and prepubertal and adult controls [7, 8]. Further studies with larger sample sizes may help to resolve these conflicting findings. It may be important to also consider whether a difference in insulin-induced fat metabolism during puberty exists between the sexes, as girls tend to gain more fat mass and boys gain more fat-free mass during this time17.

## HORMONAL INFLUENCES

The causes of insulin resistance during puberty have not been definitively established. Because normal pubertal development is accompanied by dramatic hormonal changes, many studies have attempted to determine the influence of these hormones on insulin secretion and activity.

### Growth Hormone/Insulin-Like Growth Factor-I Axis

Levels of GH and IGF-I both rise dramatically during puberty and return to prepubertal levels in early adulthood [18, 19]. Growth hormone promotes linear growth and protein synthesis, increases bone mineral density, and stimulates the production of IGF-I in the liver and non-hepatic tissues [20]. In turn, IGF-I mediates many of the metabolic actions of GH and provides feedback regulation of GH at the pituitary gland. Pubertal GH release is triggered by both estrogens and androgens, with androgenic stimulation occurring through secondary aromatization of androgens to estrogens. GH and IGF-I act in concert with the sex steroids to enhance somatic growth during puberty [21].

Because the rise and fall in GH and IGF-I levels parallel changes in insulin resistance during puberty, and because GH is a known insulin antagonist, the GH/IGF-I axis is likely a contributor to insulin resistance. In one study, the insulin resistance of diabetic and non-diabetic children was measured by the euglycemic insulin-clamp technique and compared between prepubertal and pubertal groups. Insulin stimulated glucose metabolism decreased during puberty in both diabetics and non-diabetics, and this change was inversely correlated with 24-hour levels of growth hormone [1].

Since GH secretion is difficult to measure as its pulsatile nature requires frequent blood sampling, serum IGF-I levels are often used to approximate GH secretion. IGF-I levels have been shown to reflect GH secretion in healthy children and adolescents [22]. Several studies have shown a significant relationship between IGF-I levels and insulin resistance during puberty. [6, 9, 19, 23, 24] The largest of these studies used the euglycemic insulin clamp technique to compare insulin resistance with levels of IGF-I at each Tanner stage in a group of 357 boys and girls [19]. IGF-I levels rose and fell during the course of puberty in a pattern similar to that of insulin resistance. There was a significant relationship between insulin resistance and IGF-I levels seen in both boys and girls (Figure 5).

In addition to its anabolic effects, GH influences glucose metabolism by stimulating hepatic gluconeogenesis, inhibiting peripheral glucose utilization, and increasing lipolysis [25]. Treating growth hormone deficient children with exogenous GH has been shown to significantly increase fasting insulin concentrations [26, 27]. Eight children with short stature were treated with exogenous GH over six months and evaluated before and after treatment using the hyperglycemic clamp technique [27]. Fasting insulin levels were significantly higher and insulin sensitivity was reduced after GH therapy. Despite reduced insulin sensitivity, there was greater inhibition of protein breakdown in the GH treated patients, presumably due to the direct protein anabolic effect of GH. These results indicate that increased levels of GH during puberty result in insulin resistance and a compensatory hyperinsulinemia. The effect of higher circulating levels of both GH and insulin may serve a beneficial role by synergistically augmenting protein anabolism to promote pubertal growth.

IGF-I is synthesized by the liver in response to stimulation primarily by GH but also by insulin [28]. Higher levels of insulin secretion during puberty may further augment growth by stimulating IGF-I secretion. Most of the circulating IGF-I is bound to one of six binding proteins that direct IGF-I activity. Of these, more than 95 percent of serum IGF-I is bound to IGFBP-3. IGFBP-3 levels reflect GH secretion by virtue of its dependence on GH [22, 28]. As IGF-I levels rise during puberty, the levels of IGFBP-3 rise in a similar fashion [19, 29, 30]. In contrast, the binding protein IGFBP-1 is GH independent [31]. Hepatic transcription of IGFBP-1 is inhibited by insulin, and as a result IGFBP-1 levels fall when plasma insulin levels are acutely or chronically elevated [32, 33]. These relations persist during the hyperinsulinemic state of puberty [19, 29-31]. A steady decline in IGFBP-1 levels is seen between Tanner stages II and V, and IGFBP-1 levels are inversely correlated with insulin resistance during puberty [19].

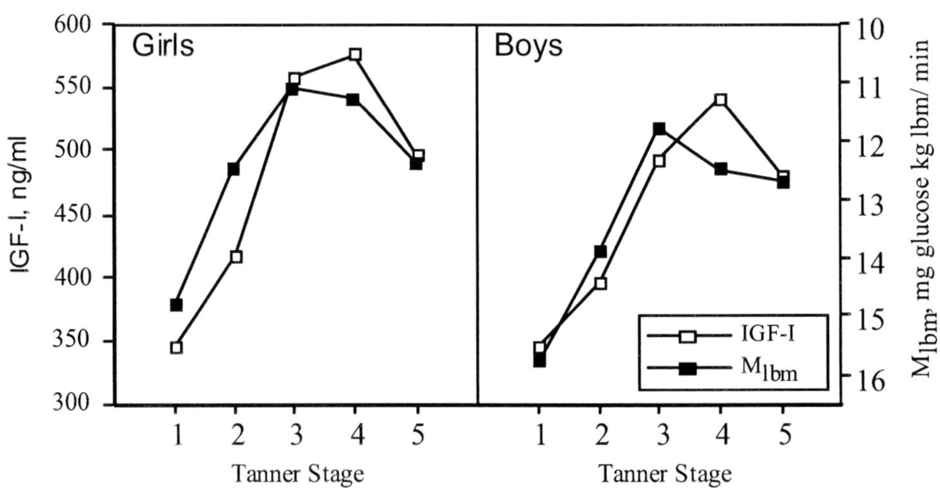


Fig. 5. Changes in IGF-I and $M_{lbm}$ from T1 to T5 in boys and girls. Note that the $M_{lbm}$ axis is inverted to better show the similar pattern for IGF-I and insulin resistance. A lower $M_{lbm}$ value indicates greater insulin resistance.

IGF-I stimulates bone formation, enhances protein synthesis, inhibits protein degradation, and promotes glucose storage in the muscle [28]. IGFBP-1 inhibits the binding of IGF-I to its receptors and, therefore, its biologic actions [34]. When IGFBP-1 levels are suppressed due to the hyperinsulemia of puberty, more bioactive free IGF-I is available [29-31]. It is possible that the rise in free IGF-I in puberty not only augments somatic growth but also offsets the diabetogenic effects of GH [19]. IGF-I is a peptide hormone with a chemical structure similar to that of insulin and has known insulin-like actions [28]. Several studies have shown that IGF-I can improve glycemic control and insulin sensitivity when given to patients with severe insulin resistance and diabetes mellitus [35]. The rise in IGF-I, particularly free IGF-I, may assist in the achievement of balanced carbohydrate metabolism during puberty. Although the exact mechanisms have not been established, current data suggest that the GH/IGF-I axis is intricately involved in the etiology, maintenance, and function of pubertal insulin resistance.

## Sex Steroids

The onset of puberty is heralded by an activation of the hypothalamic-pituitary-gonadal axis. Hypothalmic GnRH pulses increase in amplitude signaling an increased pulsatile release of LH and FSH from the pituitary gonadotropes, particularly at night [36]. The gonadotropins, in turn, trigger a marked increase in gonadal steroid production. Sex steroid levels, which are barely detectable in early childhood, rise to adult levels by the end of puberty. Estrogen is secreted by the ovaries in females and created by peripheral conversion of androgen in both males and females. Estrogen is responsible for breast enlargement and maturation of vaginal mucosa in females, and growth acceleration and skeletal maturation in both sexes. Androgen production occurs in the testes in males, the ovaries in females, and the adrenal glands in both sexes. Androgens induce secondary hair growth, genital maturation in males, bone growth and maturation, and an increase in muscle strength [37].

Because puberty is marked by dramatic changes in gonadal sex steroid production, it is intriguing to consider whether or not these hormones influence the insulin resistance seen in puberty. The observation that sex steroid levels rise rapidly during puberty and remain elevated in adulthood, while insulin sensitivity falls and then recovers, makes a direct relationship seem unlikely [1, 5]. Several studies that established reductions in insulin sensitivity during puberty also measured estrogen and testosterone levels in their subjects, and found no significant correlation between the changes in insulin resistance and changes in sex steroid levels [3, 5, 6]. Furthermore, in a study where boys with constitutional delay were treated with either testosterone and a placebo or testosterone and an aromatase inhibitor (to prevent conversion of testosterone to estrogen), neither androgens nor estrogen contributed to insulin resistance [23].

The literature evaluating the influence of the menstrual cycle on insulin resistance in adult women provides various conclusions on the relation between sex steroid levels and insulin resistance. Some studies find that insulin-mediated glucose metabolism is not affected by the phase of the menstrual cycle in female subjects, despite large fluctuations in estrogen and progesterone levels during the follicular and luteal phases [38, 39]. In contrast, other studies demonstrate decreased glucose utilization during the high-estrogen luteal phase of menstruation in diabetic and non-diabetic adult women [40, 41]. While some of these studies indicate that sex steroids influence insulin resistance, they were performed in adult women and their possible relevance in adolescent women is not known.

While current research fails to find a direct relationship between insulin resistance and the gonadal sex steroids during puberty, there is conflicting evidence regarding the role of adrenal androgens. It has been reported that the rise in pubertal androstendione levels is significantly related to the increased acute insulin response observed during puberty [5], and that adrenal androgen DHEA-S levels correlate with changes in insulin sensitivity during puberty in girls but not in boys [24]. However, others have not observed a correlation between DHEA-S and pubertal insulin resistance [6].

It is known that conditions of hyperandrogenism in females, such as polycystic ovary syndrome (PCOS), are associated with hyperinsulinemia and insulin resistance [42]. Furthermore, insulin has been found to increase adrenal sensitivity to ACTH in hyperandrogenic women [43], and a sexual dimorphism in the regulation of adrenal androgen metabolism has been suggested in the literature [42]. Therefore, it is possible that there is an interaction between physiologic insulin resistance and hyperinsulinemia in early puberty and adrenal androgens in girls [24]. This relationship is not completely understood and deserves further study.

### Stress

Adolescence is a time of important social and emotional development. While establishing a sense of personal identity, dealing with issues of self-esteem, sexuality, and independence can be quite stressful for many adolescents. In both laboratory and clinical studies, psychological stress has been shown to elevate levels of catecholamines and cortisol [44]. Catecholamines and cortisol are known to counter-regulate hypoglycaemia and have anti-insulin effects [13]. Therefore, one might postulate that the stress of adolescence could lead to elevated catecholamine and cortisol levels which could in turn contribute to insulin resistance. However, studies that have demonstrated insulin resistance during puberty have not shown differences in levels of cortisol [5, 7] or catecholamines [5] between their prepubertal and pubertal children. This observation counters the hypothesis that stress is involved in the mechanism of insulin resistance during puberty.

## Influences of Gender and Body Fat

Insulin resistance has been shown to closely correlate with total body fat during puberty, as in adults [2-4, 10, 31, 45]. In contrast to adults, there appears to be a less significant relationship to body fat distribution (abdominal visceral, muscular, and subcutaneous fat) [45]. Adiposity steadily increases throughout puberty in girls even in late puberty when insulin resistance is falling, and insulin resistance occurs in boys during the middle and late stages of puberty as adiposity is decreasing. Thus, although fatness contributes significantly to insulin resistance during puberty, it does not entirely explain the phenomenon of the physiologic insulin resistance of puberty.

Girls are more insulin resistant than boys throughout puberty. It has been suggested that one reason adolescent girls are more insulin resistant than adolescent boys is that girls have more body fat. There are clear gender differences in developmental changes in body composition as boys and girls go through puberty. BMI increases throughout puberty in both sexes, but it increases to a greater degree in girls [2]. The percentage of body fat increases as girls progress through puberty whereas it decreases in boys; likewise, the percentage of fat-free mass at the end of puberty is lower in females [3, 17, 31, 45]. In clamp studies of 357 youth, however, only half of the sex-related difference in insulin resistance appeared to be explained by differences in adiposity as measured by skinfold thickness, and there was still a significant difference in insulin resistance between the sexes when adjustment for these factors was made [2]. Adjustment for BMI, waist circumference, or hip circumference also had little effect on sex differences in insulin sensitivity. Therefore, hormonal or other factors must also play a role.

Interestingly, the sexual dichotomy in insulin resistance during puberty disappeared in very obese subjects [2]. For a given BMI, insulin resistance was significantly greater in girls than boys when the BMI was less than 27 kg/m$^2$, but the gender difference was not present in youth whose BMI was greater than or equal to 27 kg/m$^2$. In obesity, sex differences in insulin resistance may be obscured by the influence of extreme adiposity. Because body fat contributes to insulin resistance during puberty in normal weight children, it is not surprising that insulin resistance is further impaired in pubertal children who are obese [30]. Obesity is a well known risk factor for insulin resistance, although the mechanisms by which adipose tissue alters glucose metabolism are complex and not fully understood. Further investigation of transcription factors that regulate fat cell function and of other factors secreted by adipocytes, such as leptin, TNF-α, and adiponectin, will contribute to the understanding of obesity and insulin resistance [46, 47].

## Race and Insulin Resistance during Puberty

African American adults have a significantly higher incidence of type 2 diabetes than white Americans [48]. Black children have also represented a disproportionate number of those affected by the epidemic of type 2 diabetes seen in children over the past decade [49]. Even at an early age, black children have been shown by some investigators to be more insulin resistant than their white peers [50, 51]. Because of potential racial differences in insulin resistance prior to puberty and the subsequent risk of developing type 2 diabetes, it is important to consider what effects the physiologic insulin resistance of puberty have on black children.

In the Bogalusa Heart Study, 377 children aged 5 to 17 selected from a biracial community had plasma glucose and insulin levels measured during an oral glucose tolerance test. Insulin levels increased in the pubertal age group for both races. However, the insulin response was significantly greater for black children than their white counterparts at all Tanner stages, particularly in black females [52]. These results were confirmed in another study that found black adolescents had higher first- and second-phase insulin concentrations than white subjects when evaluated by hyperglycemic clamp [53]. Recently, the same investigators evaluated a group of prepubertal black children with both hyperinsulinemic euglycemic and hyperglycemic clamps and determined that the hyperinsulinemia observed in black children is due to a combination of higher insulin secretion and lower insulin clearance compared to their white peers [51]. Another study evaluating differences between prepubertal Hispanic, African American and Caucasian children using the frequent sampled IV glucose tolerance test found that both Hispanic and African American children demonstrated higher acute insulin response compared to Caucasian youth, but that the second phase insulin secretion was higher in Hispanics than African Americans, and the persistent elevation of insulin in African American children was also due to lower insulin clearance. These studies demonstrate that mechanisms whereby insulin resistance and glucose intolerance develop may differ between racial groups [52].

In contrast to the data presented above, a cohort of black children studied with euglycemic clamp methodology were not found to be more insulin resistant than whites during puberty [2]. Seventy-three black youth were not more insulin resistant than 284 white youth, and in fact, the black males were more insulin sensitive than the white males. The black youth in this study, and in particular the black males, were slender and had very high physical activity levels, while those in several other studies were overweight and may have been less active.

Racial differences may exist in the GH/IGF-I axis, which may influence insulin resistance. In a study where black prepubertal children were found to be more insulin resistant than white children, higher levels of IGF-I were also found [50]. Black female subjects were shown by another investigator to have higher fasting insulin, higher free IGF-I, and lower serum IGFBP-1 than white females during puberty. In addition, the black females were sexually more mature according to Tanner staging and had higher fat mass than their white counterparts [53]. This tendency toward greater weight and earlier maturation in black girls has been reported elsewhere in the literature [54]. Thus, it is important to consider differences in body composition and sexual maturity when evaluating racial differences in insulin resistance.

## Conclusion

As part of normal development, pubertal children experience a transient insulin resistant state. Glucose homeostasis is maintained during this time, likely due to a corresponding elevation in insulin secretion during puberty. The physiologic purpose of insulin resistance and increased insulin production during puberty may be to promote rapid growth by augmenting protein anabolism, as suggested by an impairment of glucose but not protein metabolism. While the mechanism of insulin resistance during puberty is uncertain, growth hormone and IGF-I activity appear to play an important role in this phenomena. Though sex steroid levels rise during puberty, an association with insulin resistance has not been established. Girls are more insulin resistant than boys during puberty, and this is likely due differences in adiposity. The impact of body fat and race on the severity of insulin resistance during puberty should be considered as these factors also influence the risk of developing type 2 diabetes and metabolic syndrome.

## References

[1] Amiel SA, Sherwin RS, Simonson DC, Lauritano AA, Tamborlane WV. Impaired insulin action in puberty: a contributing factor to poor glycemic control in adolescents with diabetes. *N Engl J Med* 1986; 315:215-9.

[2] Moran AM, Jacobs Jr. DR, Steinberger J, Hong C-P, Prineas R, Luepker R, Sinaiko AR. Insulin resistance during puberty: results from clamp studies in 357 children. *Diabetes* 1999; 48:2039-44.

[3] Travers SH, Jeffers BW, Bloch CA, Hill JO, Eckel RH. Gender and tanner stage differences in body composition and insulin sensitivity in early pubertal children. *J Clin Endocrinol Metab* 1995; 80:172-8.

[4] Cook JS, Hoffman RP, Stene MA, Hansen JR. Effects of maturational stage on insulin sensitivity during puberty. *J Clin Endocrinol Metab* 1993; 77:725-30.

[5] Goran MI, Gower BA. Longitudinal study on pubertal insulin resistance. *Diabetes* 2001; 50:2444-9.

[6] Caprio S, Plewe G, Diamond MP, Simonson DC, Boulware SD, Sherwin RS, Tamborlane WV. Increased insulin secretion in puberty: a compensatory response to reductions in insulin sensitivity. *J Pediatr* 1989; 114:963-7.

[7] Amiel SA, Caprio S, Sherwin RS, Plewe G, Haymond MW, Tamborlane WV. Insulin resistance of puberty: a defect restricted to peripheral glucose metabolism. *J Clin Endocrinol Metab* 1991; 72:277-82.

[8] Caprio S, Cline G, Boulware SD, C. P, G.I. S, Sherwin RS, Tamborlane WV. Effects of puberty and diabetes on metabolism of insulin-sensitive fuels. *Am J Physiol* 1994; 266:E885-91.

[9] Potau N, Ibanez L, Rique S, Carrascosa A. Pubertal changes in insulin secretion and peripheral insulin sensitivity. *Horm Res* 1997; 48:219-26.

[10] Arslanian S, Suprasongsin C. Insulin sensitivity, lipids, and body composition in childhood: is "Syndrome X" present? *J Clin Endocrinol Metab* 1996; 81:1058-62.

[11] Bratusch-Marrain PR, Waldhausl WK, Gasic S, Hofer A. Hepatic disposal of biosynthetic human insulin and porcine c-peptide in humans. *Metabolism* 1984; 33:151-7.

[12] Rudolf MCJ, Sherwin RS, Markowitz R, Bates SE, Genel M, Hochstadt J, Tamborlane WV. Effect of intensive insulin treatment on linear growth in the young diabetic patient. *J Pediatr* 1982; 101:333-9.

[13] Seaquist ER. Pancreatic Islet Hormones, Diabetes Mellitus, and Hypoglycaemia. In: Niewoehner CB, ed. *Endocrine Pathophysiology*, 1st ed. Madison, CT: Fence Creek Publishing, 1998:117-39.

[14] Freymond D, Bogardus C, Okubo M, Stone K, Mott D. Impaired insulin-stimulated muscle glycogen synthase activation in vivo in man is related to low fasting glycogen synthase phosphatase activity. *J Clin Invest* 1988; 82:1503-9.

[15] Arslanian S, Kalhan SC. Correlations between fatty acid and glucose metabolism: potential explanation of insulin resistance of puberty. *Diabetes* 1994; 43:908-14.

[16] Randle PJ, Garland PB, Hales CN, Newsholme EA. The glucose fatty-acid cycle: its role in insulin sensitivity and the metabolic disturbances of diabetes mellitus. *Lancet* 1963:785-9.

[17] Hergenroeder A, Klish W. Body composition in adolescent athletes. *Pedriatric Clinics of North America* 1990; 37:1057-1080.

[18] Martha Jr. PM, Rogol AD, Veldhuis JD, Kerrigan JR, Goodman DW, Blizzard RM. Alterations in the pulsatile properties of circulating growth hormone concentrations during puberty in boys. *J Clin Endocrinol Metab* 1989; 69:563-70.

[19] Moran AM, Jacobs Jr. DR, Steinberger J, Cohen P, Hong C-P, Prineas R, Sinaiko AR. Association between the insulin resistance of puberty and the insulin-like growth factor-I/growth hormone axis. *J Clin Endocrinol Metab* 2002; 87:4817-20.

[20] Eugster EA, Sockalosky JJ. Growth. In: Niewoehner CB, ed. *Endocrine Pathophysiology*, 1st ed. Madison, CT: Fence Creek Publishing, 1998:211-36.

[21] Mauras N, Rogol AD, Haymond MW, Veldhuis JD. Sex steroids, growth hormone, insulin-like growth factor-1: neuroendocrine and metabolic regulation in puberty. *Horm Res* 1996; 45:74-80.

[22] Blum WF, Albertsson-Wikland K, Rosberg S, Ranke MB. Serum levels of insulin-like growth factor I (IGF-I) and IGF binding protein 3 reflect spontaneous growth hormone secretion. *J Clin Endocrinol Metab* 1993; 76:1610-6.

[23] Wickman S, Saukkonen T, Dunkel L. The role of sex steroids in the regulation of insulin sensitivity and serum lipid concentrations during male puberty: a prospective study with a P450 aromatase inhibitor. *European Journal of Endocrinology* 2002; 146:339-46.

[24] Guercio G, Rivarola MA, Chaler E, Maceiras M, Belgorosky A. Relationship between the growth hormone/insulin-like growth factor-I axis, insulin sensitivity, and adrenal androgens in normal prepubertal and pubertal girls. *J Clin Endocrinol Metab* 2003; 88:1389-93.

[25] Davidson MB. Effect of growth hormone on carbohydrate and lipid metabolism. *Endocr Rev* 1987; 8:115-31.

[26] Seminara S, Merello G, Masi S, Filpo A, La Cauza F, D'Onghia G, Martelli E, Loche S. Effect of long-term growth hormone treatment on carbohydrate metabolism in children with growth hormone deficiency. *Clin Endocrinol (Oxf)* 1998; 49:125-30.

[27] Heptulla RA, Boulware SD, Caprio S, Silver D, Sherwin RS, Tamborlane WV. Decreased insulin sensitivity and compensatory hyperinsulinemia after hormone treatment in children with short stature. *J Clin Endocrinol Metab* 1997; 82:3234-8.

[28] Le Roith D. Insulin-like growth factors. N Engl J Med 1997; 336:633-40.

[29] Caprio S. Insulin: the other anabolic hormone of puberty. *Acta Paediatr* 1999; Suppl 433:84-7.

[30] Attia N, Tamborlane WV, Heptulla RA, Maggs D, Grozman A, Sherwin RS, Caprio S. The metabolic syndrome and insulin-like growth factor I regulation in adolescent obesity. *J Clin Endocrinol Metab* 1998; 83:1467-71.

[31] Travers SH, Labarta JI, Gargosky SE, Rosenfeld RG, Jeffers BW, Eckel RH. Insulin-like growth factor binding protein-I levels are strongly associated with insulin sensitivity and obesity in early pubertal children. *J Clin Endocrinol Metab* 1998; 83:1935-9.

[32] Suwanichkul A, Allander SV, Morris SL, Powell DR. Glucocorticoids and insulin regulate expression of the human gen for insulin-like growth factor-binding protein-1 through proximal promoter elements. *J Biol Chem* 1994; 269:30835-41.

[33] Lee PDK, Jensen MD, Divertie GD, Heiling VJ, Katz HH, Conover CA. Insulin-like growth factor-binding protein-1 response to insulin during suppression of endogenous insulin secretion. *Metabolism* 1993; 42:409-14.

[34] Ritvos O, Ranta T, Jalkanen J, Suikkari A-M, Voutilainen R, Bohn H, Rutanen E-M. Insulin-like growth factor (IGF) binding protein from human decidua inhibits the binding and biological action of IGF-I in cultured choriocarcinoma cells. *Endocrinology* 1988; 122:2150-7.

[35] Clemmons DR, Moses AC, McKay MJ, Sommer A, Rosen DM, Ruckle J. The combination of insulin-like growth factor I and insulin-like growth factor-binding

protein-3 reduces insulin requirements in insulin-dependent type 1 diabetes: evidence for *in vivo* biologic activity. *J Clin Endocrinol Metab* 2000; 85:1518-24.

[36] Jakacki RI, Kelch RP, Sauder SE, Lloyd JS, Hopwood NJ, Marshall JC. Pulsatile secretion of luteinizing hormone in children. *J Clin Endocrinol Metab* 1982; 55:453-8.

[37] Eugster EA, Moran A. Sexual Determination, Sexual Differentiation, and Puberty. In: Niewoehner CB, ed. *Endocrine Pathophysiology, 1st ed.* Madison, CT: Fence Creek Publishing, 1998:237-55.

[38] Yki-Jarvinen H. Insulin sensitivity during the menstrual cycle. *J Clin Endocrinol Metab* 1984; 59:350-3.

[39] Toth EL, Suthijumroon A, Crockford PM, Ryan EA. Insulin Action Does Not Change During the Menstrual Cycle in Normal Women. *J Clin Endocrinol Metab* 1987; 64:74-80.

[40] Diamond MP, Simonson DC, DeFronzo RA. Menstrual cyclicity has a profound effect on glucose homeostasis. *Fertil Steril* 1989; 52:204-208.

[41] Widom B, Diamond MP, Simonson DC. Alterations in Glucose Metabolism During Menstrual Cycle in Women with IDDM. *Diabetes Care* 1992; 15:213-220.

[42] Dunaif A. Insulin resistance and the polycystic ovary syndrome: mechanism and implications of pathogenesis. *Endocr Rev* 1997; 18:774-800.

[43] Moghetti P, Castello R, Negri C, Tosi F, Spiazzi GG, Brun E, Balducci R, Toscano V, Muggeo M. Insulin infusion amplifies 17α–hydroxycorticosteroid intermediates response to adrenocorticotropin in hyperandrogenic women: apparent relative impairment of 17,20-lyase activity. *J Clin Endocrinol Metab* 1996; 81:881-6.

[44] Biondi M, Picardi A. Psychological stress and neuroendocrine function in humans: the last two decades of research. *Psychother Psychosom* 1999; 68:114-50.

[45] Roemmich J, Clark P, Lusk M, Friel A, Weltman A, Epstein L, Rogol AD. Pubertal alterations in growth and body composititon VI. Pubertal insulin resistance: relation to adiposity, body fat distribution and hormone release. *Int J Obes* 2002; 26:701-709.

[46] Holst D, Grimaldi PA. New factors in the regulation of adipose differentiation and metabolism. *Curr Opin Lipidol* 2002; 13:241-245.

[47] Kahn BB, Flier JS. Obesity and insulin resistance. J Clin Invest 2000; 106:473-481.

[48] Harris MI. Noninsulin-dependent diabetes mellitus in black and white Americans. *Diabetes Metab Rev* 1990; 6:71-91.

[49] Arslanian S, Danadian K. Insulin secretion, insulin sensitivity and diabetes in black children. *Trends in Endorinology and Metabolism* 1988; 9:194-9.

[50] Arslanian S, Suprasongsin C, Janosky JE. Insulin secretion and sensitivity in black *versus* white prepubertal healthy children. *J Clin Endocrinol Metab* 1997; 82:1923-7.

[51] Danadian K, Balasekaran G, Lewy V, Meza MP, Robertson R, Arslanian S. Insulin sensitivity in African-American children with and without family history of type 2 diabetes. *Diabetes Care* 1999; 22:1325-9.

[52] Svec F, Nastasi K, Hilton C, Bao W, Srinivasan SR, Berenson GS. Black-white contrasts in insulin levels during pubertal development. The Bogalusa Heart Study. *Diabetes* 1992; 41:313-7.

[53] Arslanian S, Suprasongsin C. Differences in the in vivo insulin secretion and sensitivity of healthy black versus white adolescents. *J Pediatr* 1996; 129:140-3.

In: Insulin Resistance in Children and Adolescents ISBN 1-59454-215-5
Editors: D. Daneman and J. Hamilton, pp. 103-119 

*Chapter 5*

# THE METABOLIC PHENOTYPE OF PRE-DIABETES IN OBESE YOUTH

***Ram Weiss, Catherine W. Yeckel, Sara E. Taksali and Sonia Caprio***
The Department of Pediatrics, Yale University School of Medicine, New Haven, CT.

## ABSTRACT

The prevalence of obesity is increasing alarmingly among children and adolescents in the U.S. Many of the metabolic and cardiovascular complications that are commonly associated with adult obesity have their onset in childhood. These metabolic correlates of obesity are closely coupled with the presence of insulin resistance and hyperinsulinemia. In a large multiethnic cohort of obese children and adolescents, we found insulin resistance to be the best predictor of impaired glucose tolerance (IGT) and type 2 diabetes.

Here, we have described studies that examined the underlying mechanisms relevant to the putative changes in insulin sensitivity and secretion in the early stages of diabetes in youth. Furthermore, we have described whether alterations in the partitioning of myocellular and abdominal fat relates to abnormalities in glucose homeostasis in obese adolescents with pre-diabetes.

## INTRODUCTION

Childhood obesity affects one in five children in the U.S. [1] and is among the most serious and urgent public health problems facing many countries today. It is a chronic disorder that tends to track throughout life and is associated with metabolic and cardiovascular complications [2]. In addition, approximately 60% of overweight five- to ten-year-old children have one associated biochemical or clinical cardiovascular risk factor [3], such as hyperinsulinemia/insulin resistance [4], hyperlipidemia [5], or elevated blood pressure [3], and 25% of them have two or more complications [3]. This secular trend in childhood obesity parallels a concurrent increase in obesity among adults [6]. As a consequence of the increasing obesity in both adults and children, the prevalence rates of type 2 diabetes have increased significantly [7,8]. Current approaches to the obesity problem have failed to reverse or prevent it, creating a healthcare challenge never encountered previously. One dire prediction from the Center for Disease Control and Prevention (CDC) estimated that, if current rates continue, one in three babies born in 2000 will eventually develop diabetes [9]. The rates are even higher in African-American and Hispanic children.

In this review, we examine the impact of childhood and adolescent obesity on glucose homeostasis. Risk factors associated with impaired glucose tolerance (IGT) and type 2 diabetes in youth are discussed. We also describe studies that have been performed to define the underlying mechanisms relevant to the putative changes in insulin sensitivity and secretion in the early stages of diabetes in youth. Potential key modulators of insulin action in obese children and adolescents are presented as well.

## Defining the Metabolic Syndrome in Youth

Reaven and colleagues [10] described the link between insulin resistance and hypertension, dyslipidemia, type 2 diabetes and other metabolic abnormalities in adults a number of years ago. This constellation of co-morbid conditions has become known as the "metabolic syndrome" and is associated with an increased risk of morbidity and mortality from cardiovascular disease [11]. More recent studies suggest that the pathophysiologic defects leading to the development of the metabolic syndrome in adults may begin as early as the intra-uterine period [12, 13].

In children, obesity is by far the most common cause of insulin resistance [14, 15] and is frequently associated with dyslipidemia [16], type 2 diabetes [17] and long-term microvascular and macrovascular complications [18-20]. Using data collected between 1988-1994 on a nationally representative sample of U.S. adolescents (NHANES III), Cook et al [21] reported a prevalence of the metabolic syndrome of 6.8% in overweight and 28.7% in obese adolescents. However, these rates may underestimate the current magnitude of the problem, in view of the growing epidemic of obesity in children and adolescents. It is also important to note that the degree, as well as the prevalence, of childhood obesity has been increasing over time [22].

The criteria for diagnosing the metabolic syndrome that we use are a modification of the National Cholesterol Education Program Adult Treatment Panel [23] and WHO criteria [24], with adjustment for developmental differences in the evolution of metabolic abnormalities in obese children{Weiss, 2004 NEJM}. Since body proportions normally change dramatically during childhood and pubertal development and may vary between different ethnic backgrounds, definitions of central obesity based on measurements of waist-to-hip ratios are difficult to interpret in children. We elected instead to define obesity based on a threshold of BMI Z-score > 2, adjusted for age and gender. Elevated systolic or diastolic blood pressure was defined as greater than the $95^{th}$ percentile for age and gender. Abnormalities in fasting triglyceride and HDL-C levels were also adjusted for age and gender. A threshold of above the $95^{th}$ percentile was chosen for triglycerides and below the $5^{th}$ percentile for HDL-C. We used impaired glucose tolerance (IGT), defined according to the American Diabetes Association guidelines as a 2-hour glucose > 140 mg/dl and < 200 mg/dl [25], as our element of altered glucose metabolism in the definition of the metabolic syndrome in youth. In contrast to the adults, where fasting glucose levels are used as the criterion for the metabolic syndrome, impaired fasting glucose is rare in pediatrics and, even when present, fails to detect the majority of patients with impaired glucose tolerance.

In adults, diagnosis of the metabolic syndrome requires the presence of three or more diagnostic components. Similarly, subjects in this study were classified as having the metabolic syndrome when they met three or more of the criteria shown in Table 1. When testing these criteria in a cohort of 439 obese, 31 overweight and 20 lean children and adolescents, the prevalence of the metabolic syndrome phenotype in obese youth proved to be more common than previously reported and increases with increasing degrees of obesity. Indeed, 40-50% of severely obese Caucasian and Hispanic youth in our sample were classified as having the metabolic syndrome, while none of the overweight or lean youngsters met the criteria. We further demonstrated a worsening of each element of the syndrome across a spectrum of degrees of obesity, from overweight to severe obesity. As observed in adults [26, 27], insulin resistance is strongly associated with the development of specific adverse metabolic components in these obese children.

**Table 1. Modified Metabolic Syndrome Criteria for Children and Adolescents**

Three or more of:

- BMI > 97th percentile for age and gender (BMI Z-score > 2)
- Triglycerides > 95th percentile for age, gender
- HDL-C < 5th percentile for age, gender
- Systolic blood pressure and/or diastolic blood pressure > 95% percentile for age and gender
- Impaired glucose tolerance (IGT)

## Epidemiology of Impaired Glucose Tolerance in Obese Children and Adolescents

In adults, type 2 diabetes develops over a long period. Most, if not all, patients initially have impaired glucose tolerance (IGT), which is an intermediate stage in the natural history of type 2 diabetes [10] and predicts the risk of the development of diabetes [11] and cardiovascular disease [12]. With appropriate changes in lifestyle, progression from IGT to frank diabetes can be delayed or prevented [13, 14]. Thus, great emphasis has recently been placed on the early detection of IGT in adults.

Although severe obesity has a prominent role in the pathogenesis of type 2 diabetes in children and adolescents, it is unknown whether it is a risk factor for IGT. We undertook a study to determine the prevalence of IGT in a multiethnic cohort of obese children and adolescents. Using a clinic-based population of 55 obese children and 112 obese adolescents, IGT was detected in 25% of the obese children and 21% of the obese adolescents, and silent type 2 diabetes was identified in 4% of the obese adolescents [7]. Children and adolescents with IGT included both white and minority children. Higher prevalence rates of IGT have been also reported in obese children from Thailand and the Philippines [15, 16] and in Latino children living in the U.S. [17], while lower prevalence rates of 15% were found in obese children in France [18]. The best predictors of IGT in our study were, in order of importance:

- Insulin resistance index (HOMA-IR);
- Fasting proinsulin;
- 2-hr insulin levels; and
- Fasting insulin levels

How obesity relates to diabetes risk is not clear. The majority, if not all, children and adolescents with IGT and type 2 diabetes have a significant degree of insulin resistance. This may be due to obesity, a sedentary lifestyle, ethnicity, pubertal stage of development and/or a family history of diabetes. Simple surrogate measures of adiposity, such as body mass index, do not significantly predict IGT in obese children and adolescents (REF: NEJM 2002 Sinha).

## The Metabolic Phenotype of Pre-Diabetes in Obese Youth

Having found a high prevalence rate of IGT in obese youth and that insulin resistance was the best predictor of this prediabetic state, we performed a series of studies to examine the underlying mechanisms relevant to the putative changes in insulin sensitivity (REF: Lancet paper Sept 2003). We used the euglycemic-hyperinsulinemic clamp [19] in combination with 6,6 $^2H_2$-glucose and $^2H_2$-glycerol and indirect calorimetry to examine the role of insulin resistance in obese youngsters with IGT. Beta-cell function was assessed separately by using the hyperglycemic clamp technique [19].

### Insulin Resistance - A Defect of Non-oxidative Glucose Disposal

In a cross-sectional analysis, the responses in IGT obese adolescents were compared to those in obese adolescents with normal glucose tolerance (NGT) of similar ages, gender and degree of obesity (REF: Lancet paper Sept 2003). This study design allowed an assessment of differences in insulin sensitivity and fat partitioning independent of total body adiposity. Insulin-stimulated glucose disposal was significantly reduced in the obese adolescents with IGT compared with those with NGT (Figure 1). This defect was mainly accounted for by a reduction in non-oxidative glucose disposal (storage), since rates of glucose oxidation did not differ significantly between the groups. Similar metabolic defects have been described in adults with overt type 2 diabetes [20]. Co-infusion of labeled glucose and glycerol during the clamp provided a means of assessing the effects of insulin on hepatic glucose production and lipolysis. Baseline hepatic glucose production rates, plasma fatty acid and glycerol levels, as well as glycerol turnover rates were similar in the two groups. During the insulin clamp, suppression of lipolysis and hepatic glucose production was of similar magnitude in both groups. These results argue against an impaired anti-lipolytic effect of insulin in pre-diabetes in obese youth. Furthermore, the fact that both groups had similar basal hepatic glucose production rates suggest that hepatic insulin resistance did not have a major role in early pre-diabetes in our obese adolescents.

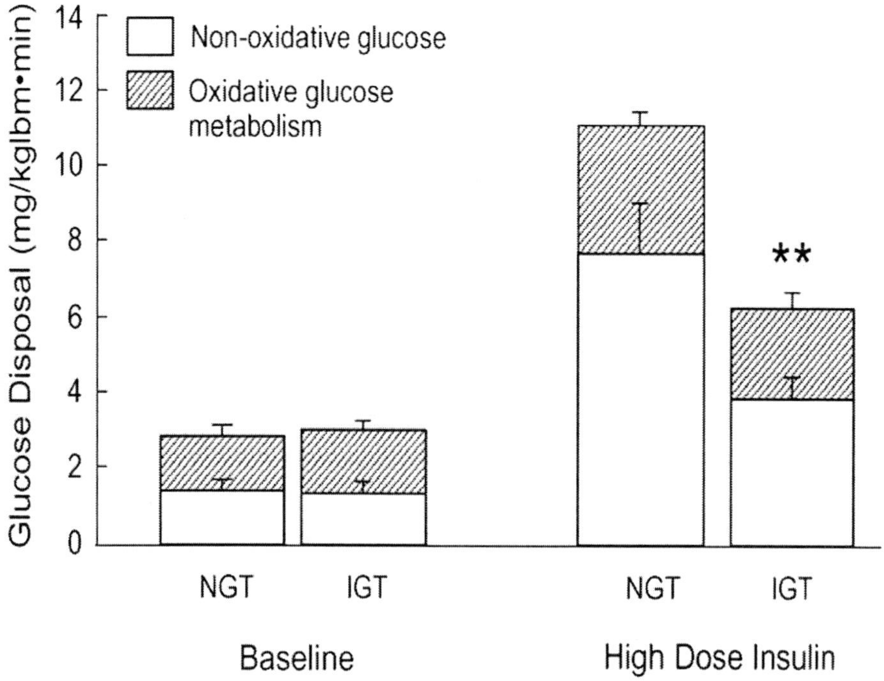


Figure 1. Total body glucose disposal in obese children and adolescents with normal (NGT) and impaired glucose tolerance (IGT) during the basal state and euglycemic insulin clamp (80 mU/m$^2$·min). Hatched bars: oxidative glucose metabolism; open bars: non-oxidative glucose metabolism.
**p<0.001.

## Muscle Lipid Deposition and Abdominal Fat Distribution

Increased insulin resistance as a function of altered myocellular and abdominal fat partitioning is increasingly being described in adults with T2DM [21, 22, 23, 24]. Consequently, to gain insights into the lipid composition of skeletal muscle, we used proton nuclear magnetic resonance ($^1$H-NMR) spectroscopy to quantify non-invasively the intramyocellular (IMCL) and extramyocellular (EMCL) lipid content of the soleus muscle (REF: Lancet paper Sept 2003). Magnetic resonance imaging (MRI) was used to examine the association of visceral and subcutaneous abdominal depot-size to altered glucose metabolism. The IMCL lipid content was significantly higher in the IGT subject (3.04±0.43%) vs NGT (1.99±0.19, p<0.03). In contrast, no difference was found in the EMCL lipid depots (Figure 2). Interesting differences also emerged in the abdominal subcutaneous and visceral depots between IGT and NGT obese youngsters (Figure 3). Indeed, subcutaneous fat in IGT subjects (460±47 cm$^2$) was significantly lower compared with NGT subjects (626±39 cm$^2$, p<0.02). Visceral fat tended to be higher in the IGT group (70±11 cm$^2$) than in the NGT group (47±3 cm$^2$, p<0.07). The ratio of visceral to subcutaneous fat was 50% higher in the IGT subjects (0.15±0.02) vs. NGT (0.07±0.008, p<0.01). Shown in Figure 4 are representative transverse abdominal MRI scans and $^1$H-NMR soleus muscle spectra from a boy with NGT and one with IGT. One can readily appreciate the marked differences in both the MRI and the $^1$H-NMR spectra in these two boys with NGT and IGT (Figure 4).

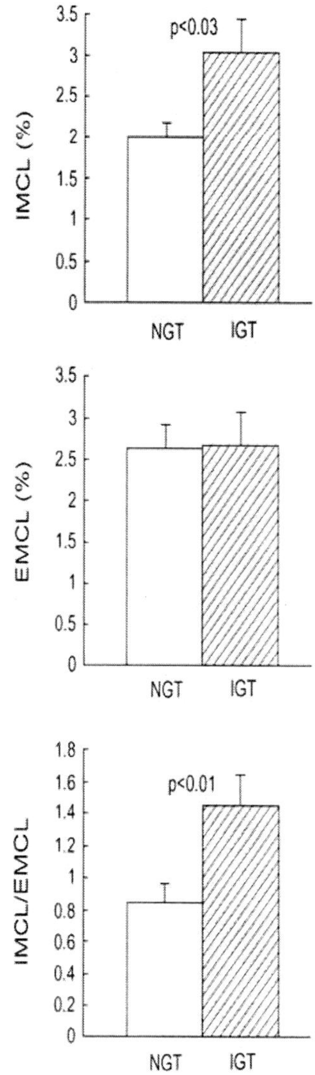


Figure 2. Differences in intramyocellular (IMCL) and extramyocellular (EMCL) lipid content and the IMCL-to-EMCL ratio in obese children and adolescents with normal (NGT) and impaired glucose tolerance (IGT).

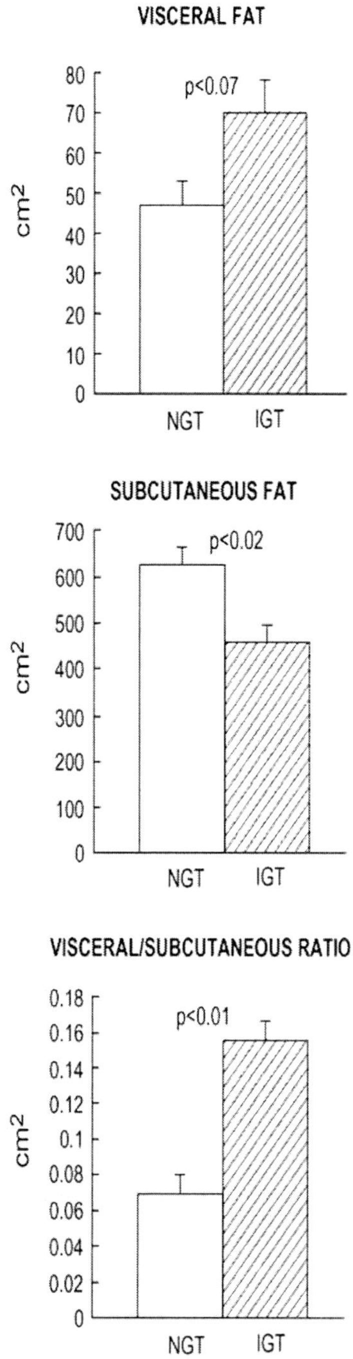


Figure 3. Differences in visceral and subcutaneous abdominal fat and the visceral-to-subcutaneous ratio in obese children and adolescents with normal (NGT) and impaired glucose tolerance (IGT).

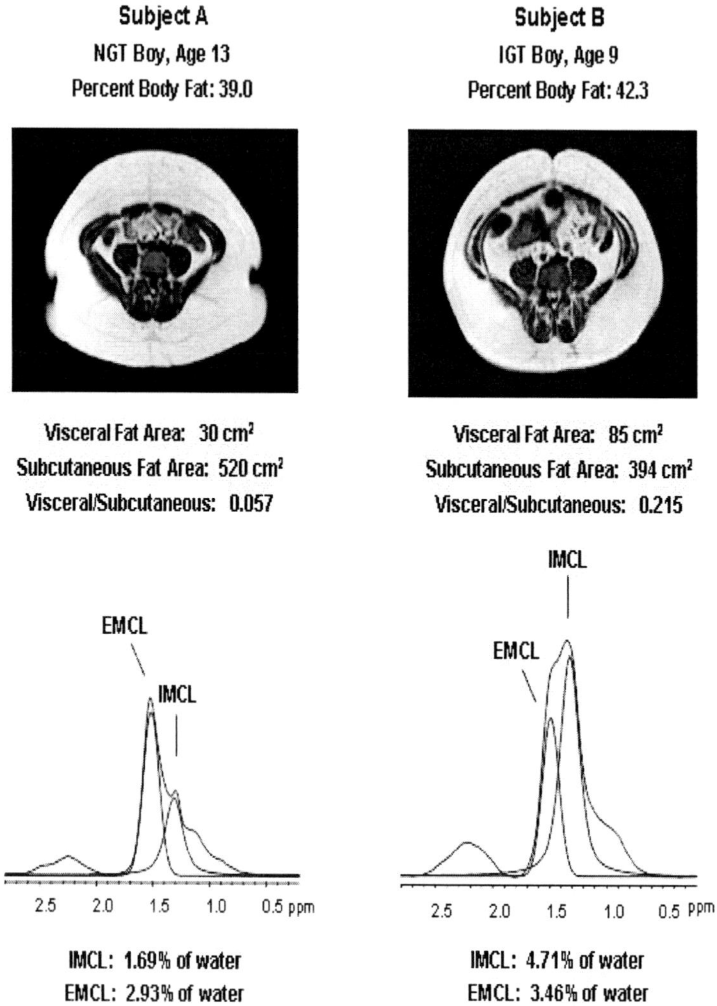


Figure 4. Transverse abdominal MRI scans (L4 vertebral level 1, fat appears white with T1 weighting) and $^1$H-NMR soleus muscle spectra from an obese boy with NGT (Subject A) and one with IGT (Subject B). The subjects have equivalent amounts of total body fat, but there is more visceral fat and less subcutaneous fat in the subject with IGT (B) compared with the matched control (A). Muscle lipid partitioning was also substantially different, with an increased IMCL and reduced EMCL in the IGT subject (B) compared with the respective control (A).

We used univariate analysis to examine the relationships between IMCL and visceral fat with insulin resistance and the 2-hr plasma glucose levels during the OGTT. We found that IMCL and visceral fat content were inversely correlated with the glucose disposal ($r=-0.51$ and $r=-0.63$, $p<0.01$, respectively) and with non-oxidative glucose metabolism in the two groups together ($r=-0.45$ and $r=-0.47$, $p<0.03$, respectively). A positive relationship was found between IMCL, as well as the visceral-to-subcutaneous fat ratio, and the 2-hr plasma glucose during the OGTT in the two groups together ($r=-0.38$ and $r=-0.57$, $p<0.04$, respectively). In contrast, no significant relationships were found between EMCL and subcutaneous fat with glucose disposal and non-oxidative glucose disposal.

This study offered a novel insight into the pathogenesis of pre-diabetes in obese children and adolescents, namely that changes in glucose homeostasis are closely linked with altered partitioning of fat in both skeletal muscle and adipose tissues.

It is not entirely clear at the present time what leads to an over-accumulation of lipid in skeletal muscle tissues. Defects in muscle fatty acid oxidation and increased fatty acid flux to muscle have both been considered as potential players [25]. Triglyceride accumulation *per se* in muscle does not cause insulin resistance. Rather, over-accumulation of various lipid moieties in myocytes, such as long chain fatty acyl-CoA, have been shown to interfere directly with insulin signaling and glucose transport [26, 27, 28, 29]. Depletion of IMCL stores was found to restore normal insulin sensitivity in obese adults [30].

Visceral fat accumulation is known to be associated with features of the insulin resistance syndrome in adults and obese children [21], although the nature of this relationship and the relative importance of visceral vs. subcutaneous abdominal fat remains a matter of debate. An important feature of the present study is that altered distribution of fat between the subcutaneous and intra-abdominal compartment is associated with the development of IGT. The IGT subjects had relatively more visceral fat and less subcutaneous fat than the NGT subjects. Therefore, the visceral-to-subcutaneous ratio was significantly greater in the IGT than in the NGT group. Both the enlarged visceral depot ($r=-0.63$, $p<0.01$) and the visceral-to-subcutaneous ratio ($r=-0.66$, $p<0.01$) were inversely related to the insulin-stimulated glucose metabolism. Our study therefore implies that insulin resistance is the result of the imbalance of fat distribution in both the abdominal adipose and skeletal muscle tissues. Furthermore, our data are consistent with results obtained in both human and animal models of lipodystrophy, in which there is an absence of subcutaneous adipose tissue, leading to increased circulation of lipids and their accumulation in both myocytes and the visceral depot [31, 32]. Thus, it appears that the ability of peripheral subcutaneous fat tissue to vary its storage capacity is critical for regulating insulin sensitivity and ultimately protecting against diabetes. Consistent with this hypothesis is the evidence derived from the use of thiazolidinediones, which improve insulin sensitivity while increasing subcutaneous abdominal fat, but decreasing the visceral and liver fat depots [33, 34, 35].

## Pancreatic Beta-Cell Function

Basal plasma insulin levels were significantly greater in IGT children (43±5 μU/ml) vs. NGT (32±3 μU/ml), $p<0.02$); however, basal plasma glucose levels were identical in the two groups (REF: Lancet paper Sept 2003). To determine whether defects in first- and second-phase insulin secretion are present early in the development of T2DM in obese youth, we used the hyperglycemic clamp, as previously described [19]. These studies revealed that both first- and second-phase plasma insulin levels and insulin secretion rates were not different in the two groups (Figure 5). However, when estimating insulin secretion in the context of the "resistant milieu" of the IGT subjects, and thus using the disposition index, we found that the IGT group had a significantly lower disposition index (Figure 5) than the NGT group. The lower DI indicates that the secretion of insulin was not able to compensate for the increased resistance, resulting in a marked decrease in insulin-stimulated glucose metabolism in the IGT subjects. One may view this phenomenon as a "relative" beta-cell failure due to the inability of the subjects to overcome the extraordinary insulin resistance. Contrasting results on first-phase insulin levels have been reported by Arslanian *et al.* in a group of obese adolescent girls with polycystic ovary syndrome [36]. Differences in the stage of diabetes and type of population studied are likely to account for these disparities.

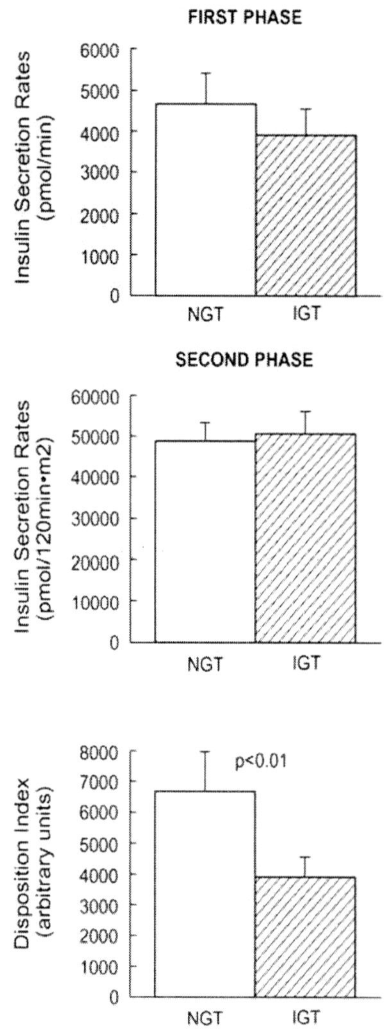


Figure 5. First and second phase insulin secretion rates and the disposition index in obese children and adolescents with normal (NGT) and impaired glucose tolerance (IGT).

## Adiponectin, Insulin Sensitivity and Intramyocellular Lipid in Obese Adolescents

The adipose tissue is known to secrete several proteins that act as potential regulators of glucose and lipid homeostasis [37]. These proteins have been collectively referred to as a adipocytokines because of their structural similarity with cytokines [37]. Among these adipocytokines, the Acrp30, known as adiponectin, is unique because, in contrast to the markedly increased levels of many other adipocytokines (e.g. leptin [38] and TNF-alpha [39]), its level is reduced in obesity [40]. Of note, the decline in circulating adiponectin levels coincided with the onset of insulin resistance and the development of diabetes in monkeys [41].

Using different measures of insulin sensitivity (M), several groups have found that adiponectin gene expression and plasma levels correlated with the insulin-sensitive stage in both rodents and obese adults [42, 43, 44]. Administration of adiponectin to mice consuming a high-fat diet led to an improvement of M, which was associated with decreased muscle and liver triglyceride content and increased fat oxidation in muscle [45, 46]. Thus, dysregulation in the synthesis and/or secretion of adiponectin from the adipose tissue may play a role in the pathogenesis of insulin resistance in both obesity and type 2 diabetes.

Most studies regarding the link between adiponectin and insulin resistance have been performed in rodents, nonhuman primates, and adult subjects with obesity and type 2 diabetes. There is little information on circulating levels of adiponectin in pediatrics. Given that adolescent obesity profoundly affects insulin and glucose metabolism, we quantitated this protein in a group of nonobese and obese adolescents with and without IGT and explored the relationship between adiponectin and whole body M (assessed by the insulin clamp technique) and muscle lipid content (determined by $^{1}H$-NMR) REF: this should be the adiponectin paper—JCEM 2003. As shown in Figure 6, we found that circulating plasma adiponectin levels were lower in obese (9±1 μg/ml) than in non-obese adolescents (14±1.6) ($p<0.01$). A further reduction, however, was seen in the obese adolescents with IGT (5±0.8 μg/ml, $p<0.01$) Ref: Lancet 2003. These differences were associated with reduced insulin sensitivity in the obese subjects with NGT and IGT, whereas the opposite was observed for the IMCL content. It is unknown at the present time what might be the cause of the reduction in adiponectin levels in obesity and type 2 diabetes and what the factors are that regulate this protein.

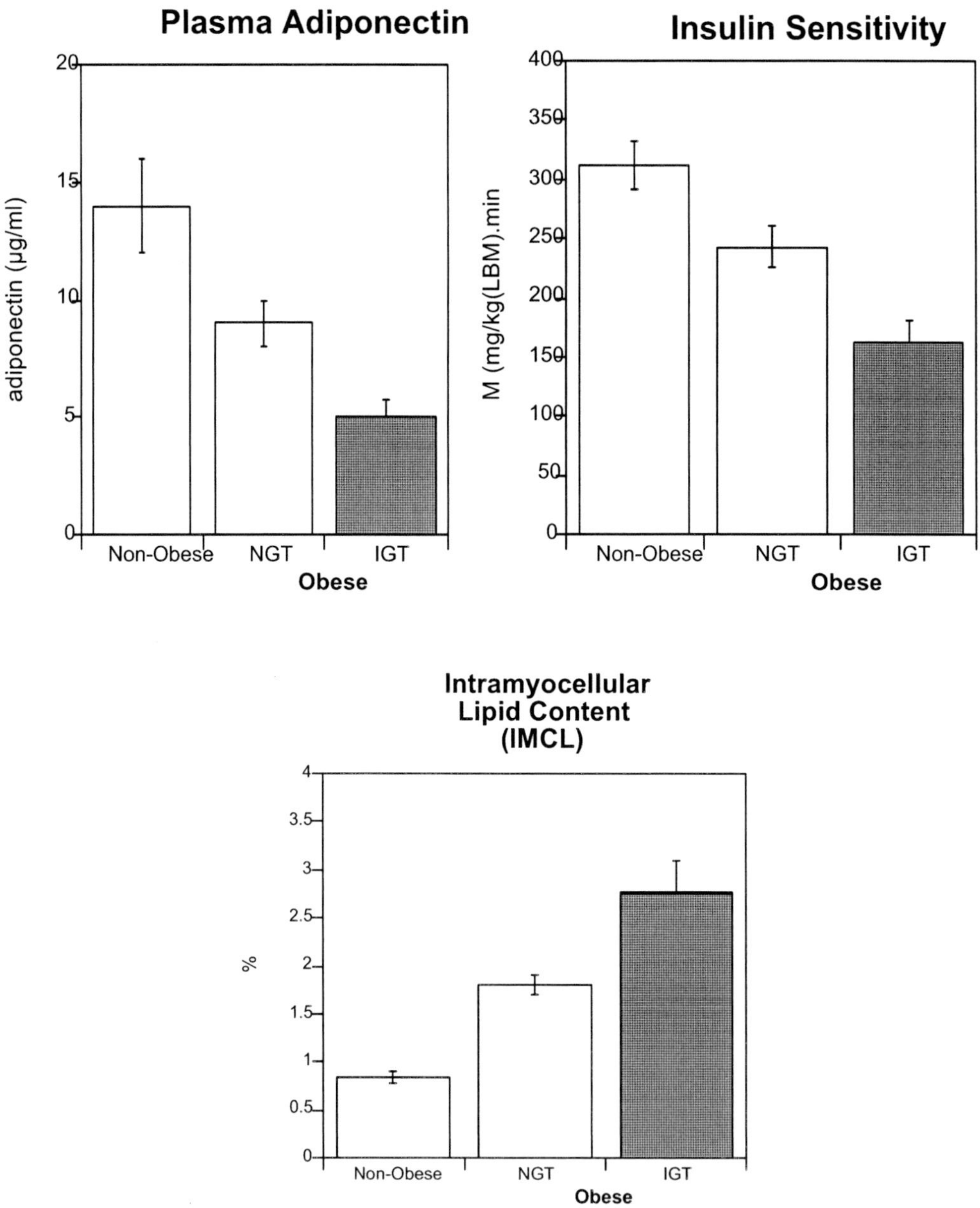


Figure 6. Plasma adiponectin levels (top left), insulin sensitivity (top right), and intramyocellular lipid content (IMCL) (bottom) for Non-Obese, Obese NGT and Obese IGT youth. Adiponectin levels were decreased in obese vs. non-obese subjects ($p<0.001$). Obese IGT subjects had further reduced levels ($p<0.02$). Insulin sensitivity was also lower in the IGT subjects ($p<0.001$). IMCL was greater in the obese vs. non-obese subjects ($p<0.001$). Among the obese subjects, the IGT had the highest levels of IMCL ($p<0.01$).

## The Whole Body Insulin Sensitivity Index: A Valuable Index Of Insulin Resistance

The increased prevalence of pre-diabetes and type 2 diabetes in obese children and adolescents is strongly influenced by increases in insulin resistance. The standard for measuring insulin sensitivity is the euglycemic-hyperinsulinemic clamp [19]. However, this method is labor intensive, costly, and relatively invasive; therefore, the development of relatively noninvasive testing strategies for assessing insulin resistance in high-risk children and adolescents is critical.

The use of the more common OGTT test procedure to ascertain the degree of insulin sensitivity in a pediatric population could be invaluable, especially due to the inherent limitations to performing the more invasive "clamp" measurements in this cohort. The OGTT is simpler to perform in larger groups of people when the efficacy of a therapeutic strategy is being considered for more general application.

Matsuda *et al.* developed a composite whole body insulin sensitivity index (WBISI) from the OGTT and found that this index correlates well with the "M" value from the insulin clamp in adults with a range of insulin sensitivities [47]. Yeckel *et al.* in our group validated the WBISI in a large cohort of obese children and adolescents of diverse ethnic backgrounds, with normal and impaired glucose tolerance [48]. A significant relationship was found between the WBISI (OGTT) and the "M" value (clamp) taken in the same individuals on separate visits ($r=0.78$, $p<0.0001$). This validation in the obese pediatric population now allows for a simple assessment of stimulated insulin sensitivity while simultaneously determining the glucose tolerance status. This index proved to be very sensitive and able to clearly differentiate individuals with different degrees of insulin resistance in the pediatric population.

Using the WBISI, we divided an obese cohort of 312 children and adolescents with NGT into tertiles and compared it to a group of 56 obese children and adolescents with IGT [48] The clinical and biochemical characteristics of interest are shown in Table 2. As can be seen from the lowest tertile of insulin sensitivity, the NGT and IGT children have equivalent WBISI values and are not significantly different in any metabolic category, except HDL cholesterol, glucose at 120 minutes, and the insulinogenic index ($p<0.05$). The individuals in the lowest tertile of WBISI displayed a high prevalence of metabolic syndrome characteristics, along with higher levels of obesity, dyslipidemia and insulin resistance. Therefore, the most clinically relevant pediatric population in terms of high-risk for type 2 diabetes and metabolic syndrome can be effectively examined for stimulated insulin sensitivity through the use of a simple OGTT.

## Conclusion

Pre-diabetes in obese children and adolescents represents a complex metabolic phenotype, characterized by severe peripheral insulin resistance and altered lipid partitioning. These youngsters are at risk for deterioration to overt diabetes, as well as for early development of adverse cardiovascular outcomes related to the metabolic syndrome. Further research is warranted for elucidation of potential interventions to reverse this phenotype.

**Table 2. Metabolic risk profile based on level of insulin sensitivity**

| | IGT | NGT | | |
|---|---|---|---|---|
| tertile of insulin resistance # | **0** | 1 | 2 | 3 |
| **N** | 56 | 102 | 103 | 107 |
| **WBISI** | $1.02 \pm .09^{2,3}$ | $1.01 \pm 0.03^{2,3}$ | $1.82 \pm 0.02^{0,1,3}$ | $3.38 \pm 0.11^{0,1,2}$ |
| **BMI (kg/m²)** | $36.7 \pm 0.8$ | $38.6 \pm 0.7^{3}$ | $36.4 \pm 0.8$ | $34.6 \pm 0.7^{1}$ |
| **fasting glucose (mg/dl)** | $92 \pm 1.3^{3}$ | $91 \pm 0.72^{3}$ | $89 \pm 0.74$ | $88 \pm 0.63^{0,1}$ |
| **fasting insulin (μU/ml)** | $51 \pm 3.9^{2,3}$ | $51 \pm 2.8^{2,3}$ | $28 \pm 0.6^{0,1,3}$ | $17 \pm 0.58^{0,1,2}$ |
| **HOMA** | $11.8 \pm 0.92^{2,3}$ | $11.5 \pm 0.54^{2,3}$ | $6.2 \pm 0.15^{0,1,3}$ | $3.8 \pm 0.13^{0,1,2}$ |
| **OGTT** | | | | |
| **Glucose 120 (mg/dl)** | $155 \pm 2.0^{1,2,3}$ | $116 \pm 1.6^{0,3}$ | $112 \pm 1.5^{0,3}$ | $103 \pm 1.6^{0,1,2}$ |
| **mean insulin (μU/ml)** | $388 \pm 39^{2,3}$ | $297 \pm 12^{2,3}$ | $157 \pm 5^{0,1,3}$ | $95 \pm 3^{0,1,2}$ |
| **IGI (μU/ml/mg/dl)** | $4.1 \pm 0.37^{1}$ | $5.6 \pm 0.9^{0,3}$ | $5.3 \pm 0.44^{3}$ | $5.1 \pm 1.6^{1,2}$ |
| **Lipids** | | | | |
| **T-CHOL (mg/dl)** | $162 \pm 4.5$ | $160 \pm 3.6$ | $167 \pm 3.6$ | $161 \pm 3.4$ |
| **HDL (mg/dl)** | $37 \pm 0.89^{1,2,3}$ | $39 \pm 0.84^{0,3}$ | $40 \pm 0.78^{0,3}$ | $44 \pm 1.1^{0,1,2}$ |
| **LDL (mg/dl)** | $99 \pm 3.7$ | $94 \pm 2.5$ | $102 \pm 3.3$ | $97 \pm 2.9$ |
| **TG (mg/dl)** | $138 \pm 11^{3}$ | $128 \pm 7.3^{3}$ | $114 \pm 6.2^{3}$ | $95 \pm 8.7^{0,1,2}$ |

NGT population subdivided by tertile of insulin sensitivity (WBISI). Numbers for comparisons refer to the level of insulin sensitivity: IGT (0); NGT lowest sensitivity (1) to highest sensitivity (3). For example, a superscript 1 in the IGT column indicates a significant difference between the IGT group and the NGT group of lowest sensitivity. Significance based on Tukey multiple comparisons $p < 0.05$. Conversion factors for SI units: glucose (mmol/l) = 0.05551; insulin (pmol/l) = 6.0; all cholesterol classes (mmol/l) = 0.02586; triglyceride (mmol/l) = 0.0116. Normal Glucose Tolerance (NGT); Impaired Glucose Tolerance (IGT); Oral Glucose Tolerance Test (OGTT).

## ACKNOWLEDGEMENTS

This chapter is Supported by grants R01 HD 40787 and R01 HD 28016 to Dr. Caprio, M01 RR-00125 and MO1 RR-06022 from the National Institutes of Health, and The Stephen I. Morse Pediatric Diabetes Research Fund to Dr. Weiss; Dr. Caprio is a recipient of a K24 HD 01464 Award for Patient-Oriented Research.

## REFERENCES

[1] Ogden CL, Flegal KM, Carroll MD, Johnson CL. Prevalence and trends in overweight among US children and adolescents, 1999-2000. *Jama* 2002; 288:1728-32.

[2] Freedman DS, Dietz WH, Srinivasan SR, Berenson GS. The relation of overweight to cardiovascular risk factors among children and adolescents: the Bogalusa Heart Study. *Pediatrics* 1999; 103:1175-82.

[3] Must A, Spadano J, Coakley EH, Field AE, Colditz G, Dietz WH. The disease burden associated with overweight and obesity. *Jama* 1999; 282:1523-9.

[4] Caprio S, Hyman LD, Limb C, et al. Central adiposity and its metabolic correlates in obese adolescent girls. *Am J Physiol* 1995; 269:E118-26.

[5] Caprio S, Tamborlane WV, Silver D, et al. Hyperleptinemia: an early sign of juvenile obesity. Relations to body fat depots and insulin concentrations. *Am J Physiol* 1996; 271:E626-30.

[6] Flegal KM, Carroll MD, Ogden CL, Johnson CL. Prevalence and trends in obesity among US adults, 1999-2000. *Jama* 2002; 288:1723-7.

[7] Sinha R, Fisch G, Teague B, et al. Prevalence of impaired glucose tolerance among children and adolescents with marked obesity. *N Engl J Med* 2002; 346:802-10.

[8] Rosenbloom AL, Joe JR, Young RS, Winter WE. Emerging epidemic of type 2 diabetes in youth. *Diabetes Care* 1999; 22:345-54.

[9] Narayan KM, Boyle JP, Thompson TJ, Sorensen SW, Williamson DF. Lifetime risk for diabetes mellitus in the United States. *Jama* 2003; 290:1884-90.

[10] Polonsky KS, Sturis J, Bell GI. Seminars in Medicine of the Beth Israel Hospital, Boston. Non-insulin-dependent diabetes mellitus - a genetically programmed failure of the beta cell to compensate for insulin resistance. *N Engl J Med* 1996; 334:777-83.

[11] Edelstein SL, Knowler WC, Bain RP, et al. Predictors of progression from impaired glucose tolerance to NIDDM: an analysis of six prospective studies. *Diabetes* 1997; 46:701-10.

[12] Haffner SM, Stern MP, Hazuda HP, Mitchell BD, Patterson JK. Cardiovascular risk factors in confirmed prediabetic individuals. Does the clock for coronary heart disease start ticking before the onset of clinical diabetes? *Jama* 1990; 263:2893-8.

[13] Knowler WC, Barrett-Connor E, Fowler SE, et al. Reduction in the incidence of type 2 diabetes with lifestyle intervention or metformin. *N Engl J Med* 2002; 346:393-403.

[14] Tuomilehto J, Lindstrom J, Eriksson JG, et al. Prevention of type 2 diabetes mellitus by changes in lifestyle among subjects with impaired glucose tolerance. *N Engl J Med* 2001; 344:1343-50.

[15] Keamseng C, Likitmaksul S, Kiattisakthavee P, et al. Risk of metabolic disturbance and diabetes development in Thai obese children, *29th Annual Meeting of the International Society for Pediatric and Adolescent Diabetes*, Saint-Malo, France, September 3-6, 2003.

[16] Lee W, Tang J, Karim H, et al. Abnormalities of glucose tolerance in severely obese Singapore children, *29th Annual Meeting of the International Society for Pediatric and Adolescent Diabetes*, Saint-Malo, France, September 3-6, 2003.

[17] Cruz M, Weigensberg M, Goran M. Prevalence of the metabolic syndrome in overweight Latino youth. *Diabetes* 2003; 52(Suppl 1):A399, 1734-P.

[18] Tounian P, Aggoun Y, Dubern B, et al. Presence of increased stiffness of the common carotid artery and endothelial dysfunction in severely obese children: a prospective study. *Lancet* 2001; 358:1400-4.

[19] DeFronzo RA, Tobin JD, Andres R. Glucose clamp technique: a method for quantifying insulin secretion and resistance. *Am J Physiol* 1979; 237:E214-23.

[20] Shulman GI, Rothman DL, Jue T, Stein P, DeFronzo RA, Shulman RG. Quantitation of muscle glycogen synthesis in normal subjects and subjects with non-insulin-dependent diabetes by 13C nuclear magnetic resonance spectroscopy. *N Engl J Med* 1990; 322:223-8.

[21] Montague CT, O'Rahilly S. The perils of portliness: causes and consequences of visceral adiposity. *Diabetes* 2000; 49:883-8.

[22] McGarry JD. Banting lecture 2001: dysregulation of fatty acid metabolism in the etiology of type 2 diabetes. *Diabetes* 2002; 51:7-18.

[23] Krssak M, Falk Petersen K, Dresner A, et al. Intramyocellular lipid concentrations are correlated with insulin sensitivity in humans: a 1H NMR spectroscopy study. *Diabetologia* 1999; 42:113-6.

[24] Kelley DE, Williams KV, Price JC, McKolanis TM, Goodpaster BH, Thaete FL. Plasma fatty acids, adiposity, and variance of skeletal muscle insulin resistance in type 2 diabetes mellitus. *J Clin Endocrinol Metab* 2001; 86:5412-9.

[25] Kelley DE, Goodpaster BH, Storlien L. Muscle triglyceride and insulin resistance. *Annu Rev Nutr* 2002; 22:325-46.

[26] Itani SI, Ruderman NB, Schmieder F, Boden G. Lipid-induced insulin resistance in human muscle is associated with changes in diacylglycerol, protein kinase C, and IkappaB-alpha. *Diabetes* 2002; 51:2005-11.

[27] Dresner A, Laurent D, Marcucci M, et al. Effects of free fatty acids on glucose transport and IRS-1-associated phosphatidylinositol 3-kinase activity. *J Clin Invest* 1999; 103:253-9.

[28] Griffin ME, Marcucci MJ, Cline GW, et al. Free fatty acid-induced insulin resistance is associated with activation of protein kinase C theta and alterations in the insulin signaling cascade. *Diabetes* 1999; 48:1270-4.

[29] Yu C, Chen Y, Cline GW, et al. Mechanism by which fatty acids inhibit insulin activation of insulin receptor substrate-1 (IRS-1)-associated phosphatidylinositol 3-kinase activity in muscle. *J Biol Chem* 2002; 277:50230-6.

[30] Greco AV, Mingrone G, Giancaterini A, et al. Insulin resistance in morbid obesity: reversal with intramyocellular fat depletion. *Diabetes* 2002; 51:144-51.

[31] Petersen KF, Oral EA, Dufour S, et al. Leptin reverses insulin resistance and hepatic steatosis in patients with severe lipodystrophy. *J Clin Invest* 2002; 109:1345-50.

[32] Kim JK, Gavrilova O, Chen Y, Reitman ML, Shulman GI. Mechanism of insulin resistance in A-ZIP/F-1 fatless mice. *J Biol Chem* 2000; 275:8456-60.

[33] Miyazaki Y, Mahankali A, Matsuda M, et al. Effect of pioglitazone on abdominal fat distribution and insulin sensitivity in type 2 diabetic patients. *J Clin Endocrinol Metab* 2002; 87:2784-91.

[34] Shadid S, Jensen MD. Effects of pioglitazone versus diet and exercise on metabolic health and fat distribution in upper body obesity. *Diabetes Care* 2003; 26:3148-52.

[35] Neuschwander-Tetri BA, Brunt EM, Wehmeier KR, Sponseller CA, Hampton K, Bacon BR. Interim results of a pilot study demonstrating the early effects of the PPAR-gamma ligand rosiglitazone on insulin sensitivity, aminotransferases, hepatic steatosis and body weight in patients with non-alcoholic steatohepatitis. *J Hepatol* 2003; 38:434-40.

[36] Arslanian SA, Lewy VD, Danadian K. Glucose intolerance in obese adolescents with polycystic ovary syndrome: roles of insulin resistance and beta-cell dysfunction and risk of cardiovascular disease. *J Clin Endocrinol Metab* 2001; 86:66-71.

[37] Saltiel AR. You are what you secrete. *Nat Med* 2001; 7:887-8.

[38] Zhang Y, Proenca R, Maffei M, Barone M, Leopold L, Friedman JM. Positional cloning of the mouse obese gene and its human homologue. *Nature* 1994; 372:425-32.

[39] Hotamisligil GS. The role of TNFalpha and TNF receptors in obesity and insulin resistance. *J Intern Med* 1999; 245:621-5.

[40] Arita Y, Kihara S, Ouchi N, et al. Paradoxical decrease of an adipose-specific protein, adiponectin, in obesity. *Biochem Biophys Res Commun* 1999; 257:79-83.

[41] Hotta K, Funahashi T, Bodkin NL, et al. Circulating concentrations of the adipocyte protein adiponectin are decreased in parallel with reduced insulin sensitivity during the progression to type 2 diabetes in rhesus monkeys. *Diabetes* 2001; 50:1126-33.

[42] Hu E, Liang P, Spiegelman BM. AdipoQ is a novel adipose-specific gene dysregulated in obesity. *J Biol Chem* 1996; 271:10697-703.

[43] Weyer C, Funahashi T, Tanaka S, et al. Hypoadiponectinemia in obesity and type 2 diabetes: close association with insulin resistance and hyperinsulinemia. *J Clin Endocrinol Metab* 2001; 86:1930-5.

[44] Comuzzie AG, Funahashi T, Sonnenberg G, et al. The genetic basis of plasma variation in adiponectin, a global endophenotype for obesity and the metabolic syndrome. *J Clin Endocrinol Metab* 2001; 86:4321-5.

[45] Yamauchi T, Kamon J, Waki H, et al. The fat-derived hormone adiponectin reverses insulin resistance associated with both lipoatrophy and obesity. *Nat Med* 2001; 7:941-6.

[46] Fruebis J, Tsao TS, Javorschi S, et al. Proteolytic cleavage product of 30-kDa adipocyte complement-related protein increases fatty acid oxidation in muscle and causes weight loss in mice. *Proc Natl Acad Sci U S A* 2001; 98:2005-10.

[47] Matsuda M, DeFronzo RA. Insulin sensitivity indices obtained from oral glucose tolerance testing: comparison with the euglycemic insulin clamp. *Diabetes Care* 1999; 22:1462-70.

[48] Yeckel C, Weiss R, Dziura J, et al. Validation of insulin sensitivity indices from oral glucose tolerance test parameters in obese children and adolescents. *J Clin Endocrinol Metab* 2004; 89(3): 1096-101.

In: Insulin Resistance in Children and Adolescents ISBN 1-59454-215-5
Editors: D. Daneman and J. Hamilton, pp. 121-161 

*Chapter 6*

# TYPE 2 DIABETES IN CHILDREN AND ADOLESCENTS

***Susan A. Phillips, Asheesh K. Dewan and Kenneth Lee Jones***
Department of Pediatrics, University of California, San Diego

## INTRODUCTION

Type 2 diabetes mellitus (T2DM) is the disease most commonly associated with insulin resistance and most clearly resulting from it.

In this chapter we address the epidemiology of T2DM in childhood, briefly mention issues of pathophysiology, and review cellular mechanisms of insulin resistance and diabetes development.

We then address diagnosis of T2DM and it's differentiation from other forms of diabetes in children including mixed or "hybrid" forms of diabetes. "Hybrid" diabetes can be described as features of more than one recognized type of diabetes present simultaneously in the same individual.

Finally, we review approaches to therapy of T2DM and its comorbid conditions, and briefly address the prevention of T2DM in the young.

## EPIDEMIOLOGY OF T2DM

Although it appears that type 2 diabetes has been "discovered" in children only over the last two decades, documentation of its presence is not new. In 1968, Paulson et al studied a group of 66 obese children utilizing measurement of plasma insulin and oral glucose tolerance (OGTT). [1] When the data on these children are re-analyzed using current classification criteria, [2] 5 had diabetes and 7 impaired glucose tolerance (IGT). In this early publication, the importance of a family history of diabetes in diagnosis of T2DM in the young was first established. Four of the five individuals with diabetes had diabetes in their families. When the mean values of glucose and insulin following OGTT were plotted, based on positive or negative family history, the controls showed the lowest blood glucose, next were the obese children without family history of T2DM, and highest were those with positive family histories. Analysis of plasma insulin showed a similar pattern, with the lowest insulin responses in the controls and the highest in those obese subjects belonging to families with individuals with T2DM.

This report by Paulson et al. was either overlooked or discounted, and T2DM in children received little attention in the "Western" world again until the last decade of the last century. Although there had been reports of T2DM in children from the Pima Indian study in Arizona [3] and from "North American" Indians or Indigenous People in Canada, [4] it was not until a series of case reports from large cities in the United States began to appear, that T2DM in children received appropriate attention

Most of the epidemiologic and case report information, available from North America before and through the 1990's, was reviewed by Fagot-Campana et al. [5] In the Pima Indian population, aged 15-19 years, the prevalence of T2DM was 50.9 per 1,000. This compared to 4.5/1,000 for all American Indians and 2.3/1,000 for the Ojibwa-Cree, in Canada. These numbers were much higher than the incidence $7.2/10^5$ found in 1994 in a mixed race American urban population and reported from the Cincinnati Children's Hospital. The trend seen in Cincinnati, however, seemed ominous, as the incidence had increased from $0.7/10^5$ in 1982 and $1.2/10^5$ in 1992. [6] This paper also reported that, in 1994, 33% of the children aged 10-19 years presenting with new onset diabetes had T2DM. This represented an increase from 3-10% in the period from 1982-92. A similar trend of increased recognition of T2DM was subsequently reported from other pediatric referral centers. [7, 8, 9]

The increasing occurrence of T2DM in children has not been purely a North American problem. In fact, studies from Kitagawa's group in Japan constituted one of the first reports identifying type 2 diabetes in children and found it was more common in their population than type 1. [10] At about the same time the U.S. series were being published, Braun et al, in Australia, reported glucose, insulin, C-peptide, and lipids in a cohort of 100 aboriginal children, studied first in 1989. Seventy four were restudied in 1994. [11] Obesity increased from 2.7% initially to 17.6% on follow-up. By the second examination, 8.1% had impaired glucose tolerance (IGT) and 2.7% diabetes. Wei et al have recently reported a surveillance study of Taiwanese children, in which they found a rate of newly diagnosed diabetes of $9.0/10^5$ in boys and $15.3/10^5$ in girls. [12] When evaluated 3 years after the initial survey, of the 253 children with new onset diabetes, 9.5% had T1DM and 54.2% had T2DM. The estimated rate of T2DM in this population was $6.5/10^5$.

This evidence suggests that T2DM is a significant health problem in children and that, though more prevalent in some populations than in others, it is a problem throughout the world.

## PATHOPHYSIOLOGY

It is helpful to review the pathophysiology of T2DM in the context of insulin resistance. Although etiologic primacy of β-cell failure versus insulin resistance is still debated, [13, 14] many, if not most, investigators believe that the latter is the major causative factor in the evolution of T2DM. Specific evidence for this opinion has been derived from tissue specific knockouts in mice. [15] Insulin resistance, coupled with a relative deficiency of insulin secretion, produces the hyperglycaemia which defines type 2 diabetes. [16] Insulin resistance reduces insulin-mediated glucose disposal in muscle as well as insulin-mediated suppression of hepatic glucose production. These two blocks, one decreasing glucose utilization and the other increasing endogenous glucose production, contribute significantly to hyperglycaemia and comprise the current primary targets of diabetes pharmacotherapy. A third target remains enhancement of insulin secretion with secretagogues.

Normal regulation of plasma glucose depends on food intake and absorption, insulin secretion, insulin-regulated peripheral glucose uptake, and hepatic glucose output (Figure 1a). Figure 1b presents a schematic diagram of the metabolic "lesions" in T2DM. It presents a relatively simple concept of insulin resistance and compromised insulin secretion. Although this is valid, it betrays a concept which used to consider T2DM as a single disease process. Based on our improving understanding of the complexities of glucose transport and of insulin signaling, investigators are now postulating that T2DM may represent the final common pathway for a number of different metabolic defects in these pathways. We cannot clearly separate these at this time, but we will review the insulin signaling pathway, the points which represent or may represent the lesions leading to insulin resistance, and, later, the therapeutic options which may be directed at these lesions.

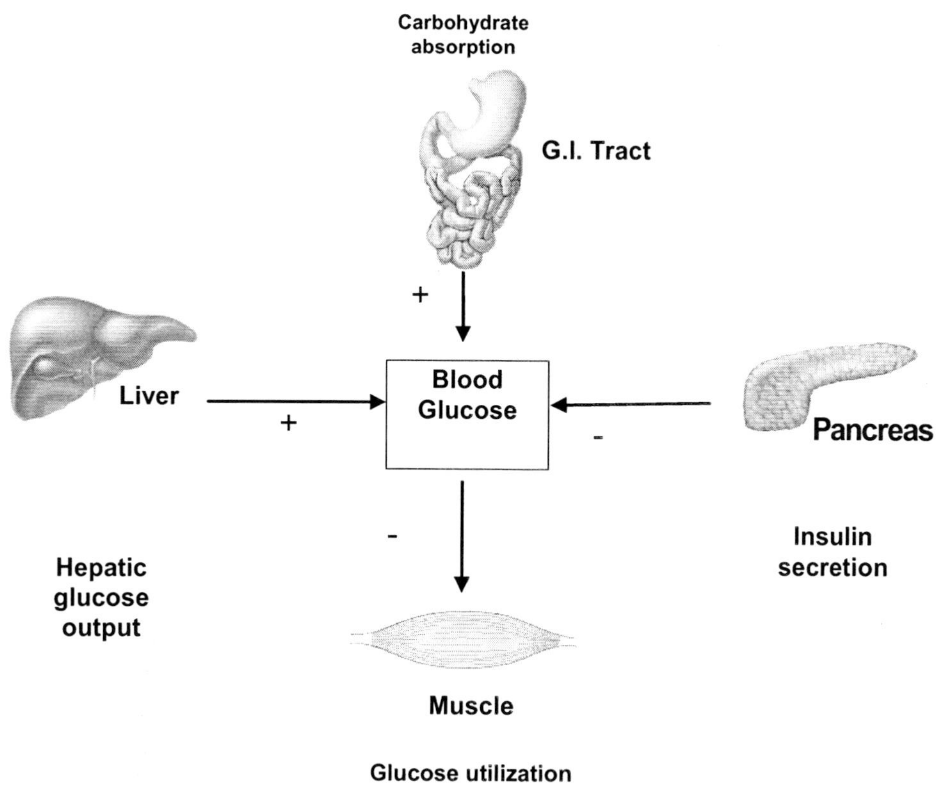


Figure 1a. Normal glucose regulation accomplished through food absorption in the gut, peripheral glucose utilization with normal insulin secretion, and fasting maintenance through hepatic glucose release and production.

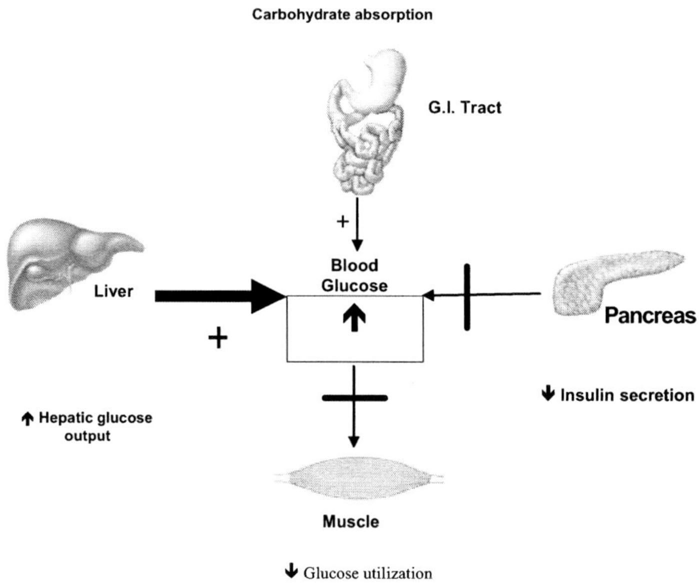


Figure 1b. Pathophysiology of type 2 diabetes. Insulin resistance decreases peripheral glucose utilization by muscle and diminishes inhibition of hepatic glucose output. Normal regulation is further compromised by decreased insulin secretion by the pancreas, resulting in increased blood glucose.

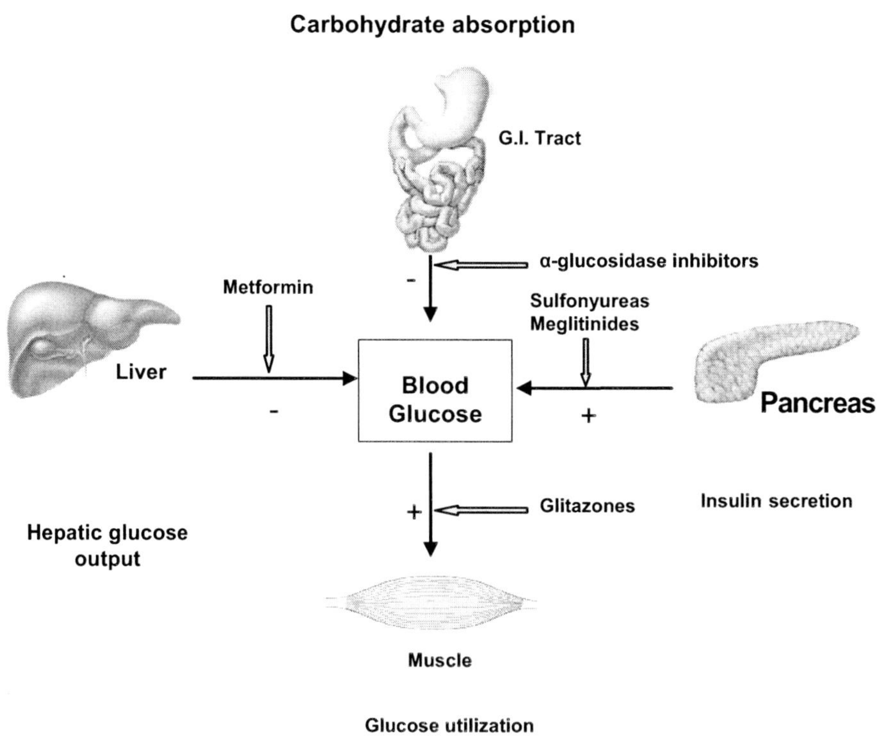


Figure 1c. Sites of action through which oral antidiabetic drugs reduce hyperglycaemia.

## Pathways Signaling Insulin Actions

Insulin signaling begins at the cell membrane upon the interaction of insulin with its receptor. [17] The insulin receptor is a transmembrane glycoprotein belonging to the receptor tyrosine kinase family. [18] Other members of the family include the insulin-like growth factor receptor-1, the epidermal growth factor receptor, and the insulin receptor-related receptor. Structurally the insulin receptor is a heterotetrameric protein consisting of two identical extracellular β-subunits that contain the ligand-binding domain and two membrane-spanning beta subunits that contain the tyrosine kinase domain. Under basal conditions the α-subunits exert tonic inhibition of the receptor's intrinsic kinase activity. Binding of insulin releases this inhibition by causing the α-subunits to move closer together thereby allowing ATP to bind and activate the intracellular kinase. Next, tyrosine residues within the receptor's juxtamembrane and C-terminal domains are phosphorylated by the activated kinase creating high affinity docking sites for insulin receptor substrates to be bound and phosphorylated. [19, 20]

Considerable progress has been made in elucidating post-receptor events that allow for the propagation of the insulin signal to both metabolic (carbohydrate, protein and lipid) and mitogenic pathways. There are essentially three major signal transduction pathways that operate in the key insulin responsive tissues of skeletal muscle, adipose tissue, and liver. The first is the IRS1/2/PI3K pathway, the second is the CAP-cbl/crkIII-C3G/TC10 pathway, and the third is the Shc/Grb2/ras/MAPK pathway. Drugs targeting these pathways represent many current and experimental approaches to the treatment of T2DM.

The IRS1/2/PI3 pathway is the primary pathway for signaling glucose transport, glycogen synthesis, and protein synthesis. The initiation of this pathway is triggered by the binding of activated IR to one of the insulin receptor substrates (IRSs). [21] The IRS family consists of four closely related proteins, IRS1-4 [22, 23, 24, 25] that share a common domain structure. [26] The N-terminal pleckstrin homology (PH) domain of IRS molecules allows for their efficient targeting to the plasma membrane in close proximity to the insulin receptor. [27] The phospho-tyrosine binding (PTB) domain of IRS molecules contains sequences that bind phospho-tyrosine residues of the activated insulin and insulin-like growth factor (IGF) receptors. [28] The C-terminal src homology-2 (SH2) domain of the IRS molecule contains numerous tyrosine residues, which when phosphorylated by the activated IR serve as specific adaptor binding sites. [26] It is the presence, within the PTB and the SH2 domains, of multiple phosphotyrosine residues in specific sequence motifs that allows for the divergence of the insulin signal. Beyond tyrosine phosphorylation, IRS can also be phosphorylated on any one of 35 putative serine and threonine phosphorylation sites, creating additional opportunities for further modulation of the insulin signal. The next step following activation of IRS is the recruitment by IRS of PI-3 kinase to the plasma membrane. [29, 30] PI-3 kinase consists of two subunits, a regulatory domain p85 and a catalytic domain p110. Once bound and activated PI-3 kinase phosphorylates membrane phosphoinositides in the 3-position producing PtdIns (3)P, PtdIns (3,4,)P2 and PtdIns (3,4,5)P3. The activation of the serine/threonine kinase PI-dependent kinase-1 (PDK-1) by PtdIns (3,4,5)P3 represents both a switch in the signaling pathway from tyrosine to serine/threonine kinases and a point of signal divergence. [31]

Substrates of PDK-1 include the atypical forms of protein kinase C (PKC) ζ and λ, [32] Akt (a product of the akt protooncogene), [33, 34] and classic PKC. [35] The atypical PKC's ζ and λ are an important class of substrates for PDK-1. When activated by PDK-1, PKC ζ and λ are associated with the activation and translocation to the plasma membrane of the muscle and fat specific glucose transporter, GLUT4. [36] The atypical PKCs are also another important source of "off signals" in the IR/IRS signaling cascade. Their phosphorylation of IRS-1 on serine residues results in decreased IRS-1/2 affinity for and activation of PI-3 kinase. [37]

Akt is a key substrate of PDK-1. [33] Phosphorylation and activation of Akt by PDK-1 results in two significant insulin-signaling events. [34] First, activated Akt phosphorylates glycogen synthase kinase (GSK) representing a primary pathway for insulin-mediated increases in glycogen synthesis. [38] Second, Akt activation leads to the enhancement of mammalian Target of Rapamycin (mTOR) activity [39] that is primarily responsible for mediating increases in protein synthesis by insulin. [40]

Glycogen is a critical source of stored cellular energy. As such the regulation of its synthesis by glycogen synthase (GS) and degradation by phosphorylase are subject to multiple levels of control. Under basal non-insulin stimulated conditions GSK-3 activity promotes glycogen breakdown through its phosphorylation and inhibition of GS. Under insulin-stimulated conditions glycogen storage is ensured via two mechanisms that increase GS activity. First, as discussed above, insulin signaling through PI-3K leads to the phosphorylation and inactivation of GSK-3, promoting the net dephosphorylation and activation of GS. Second, insulin activates serine/threonine phosphatases, especially protein phosphatase-1 (PP-1) [41] that further promote the dephosphorylation and activation of GS. Moreover, it should be noted that insulin further promotes the storage of glycogen through PP-I mediated dephosphorylation and inactivation of phosphorylase and phosphorylase kinase, enzymes mediating glycogenolysis. [41]

To summarize, phosphorylation cascades initiated at the IR and transduced via the IR/IRS/PI-3K pathway play a primary role in directing insulin mediated increases in glucose transport, glycogen synthesis and protein synthesis. Signaling via this pathway is necessarily transient, and termination signals therefore represent an important source of regulatory control. One source of termination signals is the IR itself. Activation of the signal transduction cascade results in feedback inhibition in the form of serine/threonine phosphorylation of both IR and IRS1/2. Also important in the inhibition of insulin signaling is protein tyrosine phosphatase activity. [42] Membrane associated protein phosphatases can associate with activated IR and dephosphorylate residues within the kinase domain, reducing signal transduction. [43] Likewise cytoplasmic phosphatases, including PTP-1B and SH2-containing protein phosphatase, SH-PTB2, can associate with and dephosphorylate IR and IRS1/2 to decrease signaling. [44]

The CAP-cbl pathway is a second signaling pathway important in directing insulin-stimulated glucose transport. [45] A number of studies have suggested that activation of glucose transport by insulin requires both PI-3 kinase dependent and independent pathways. For example, over-expression of constitutively active PI-3 kinase mutants only partially stimulate GLUT4 translocation, [46] moreover other growth factors that activate PI-3 kinase and its downstream kinases have no effect on glucose transport or GLUT4 translocation. [47] In the CAP-cbl pathway the adaptor protein cbl-associated protein (CAP) recruits the cbl protooncogene product to the IR. Upon tyrosine phosphorylation of cbl by the IR the CAP-cbl complex is released by the IR and moves to caveolin-enriched areas of the plasma membrane called lipid rafts to associate with the caveolar protein flotillin. Phosphorylated cbl then recruits the constitutively associated crkII-C3G complex to the lipid raft. C3G, a guanyl nucleotide-exchange protein then promotes the exchange of GDP for GTP on the G-protein TC10. Activation of TC10 appears to provide the signal for the translocation of GLUT4 and increases in glucose uptake.

The Shc/Grb2/ras/MAPK pathway is the third signaling pathway important in mediating insulin action. Unlike the primarily metabolic effects associated with activity in the IR/IRS/PI-3K and CAP-cbl pathways, activity in the Shc/Grb2/ras/MAPK pathway is associated with mitogenesis. In this pathway the key protein is Shc. Shc is phosphorylated on tyrosine residues by the activated IR allowing it to recruit the adaptor protein Grb-2. Grb-2 exists in constitutive association with the guanine nucleotide exchange factor son-of-sevenless (SOS). When Shc binds the protein complex of Grb-2 and SOS it recruits them to the membrane where SOS in brought into close proximity with the small G-protein *ras*. [48] The activation of *ras* by SOS leads through a series of serine kinases to the phosphorylation/activation of p42/p44 forms of mitogen activated protein kinases (MAPK). Activation of MAPK is associated with regulation of transcription factors and nuclear events and is the major pathway mediating the nuclear effects of insulin on gene expression. [49, 50, 51]

## Alterations of Signaling in Insulin Resistant States

For simplicity, insulin resistance may be considered to develop from one of three mechanisms. First, it may develop from the production and release of abnormal insulin molecules by the β-cell. Second, it may develop in response to a circulating insulin antagonist. And, third it may develop from target tissue defects in insulin signaling. Often, however, insulin resistance results from some combination of the above.

Conditions in which insulin resistance develops from the release of mutant insulin are rare, [52, 53] do not represent a common mechanism for the development of insulin resistance, and will not be discussed further. Circulating insulin antagonists represent a second mechanism for the development of insulin resistance and include a growing number of both hormonal and non-hormonal substances known to antagonize insulin signaling.

Hormonal antagonists include the counterregulatory hormones, namely glucocorticoids, growth hormone, glucagon and catecholamines. Although syndromes associated with excessive hormone production (pheochromocytoma, glucagonoma, acromegaly, and Cushing's disease) commonly result in insulin resistant states, insulin resistance does not generally result from excessive production of the counterregulatory hormones. It is instructive to note that the inappropriate release of glucagon, as seen with β-cell failure in T2DM, can contribute to enhanced hepatic gluconeogenesis and the worsening of hyperglycaemia. Non-hormonal insulin antagonists include free fatty acids, inflammatory cytokines, and antibodies directed against insulin and the insulin receptor. Elevations in free fatty acids (FFAs) represent a significant source of circulating insulin antagonism. Randal and colleagues reported some years ago that FFA's compete with glucose for oxidation in muscle and hypothesized that elevations of FFA's as seen with T2DM could impair glucose uptake. [54]

Indeed, increased FFA levels impair insulin signaling, [55] promote FA oxidation [56] and decrease glucose oxidation in muscle cells, [57] all changes which effectively decrease glucose uptake and decrease insulin responsiveness in muscle. Elevations in FFA also provide increased substrate for hepatic gluconeogenesis and triglyceride synthesis increasing hepatic glucose production and VLDL release. [57, 58] Hyperlipidemia is further aggravated by the inhibition of endothelial lipoprotein lipase by FFAs, decreasing clearance of triglyceride-rich lipoproteins. Lastly, elevations in FFAs are toxic to the pancreatic β-cells leading to their dysfunction and ultimate failure. [59]

Circulating cytokines including tumor necrosis factor α (TNFα), Interleukin-6 (IL-6) and resistin are another source of non-hormonal insulin antagonism. TNFα is one of many inflammatory cytokines released by skeletal muscle and adipose tissue that affects peripheral insulin sensitivity. [60] TNFα is increased in both human [61] and rodent obesity. [62] Chronic exposure of cultured cells to TNFα induces insulin resistance [63] and the infusion of soluble TNFα or neutralizing antibody ameliorates insulin resistance at least in rodents. [64] Mechanistically TNFα appears to work as an autocrine/paracrine factor. In adipose tissue, it stimulates lipolysis and enhances FFA release. In skeletal muscle TNFα exerts *direct* effects to down regulate GLUT4 [65] and in adipose tissue and skeletal muscle TNFα inhibits insulin signaling via increased serine phosphorylation of IRS-1. [66] TNFα also increases the release of cytokines such as IL-6 that aggravate peripheral insulin sensitivity while it decreases the release of cytokines, such as adiponectin that enhance sensitivity. Interleukin-6 (IL-6), a cytokine produced by both adipose tissue and contracting skeletal muscle, exerts a number of metabolic effects. [67] In human subjects receiving injections of rhIL-6, hepatic glycogen synthase activity is reduced, glycogen phosphorylase activity is enhanced [68] and hepatic glucose production is increased, resulting in elevations of fasting blood glucose concentrations. [69] IL-6 is also strongly lipolytic and increases arterial FFA concentrations. Although not an insulin antagonist, adiponectin, a cytokine released by adipose tissue, has emerged as an important circulating modulator of insulin sensitivity. [70] Concentrations of plasma adiponectin have been shown to correlate negatively with glucose, insulin, triglyceride levels and body mass index, and positively with insulin-stimulated glucose disposal. [71] Infusion of the full-length recombinant adiponectin decreases hepatic glucose production and improves insulin sensitivity in rodents. [72] Administration of the globular domain of adiponectin to rodents is associated with increased fatty acid oxidation and decreased FFAs and plasma glucose concentration. [73]

The third mechanism by which alterations of insulin signaling may develop is by means of target-tissue specific defects. These defects may take the form of genetic mutations, alterations in protein expression, or post-translational modifications. Genetic mutations of the IR or proteins associated with its signal transduction pathway are rare but may contribute to insulin resistance in a subset of subjects with T2DM. Defects in the IR can decrease receptor number and/or activity. [74] In rodents, targeted mutagenesis of the IR and of IRS1/2 is associated with the development of insulin resistance. [75] A number of polymorphisms have been described in the human IRS-1 gene [76] including some that are associated with decreased phosphorylation of IRS-1 and its subsequent activation of PI-3 kinase. [77] Polymorphisms affecting insulin sensitivity have also been reported in the p110 catalytic subunit of PI-3 kinase. In a population of Pima Indians, expression of a Met to Ile substitution at amino acid position 326 of p110 correlates with glucose intolerance. The occurrence of a mutation or a decrease in protein expression however, does not always predict the development of insulin resistance, for example, targeted disruption of the p85 regulatory subunit of PI 3-kinase results in increased insulin sensitivity. [78]

In studies preformed on skeletal muscle and adipose tissues obtained from subjects with T2DM post-translational modifications and abnormalities of protein expression in insulin signaling molecules have been described. IR number and insulin binding are commonly reduced. [79] Intrinsic and extrinsic receptor kinase activities in subjects with T2DM are also reduced resulting in impaired IR autophosphorylation [80, 81] as well impairment in the phosphorylation of IRS-1. [82, 83] Whether changes occur in IRS-1protein expression is less certain. In adipose tissue normal [84] and reduced levels of IRS-1 have been reported in diabetic subjects, [85] whereas no change in IRS-1 expression has been reported in skeletal muscle. [86] Post-translational modifications appear to play an important role in the regulation of PI-3 kinase activity. Reductions in activity of up to 50% have been reported in skeletal muscle, 83, 86, 87, 88] and adipose tissue [82] obtained from subjects with T2DM.

Downstream of PI-3 kinase is PDK-1, the serine-threonine kinase that phosphorylates and activates other important kinases such as Akt, and atypical PKCs (ζ and λ). PDK-1 activity and expression appears to be normal in diabetics. [89] The expression of Akt and its activation by PDK-1 has been measured in both human adipose and skeletal muscle tissues. In adipocytes Akt phosphorylation and activation is decreased. [90] In diabetic skeletal muscle the results have been mixed. Whereas Akt activity is reduced in diabetic muscle cultured under hyperinsulinemic conditions, [87] it is normal when cultured under physiologic conditions, despite decreased activation of IRS-1/2 and PI-3 kinase and reductions in glucose uptake and glycogen synthesis. [83] These studies suggest that important tissue specific differences exist in Akt activation and in signaling in insulin resistant states.

An important target of Akt is GSK-3, a kinase whose activity inhibits glycogen synthase (GS). In this complicated signaling cascade, insulin stimulated Akt activity results in the phosphorylation and inhibition of GSK-3. Inhibition of GSK-3 then reduces the phosphorylation and therefore increases the activation of glycogen synthase. In T2DM, GSK-3 expression and activation are increased, [91] GS activity is decreased, [92] and glycogen synthesis is impaired. Although insulin mediated activation of Akt appears to be normal in diabetic muscle (see above) it appears to be insufficient to overcome the increased expression of GSK-3 and subsequent inhibition of GS. [91]

Other targets of PDK-1 signaling are the atypical PKCs ζ and λ. Their activation is required for maximal insulin mediated glucose uptake. In skeletal muscle biopsy tissue from obese insulin resistant and diabetic subjects, expression and activation of PKCs -ζ and -λ is impaired. [93] Studies of PKC-ζ and -λ activity in human fat have not been reported.

Finally, it should be noted that tissue specific defects in GLUT4 protein content and mRNA expression have been reported in subjects with T2DM. In skeletal muscle, GLUT4 content is essentially unchanged. [94] In adipose tissue, however, GLUT4 content is reduced by 40-50%. [95] The translocation of GLUT4 to the cell surface in response to insulin also appears to be impaired in both adipose tissue and muscle of individuals with T2DM. These tissue specific differences in GLUT4 protein content are consistent with human tissue culture data showing impairments in insulin-stimulated glucose uptake in skeletal muscle, but not adipocytes are rapidly reversible following pre-incubation of tissue in media containing physiologic levels of glucose. [96]

## DIAGNOSIS AND DIFFERENTIAL DIAGNOSIS

Diagnosis of T2DM in children has evolved from a condition which was infrequent, and probably under-diagnosed, to one which is now much more prevalent and may in fact be over-diagnosed. With the epidemic of obesity affecting children throughout the world, there is a tendency to diagnose T2DM in any hyperglycemic young person who is overweight, especially if the disease affects others in their family.

The criteria for the diagnosis of diabetes are well established by the American Diabetes Association (Table 1). [2] These are based on the presence of symptoms associated with hyperglycaemia or on certain blood glucose levels obtained fasting or during an oral glucose tolerance test. These criteria were developed primarily for adults, who frequently have diabetes without persistent or symptomatic hyperglycaemia and/or acute metabolic decompensation.

**Table 1. ADA Criteria for the Diagnosis of Diabetes Mellitus**

One of Three Criteria must be Met for Diagnosis

1. Symptoms of diabetes, especially polyuria, polydipsia, and unexplained weight loss, plus random plasma glucose concentration $\geq$200 mg.dl (11.1mmol/l).
2. Fasting ($\geq$8 hours) plasma glucose $\geq$126 mg/dl (7.0 mmol/l).
3. 2 hour plasma glucose $\geq$200 mg/dl (11.1 mmol/l) during an oral glucose tolerance test.

In asymptomatic individuals, abnormal tests should be confirmed by a second test on a separate day.

The statement of the American Diabetes Association's consensus panel, convened to examine the issue of type 2 diabetes in children, mentioned clinical features which could be used to determine who should be tested for T2DM. These included obesity, a family history of T2DM, a race/ethnicity at increased risk, and signs of insulin resistance. [97] The epidemiologic data certainly substantiate that most children reported with type 2 are obese, are more likely to be of the non-Caucasian racial/ethnic groups, will most likely be adolescent rather than younger, and will probably be part of a family affected by T2DM. Also, children with T2DM present less frequently with acute decompensation and DKA than those with T1DM.

The difficulty with utilization of these guidelines is that there is disagreement about the requirements for confirming the diagnosis of T2DM in the young. With no specific test to identify T2DM, it remains a clinical diagnosis and one of exclusion. The clinical features which we use to attempt differentiation of T1DM from T2DM in our initial evaluation are listed in Table 2. In adults, especially those who are older, there are few conditions which produce diabetes which cannot be easily established as resulting from drugs, endocrinopathies, pancreatic disease, or other known causes. In younger individuals, T1DM, MODY states, or atypical diabetes (ADA type 1b) are more difficult to exclude.

**Table 2. Useful Clinical Features in the Initial Differentiation of Type 1 from Type 2 Diabetes in Children**

| T1DM | T2DM |
|---|---|
| Younger age | Usually pubertal |
| Short duration of symptoms | Longer duration and more subtle symptoms |
| Ketoacidosis common | Infrequent and/or mild ketoacidosis with more frequent hyperosmolar component |
| More frequently Caucasian | More frequently of African, Mexican or Native American, or Asian ancestry |
| Infrequent family history of T1DM | T2DM frequent in the family and in parents |
| Lean | Obese |
| May have other autoimmune disorders | Acanthosis nigricans usually present |
| | PCOS and ovarian hyperandrogenemia |

T2DM is essentially a diagnosis of exclusion, but the clinician can also be guided by therapeutic response. We separate those children fitting clearly into type 1 or 2. Those whose diagnosis is less clear, based on the presence of obesity or features of the metabolic syndrome, or who are diagnosed following mild symptoms, by random testing, or via another path which recognizes glucosuria and/or hyperglycaemia, are more intensively investigated with antibody testing, C-peptide measurement, or, if family or clinical history is suspicious, for mitochondrial or MODY mutations. We have chosen to arbitrarily classify individuals with positive immune markers as having immune-mediated T1DM. This practice can certainly be questioned, as some "normal" individuals and adults classified as type 2, have immune markers, especially directed against glutamic acid decarboxylase (anti-GAD). [98]

## TREATMENT

Defining a regimen for the treatment of type 2 diabetes in children is difficult, as there are few studies and little published experience on which to base recommendations. Treatment is further complicated by the fact that it falls to pediatricians, whose diabetes education and experience is based primarily on algorithms addressing insulinopenic states. The concept of insulin resistance as a cause of diabetes and the use of oral agents in therapy are unfamiliar. Treatment of T2DM in children is made even more complex because it is linked to several comorbid conditions, including a significant long term risk of serious coronary, cerebral, and peripheral vascular complications, which, in adults, require therapeutic interventions beyond glycemic management. The importance of, and consequences of treating these conditions in the young, is not yet established.

Due to the paucity of data in children, almost all of the information available about therapy comes from studies performed in adults. In addition to the obvious difficulty with extrapolating information from a very old population to a much younger one, there are other concerns about use, over decades, of drugs which have not been employed for such prolonged periods. The involvement of this much younger population also elevates, in importance, the need to address prevention rather than treatment alone.

The treatment of children and adolescents with T2DM offers an opportunity to investigate aspects of diabetes complications and of the chronology of their development which have been difficult to study in adults. A partial list, not necessarily in order of importance, includes: prevention of macrovascular complications, the development of dyslipidemia, preservation of islet cell function, reduction of insulin resistance, and, of course, diabetes prevention. In the older, adult population, it is estimated that about 50% of individuals with T2DM are undiagnosed, implying that many of those diagnosed have had diabetes for significant periods of time before disease discovery. [99] There is also evidence that the risk factors for associated comorbidities have been present for years before diagnosis of diabetes. As a result, in adults, any study begins with population of uncertain duration of disease, complicating the assessment of therapeutic intervention. In the young, we would anticipate that many of these processes, considered to be long term complications of diabetes, will be either non-existent or very early in their development, providing an opportunity to study their progression or their arrest by therapeutic intervention.

## Treatment of Hyperglycaemia

The therapeutic goal, regardless of diabetes type, is to maintain blood glucose concentrations as close to normal as can be done safely, without frequent and/or significant hypoglycaemia. Achieving this goal is important to delay or prevent the chronic complications of diabetes, especially microvascular complications such as retinopathy and nephropathy. [100] Also important is the correction of symptoms of hyperglycaemia, maintenance of normal nutrition and growth, and avoidance of the acute complications of ketoacidosis and/or hyperosmolar crisis.

## Lifestyle Change

Lifestyle changes have been the traditional first stage approach to therapy of T2DM in adults and are an important adjunct to any therapeutic regimen. [101, 102] These changes in lifestyle primarily involve diet/nutrition and exercise. Though this approach may initially be successful in controlling hyperglycaemia, in adult studies there is a very high rate of recidivism to old habits and weight gain, resulting in the need to add other forms of therapy to control hyperglycaemia. One of the most encouraging pieces of information about the benefit of lifestyle change in improving glucose tolerance and arresting progression to diabetes has been the publication of the findings of the Diabetes Prevention Program Research Group, discussed later. [103]

In a clinical trial evaluating metformin versus placebo in children with T2DM, described in detail later, all subjects were provided instruction in nutrition and regular exercise, but only 7.5% of those in the placebo group maintained a degree of glycemic control for the 16 week trial period which did not dictate rescue with other therapeutic intervention. [104] Beyond this study, there is little data about the success or failure of change in lifestyle in children, and most of it is anecdotal. Lifestyle therapy is successful almost exclusively in those patients who are so developmentally impaired that parents or caregivers can carefully control their diet and encourage or enforce regular exercise programs. Success can also be attained when patients are in care facilities such as group homes, in which the staff also have the ability to enforce diet and activity regimens. [105, 106] In more usual circumstances of a primarily adolescent population with an average amount of parental supervision, this form of treatment has limited effectiveness.

## Nutrition

Nutritional consultation with a dietitian familiar with both childhood nutrition *and* with T2DM is important for all patients. In addition to assessing the nutritional status and practices of the child and family, the dietitian should provide guidance and a meal plan which, at least initially, does not deviate in a major way from their usual eating practices. Additional change can be made in later appointments and contacts. General principles recommended for adults, as outlined by the ADA, can be utilized in adolescents. [107]

The dietitian providing education must be knowledgeable about the differences in counseling for type 1 and type 2 diabetes. Since obesity is a finding in most type 2 patients and since caloric restriction can result in improved glycemic control and increased insulin sensitivity, modest caloric restriction and weight loss, or maintenance in growing children, are important goals. Between meal snacks, often important in conjunction with insulin therapy in T1DM, are rarely indicated with T2DM and are to be discouraged. Correction of the dyslipidemia, which frequently accompanies T2DM, is also very important. Recommendations are that dietary fat intake be reduced to <30% of total calories, limiting saturated fat to <10%. If hyper-cholesterolemia is present, an effort should be made to limit cholesterol in the diet to <200 mg/day. Increasing monounsaturated fats to 15-20% of total calories may have beneficial effects on triglycerides and HDL. Protein should account for 15-20% of total calories, but may need to be adjusted for growth requirements. The remainder of daily calories is supplied as carbohydrate.

## Exercise

The general benefits of exercise are improved insulin sensitivity, loss or maintenance of weight, beneficial effects on blood pressure and serum lipids, and improved glycemic control. As in adults, the key to successful implementation is finding a form of exercise which the child enjoys and will do. In this age group, there is the potential for incorporation of school physical education and other supervised athletic programs. We have worked with schools to persuade patients to participate more actively in scheduled physical education programs. We have also encouraged many of our patients to increase physical activity at home or with parents, taking family walks and spending active time in parks.

## Pharmacotherapy

The philosophy underlying the use of oral antidiabetic drugs in the treatment of T2DM has been based on our improved understanding of its pathophysiology. Pharmacotherapy attacks, singly or in combination, the "blocks" of normal glucose metabolism (Figure 1c), which characterize T2DM or slow other aspects of blood glucose "peaking." Developing successful therapeutic strategies for the treatment of T2DM requires a dynamic approach.

***Insulin Signaling as a Target for Therapeutic Intervention***

Research to develop new drugs targets both the traditional clinical endpoint of diabetes-hyperglycaemia (new sulfonylurea or nonsulphonylurea derivatives, glucagon-like peptide-1 and amylin), as well as insulin action (thiazolidinediones, lipid lowering agents, glucagon antagonists).

Sulfonylureas are insulin secretagogues that exert potent hypoglycemic effects via their stimulation of the pancreatic β-cell. First-generation (tolbutamide, chlorpropamide, tolazamide, and acetohexamide) and second-generation sulfonylurea compounds (glyburide, glibenclamide, glipizide, gliclazide, and glimepiride) bind to receptors (SUR) on the β-cell membrane. The SUR together with the inward rectifier channel protein (KIR6.2) comprise the β-cell K+ATP channel. The binding of sulfonylureas leads to a series of cellular events: the closure of the K+ channel, depolarization of the cell, opening of voltage-dependent Ca+ channels that result in the exocytosis of insulin-containing secretory granules. Although most agree that the primary effect of sulfonylurea agents relates reductions in hyperglycaemia and a lowering of glucose toxicity, [108] secondary or extrapancreatic insulin sensitizing effects of the sulfonylureas have been reported in both skeletal muscle and adipose tissue [109] The development of new insulin secretagogues includes both sulfonylureas and non-sulfonylureas (meglitnides and succinate ester derivatives). The meglitnides, repaglinide and nateglinide work by binding to the ATP-sensitive K+ channel at a site distinct to that of the sulfonylureas. The effectiveness of the newer insulin secretagoges relates to improvements in both their potency and time course of action. [110] Succinate ester derivatives also represent a potential novel approach to improving beta-cell function through enhancement of insulin biosynthesis and secretion. [111]

The biguanides, phenformin and metformin, were first introduced for the treatment of T2DM in the 1950's [112] and metformin was approved for use in the United States in 1995. Although both agents are associated with an increased incidence of lactic acidosis the risk is considerably lower with metformin because, it unlike phenformin does not undergo liver metabolism. [113] Metformin decreases hepatic glucose production and improves peripheral insulin sensitivity. [124] Recently published studies have shown that AMP dependent protein kinase (AMPK) activation is required for both metformin's inhibitory effect on glucose production by hepatocytes [114] and its observed lowering of serum lipids. [115, 116] Metformin's beneficial effects on circulating lipids have also been linked to AMPK activation in hepatocytes via its suppression of SREBP-1, a key transcription factor for lipogenic enzymes. [112] The varied beneficial effects of AMPK activation suggest that the development of other drugs capable of modulating AMPK activity could prove useful for the treatment of metabolic disorders.

The alpha-glucosidase inhibitors, acarbose and miglitol were first introduced into the US market in the mid-1990s. These agents are potent inhibitors of α-glucosidase enzymes (glycoamylase, sucrase, maltase and dextranase) located in the brush border of the proximal small intestine. [117] Clinically their use results in the delayed digestion and absorption of carbohydrates by the small intestine and a delayed and prolonged postprandial rise in plasma glucose. [118]

Newly available thearapeutics targeting hyperglycaemia include agents such as glucagon-like-peptide (GLP-1) and amylin (pramlintide) agonists. GLP-1 is a gastrointestinal incretin that acts to promote glucose-dependent insulin release, slow gastric emptying, reduce inappropriately elevated glucagon levels and decrease fasting and post-prandial glucose concentrations. Given its extremely short half-life and need for parenteral administration, the development of agonists and drugs that elevate its levels are being pursued by several pharmaceutical companies. [119, 120] Exendin-4, a GLP-1 agonist with a prolonged half-life has been successfully tested in human subjects. These studies have shown it to augment insulin secretion, reduce fasting and post-prandial glycaemia, suppress inappropriate glucagon release and delay gastric emptying. [121] Development of DDP-IV, an inhibitior of the enzyme that degrades GLP-1, has been similarily successful when used in the treatment of T2DM. [122] Pramlintide, a synthetic agonist of the β-cell hormone amylin, has also been successfully employed in T2DM. Its use is associated not only with reductions in fasting and post-prandial glucose excursions and also with weight loss. [123, 124]

Troglitazone, pioglitazone and rosiglitazone are members of the insulin sensitizing family of PPAR-γ agonists, the thiazolidinediones (TZDs). These agents exert a multitude of effects that improve insulin sensitivity. [125] Although troglitazone was removed from the market due to safety concerns related to hepatotoxicity, pioglitazone and rosiglitazone remain safe and approved for use in T2DM. The TZDs are synthetic ligands for the PPAR-γ nuclear receptor, and exert their insulin sensitizing effects relative to their potency for this receptor in adipose tissue, skeletal muscle and liver.

In adipose tissue TZDs improve insulin sensitivity via a variety of mechanisms [126] Glucose transporter expression is enhanced [127], adipocyte differentiation is stimulated, [126] and release of the insulin sensitizing cytokine adiponectin is increased [128] The apparently paradoxical effects of TZDs to increase both insulin sensitivity and adiposity can be explained by the fact that TZDs increase fat mass by increasing the number of smaller more insulin sensitive fat cells. [128, 129] In addition, TZDs appear to shift fat distribution from visceral to subcutaneous depots where adipocytes are more sensitive to the antilipolytic effects of insulin. [130] In skeletal muscle and liver, TZDs exert direct [131] and indirect effects via reductions in plasma free fatty acid levels improving muscle glucose metabolism and inhibiting hepatic glucose production. [126] In cultured human skeletal muscle TZDs have been shown to upregulate the PPARγ receptor and increase glucose uptake and glycogen synthase activity. [132, 133] The TZDs also exert potent antiatherosclerotic activity, affecting endothelial function, atherogenesis, and fibrinolysis, ensuring a key role for their use in treatment of diabetic dyslipidemia. [134]

The development of novel therapeutics for the treatment of T2DM is ongoing and includes many agents capable of mimicking or potentiating the insulin signaling pathway. An orally active fungal derivative that mimics insulin action by causing phosphorylation of the IR tyrosine kinase has been shown to have anti-diabetic activity in mice. [135] Another orally active peptide under study enhances insulin stimulation IR tyrosine kinase activation and improves glucose tolerance in diabetic mice. [136, 137] Other agents under development include inhibitors of protein tyrosine phosphatase-1B (PTP-1B). PTP-1B binds and dephosphorylates both IR and IRS-1 reducing the activation of PI 3-kinase activity and mice lacking its activity have increased insulin sensitivity. [138] Lastly, GSK-3 inhibitors are emerging as promising new drugs in the treatment of T2DM. Treatment of Zucker Diabetic

Fatty (fa/fa) rats with oral GSK-3 inhibitors results in increased liver glycogen synthesis and significant improvements in oral glucose disposal. [139] In human skeletal muscle cell-permeable GSK-3 inhibitors improve insulin action and glucose metabolism via increased glucose uptake, IRS-1 protein expression and GS activity. [140] It is also of interest to note that GSK-3 is required for the nuclear functioning of NF-κB. NF-κB is key mediator of TNFα and IL-6 inflammatory cytokine signaling and its attenuation by GSK-3 inhibitors represents another mechanism by which improvements in insulin sensitivity can be achieved. [141]

# Specific Drug Use

## Insulin Secretagogues

***Sulphonylureas***

Insulin secretion is compromised in individuals with T2M, and although hyperinsulinemia is present early in the course of the disease, it is insufficient to maintain euglycaemia. Until β-cell exhaustion occurs in later stages, agents which stimulate insulin secretion can be successful in reducing blood glucose concentrations.

Sulfonylureas (SU) are the secretagogues with which there is the longest and most extensive experience. Studies in children and adolescents are in early or planning stages, but anecdotal experience is being reported. The SU's which are currently available for use are listed in Table 3.

**Table 3. Thiazolidinediones: Reported Actions and Side Effects**

| |
|---|
| **Actions** |
| Increases insulin sensitivity in muscle and liver |
| ↓ Plasma insulin levels in insulin resistance |
| ↑ Insulin-dependent glucose disposal |
| Improves dysfunctional glucose homeostasis |
| ↓ Hyperglycaemia |
| ↓ $HbA_{1c}$ values |
| ↑ HDL cholesterol |
| ↓ Triglycerides |
| **Side Effects** |
| Weight gain |
| ↑ Creatine phosphokinase levels |
| Fluid retention |
| ↑ LDL cholesterol |
| Hepatotoxicity and ↑ Serum Transaminase Levels |

These agents are effective in T2DM, lowering fasting plasma glucose (FPG) up to 70 mg/dl (3.9 mmol/L) and HbA1c by as much as 1.7%. There is, however, a primary failure rate of 20-25% in adult studies, with additional failure rates of 5-10% with each subsequent year of use. [142] The UKPDS found the effectiveness of SU therapy in glycemic control to be comparable to that of metformin. [143] Since it appears that SU failure is the result of β-cell failure, this class of anti-diabetic drugs may prove more effective in younger patients, if they have better reserve islet function. [144] Studies in adults suggest that SU's are most effective in patients who are less obese, have diabetes of shorter duration, and have relatively low insulin requirements.

The major adverse effect of SU therapy is hypoglycaemia. Although this appears to occur less frequently with second generation SU preparations, it is still relatively frequent with glyburide. [145] Glipizide [146] and glimepiride produce hypoglycemic episodes less frequently. [147] Concerns about increased frequency of death from myocardial infarction in SU treated patients have not been substantiated in subsequent studies and is not a concern in young patients. [148] SU use in T2DM has been associated with weight gain, and patients using these agents should be following concurrent diet and exercise programs.

Most SU's should be taken shortly before meals, and initial doses should begin in a low range and be gradually increased until the desired effect on blood glucose is achieved, without inducing hypoglycaemia. These drugs are metabolized primarily in the liver and, with liver dysfunction, inactivation may be slowed, increasing the risk of hypoglycemic events.

***Meglitinides***

Meglitinides, a relatively new class of secretagogues, were designed to produce peak insulin concentrations which coincide with postprandial glucose peaks, mimicking the normal physiologic response and decreasing the risk of hypoglycaemia. Currently available meglitinides include repaglinide and nateglinide. They have a shorter half-life, resulting in a more rapid return to baseline insulin concentration than is seen with sulfonylureas (Table 3). With repaglinide, insulin concentrations return to baseline within 4-6 hours [149] and, following nateglinide, within 2 hours. [150] With this shorter half-life, there is a lower incidence of late postprandial hypoglycaemia [151] than is seen with SU therapy.

As a class, meglitinides decrease fasting glucose levels by about 60 mg/dl (3.3mmol/L) and the HbA1c by 1.7 to 1.9%. [152, 153] In individuals showing a poor response to meglitinide monotherapy, combination with metformin has been proven safe and efficacious. Nateglinide, used in combination with the biguanide, has produced a decrease of 0.4% in individuals who have fairly well controlled diabetes (HbA1c <8%) and of 1.4% in those with higher baseline HbA1c (>9.5%). [154]

One disadvantage of meglitinides is their frequent dosing requirement and the resultant compliance vulnerability, which may be exaggerated in adolescents. Hypoglycaemia occurs especially in those with low HbA1c's, but less frequently than with sulfonylureas.

## Biguanides

The biguanides have one of the longest therapeutic histories of any drug used to treat diabetes. [155] They were withdrawn from use in the U.S. because of the association of phenformin with lactic acidosis. Metformin, infrequently associated with this complication, continued to be used in much of the developed world and was re-approved for use in the U.S. in 1995. A real role of metformin in cases of lactic acidosis reported in patients taking the drug has been questioned. [156] Young patients appear relatively resistant to the development of lactic acidosis, even with the unintentional ingestion of large amounts of metformin. [157]

The complex actions of metformin on glucose and lipid metabolism, although extensively studied, are still incompletely understood. Comprehensive reviews are available. [158, 159] It has been a very effective drug in trials in adults, reducing FPG by as much as 26% and HbA1C by 1.7%. About 5-10% of patients are intolerant of the drug because of gastrointestinal side effects, and its secondary failure rate parallels that described with SU. [160] Metformin has been tested in a clinical trial in children and is now approved by the FDA for use in children with T2DM.

Even before it had been subjected to a formal therapeutic trial in children and adolescents, metformin was the drug recommended by an American Diabetes Association Expert Committee for initial oral therapy of T2DM in children. [161] This recommendation was based on good but uncontrolled results obtained in children with early "off label" use by physicians. A need existed to evaluate this drug in a clinical trial in children to define its safety and efficacy, and a multi-center, randomized, double-blind, placebo-controlled trail was initiated. [104]

In order to randomize the number of patients necessary to power the study, 44 sites were utilized to screen 481 subjects. Nine of the sites were in Eastern Europe. The large rejection percent may have resulted from the requirements for inclusion, especially those which reflected patients' glycemic state at screening. For example, 76% of the referred subjects were excluded because they fell outside the inclusion criteria for fasting plasma glucose of <126 or >240 mg/dl (<7 or >13.3 mmol/L). Of the patients screened, 72% were excluded for HbA1C's <7.0%. Ten percent of those referred were excluded because they were positive for one or more of the immune markers assessed (anti-GAD, anti-ICA-512, insulin autoantibodies).

The demographic data from the enrolled group was very similar to those patients described in earlier reports and summarized by Fagot-Campana et al. [5] Approximately 70% of the patients were female, the mean age was 13-14 years, fewer than 50% were white (37.5-40.5%), and the mean BMI was increased (mean was approximately 34 kg/m$^2$). The racial/ethnic data was skewed from the usual demographics of children with T2DM reported in the U.S. because 20 of the 82 patients were from the European centers with predominantly or exclusively Caucasian populations.

This study was designed to compare patients randomized into a placebo group and a metformin group. All patients received information about therapeutic lifestyle changes, which included advice about dietary modifications and moderate exercise.

At the end of the 16 week, double blind treatment period, the mean fasting plasma glucose (FPG), adjusted for baseline, decreased by 42.9 mg/dl in the metformin treated group while increasing by 21.4 mg/dl in the placebo treated patients. This improvement was confirmed by differences in the HbA1C at the end of the double-blind period. The mean values, adjusted for the baseline mean difference, were 8.6% in the placebo patients and 7.5% in those receiving metformin. Patients receiving metformin also experienced a mean 9.7 mg/dl decrease in serum cholesterol as contrasted with a 0.7 mg/dl increase in the patients receiving placebo. There was also slightly more weight loss and decrease in BMI in the metformin group, but neither reached statistical significance.

The number of patients experiencing at least one adverse event was higher in those receiving metformin (70% vs. 60%), but the length of exposure to metformin was longer than that to placebo. As might have been predicted from experience in adults, the primary adverse events involved the GI tract. Almost twice as many patients receiving metformin reported abdominal pain and nausea and/or vomiting as did those taking placebo.

This study confirmed that metformin was safe and effective for use in glycemic management of children with T2DM. Metformin must now be considered the drug of choice in youth with T2DM.

## α-Glucosidase Inhibitors

One of the more difficult challenges in therapy of T2DM is reduction of post-meal hyperglycaemia. [162] Their use and success in diabetes management have been reviewed. [163] Because acarbose and voglibose are not absorbed, they have few adverse effects, other than occasional abdominal pain, flatulence and diarrhea, which result from the bacterial metabolism of oligosaccharides arriving undigested in the colon. [164] Miglitol is absorbed, but re-concentrated in the small intestine, so the effect is similar.

Studies in adults indicate that acarbose combined with diet can reduce HbA1C by as much as 1.3%. [165] These drugs are not generally used as primary or single drug regimens, but are more frequently employed as adjunctive therapy. [166]

## Thiazolidinediones

Thiazolidinediones (TZDs) reduce the peripheral insulin resistance which is a major pathophysiologic feature of type 2 diabetes. Their pharmacology and metabolic effects have been extensively reviewed, [167, 168] and their major actions are listed in Table 4.

Troglitazone was the first TZD to be employed in large clinical trials in adults with type 2 diabetes. The results were promising when it was used as monotherapy [169] or in combination with sulfonylurea [170] or insulin. [171] Fasting plasma glucose and HbA1C were reduced, as was insulin requirement. There were also potentially beneficial effects on lipid profiles, with increases in HDL cholesterol and decreases in triglycerides and free fatty acids. [172]

Unfortunately, the drug was found to have adverse effects on the liver, noted by increases in alanine transaminase, reversible jaundice and infrequent liver failure, [173] it was removed from use in the U.S. in March of 2000.

**Table 4. Comorbidities of Type 2 Diabetes**

- Obesity
- Hypertension
- Dyslipidemia
- Polycystic ovarian syndrome
- Sleep apnea
- Hepatic steatosis (fatty liver without elevated hepatic transaminases)
- Non-alcoholic steatogenic hepatitis (NASH)

Other TZDs have now been approved by the FDA and are in general use. Trial results with pioglitazone and rosiglitazone in adults have been published, [174, 175] and clinical trials in children are now in progress or being planned. In addition to their effects on blood glucose, rosiglitazone and pioglitazone have other effects which impact on diabetes complications and cardiovascular disease. [176, 177, 178] They have beneficial effects on dyslipidemia and may have other beneficial effects on blood pressure and fibrinolysis.

Rosiglitazone has a relatively short half-life of 4 hours and is excreted primarily in the urine. Rosiglitazone monotherapy has been very effective compared to placebo, reducing the FPG by 58 mg/dl at 4 mg/d and by an average of 76 mg/dl at 8 mg/d over a 26 week trial. At the higher dose, a reduction in HbA1C reduction of 1.5% was achieved over that in patients receiving placebo. [179] Rosiglitazone has been very effective when used in combination with SU and with metformin, reducing FPG and HbA1C in patients who were stable, but not ideally controlled with maximal doses of either drug. [180, 181] It can also be effectively employed in conjunction with insulin therapy, lowering FPG and insulin requirement. [182]

Pioglitazone, although different in some actions and in its metabolic processing, has a similar therapeutic profile to rosiglitazone. Both of these drugs have been reported to have hepatotoxic effects, but they have not been associated with the frequency or severity of adverse effects on liver seen with troglitazone. [183, 184, 185] The idiosyncratic hepatic failure associated with troglitazone was believed to be secondary to an α-tocopheral side-chain, a feature that rosiglitazone and pioglitazone do not exhibit. [184] Edema and small reductions in hemoglobin have also been reported as has weight gain. We do not know whether these effects are age related, or whether they will be present, worse, or less significant in children. A detailed comparison of these agents is beyond the scope of this chapter.

## Combination Therapy

One of the benefits of having drugs available to combat different aspects of the pathophysiology of type 2 diabetes is that they can be combined for an effect which may be additive or greater. For example, insulin secretagogues or insulin can be combined with agents which decrease hepatic glucose output or with those which decrease peripheral insulin resistance. It is also possible to combine agents such as a TZD and metformin, which, respectively, improve peripheral insulin sensitivity and decrease hepatic glucose output. A recent report has utilized metformin in combination with insulin in treating adolescents with T1DM who are also insulin resistant. [186] This combined therapy allowed reduction in insulin dose and lowered HbA1C. Our experience has produced similar effects in obese type 1 patients and has also improved erratic control in patients who were clinically insulin resistant. Combination therapy can also employ α-glucosidase inhibitors with other agents.

In general, a few cautions must be observed. When using insulin or insulin secretagogues, the risk of hypoglycemic events increases with the addition of metformin or TZDs. As a result, the frequency of blood glucose monitoring should be increased following the addition of a new drug, at least until stability is established. This concern is lessened if metformin is combined with a TZD. Excellent reviews are available for using oral agents in combination, [187, 188] or for using oral agents in combination with insulin. [189]

For those patients who fail to achieve optimal glycemic control with lifestyle change or who are initially treated with insulin, our protocol is to move to metformin as the initial monotherapy, as outlined in the algorithm (Figure 2). Our success rate is good with this drug at maximal doses, but the goal of achieving normal HbA1c's may require addition of a second agent. There are general strategies, not universally accepted, for using drug combinations in adults with T2DM. Very obese patients, who have other features suggesting significant insulin resistance, may have TZDs added to their regimens. These agents have an advantage of being associated with less weight gain than insulin or insulin secretagogues. Leaner patients, who may be less insulin resistant, can have sulfonylureas or meglitinides added in combination initially rather than a TZD. There are no guidelines in young patients, but our practice is to initially add SU to metformin. This pattern is partially dictated because there is no safety or efficacy data in children with TZDs or meglitinides. As more information becomes available and new drugs emerge, this pattern of combinations may change.

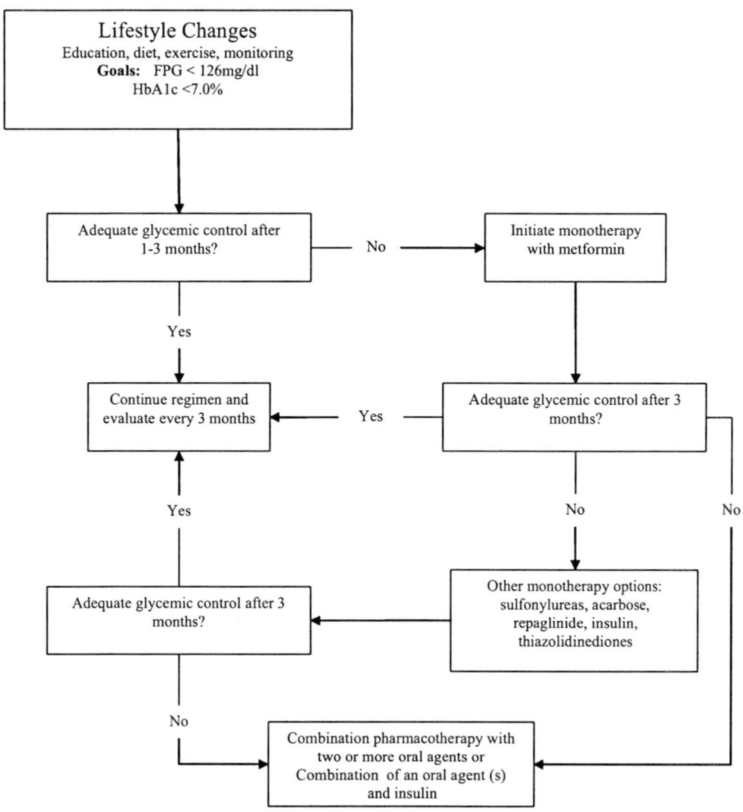


Figure 2. Proposed algorithm for therapy of type 2 diabetes in children and adolescents.

## Treatment of Patients Presenting Acutely Ill or with an Unclear Diagnosis

Presentation with acute clinical decompensation and development of ketoacidosis or a hyperosmolar state is relatively common in youth with T2DM, occurring in 10-15% of newly diagnosed patients. [190] The experience in our clinic population suggests that this presentation is frequently associated with another, concomitant, acute illness, usually infectious and occasionally related to diabetes or its comorbid conditions. Examples, in our experience, include an obese, antibody negative, African American adolescent girl who presented with ketoacidosis and severe hyperthyroidism and a morbidly obese Native American male who developed DKA associated with a severe cellulitis arising in an area of intertriginous skin breakdown. Those patients with severe hyperosmolar states frequently give a history of marked thirst, treated with soda, juice or other drinks with high sugar content.

It is important to remember that children with T2DM, because of their obesity and, usually because of genetic factors, are more insulin resistant than the usual type 1 patient with ketoacidosis. [191] They may require higher doses of insulin, either in concentration in infusions or in the number of units of subcutaneously administered doses.

In our practice, these patients, after they recover from their acute illness, are continued on insulin therapy until the specific diagnosis becomes clear. If their C-peptide returns low and there are positive immune markers, we assign a diagnosis of type 1 and treat accordingly.

As was mentioned, the differentiation between T1DM and T2DM is not always initially clear in children and adolescents, regardless of presentation. In this discussion, these unclear cases will be referred to as "hybrid" cases, but have, in the past, been called "type 1½" (between types 1 and 2), and, on occasion, "type 3," (types 1 + 2). In most of these patients, confusion arises because of clinical and/or laboratory findings which are characteristic of both type 1 and type 2. In our experience, the usual situation is the finding of immune markers in an individual who has many features of the insulin resistant syndrome (syndrome X or the metabolic syndrome [192]). This might occur in an adolescent, with one or more immune markers, who has parents and/or siblings with T2DM, and who is obese, has acanthosis nigricans, and a normal or elevated C-peptide at diagnosis. There are obvious and unanswered questions in such a patient. Is this a child with immune-mediated type 1 diabetes who presented early and atypically because of significant insulin resistance, or does he/she have T2DM, with a positive antibody, that is of little or no significance in β-cell destruction at the time of diagnosis?

With no clear solution to this question, the approach taken in our clinic is to evaluate clinically, by response to therapy, and/or biochemically by C-peptide concentrations, and to treat with insulin as type 1 or move to oral agents depending on measured insulin reserve. In these individuals, if insulin resistance is a major contributor to hyperglycaemia, oral agents will usually reduce it. If the autoimmune process contributes significantly to β-cell failure, insulin dependence will evolve and insulin therapy will be required. The classification given to the disease process in individual cases may be irrelevant to early therapy.

### *Insulin Regimens*

The regimens for insulin therapy of diabetes are familiar to most physicians who treat children, as it is the only method for successfully managing T1DM, although there are differences in the ways insulin is used in treating T2DM. Until the later stages of T2DM, most affected individuals maintain some level of endogenous insulin secretion. As a result, they do not need total replacement, but rather supplementation of this residual endogenous secretion. It should also be remembered that these patients are nearly uniformly insulin resistant, and, when they have deficient secretion, they may have insulin requirements which are relatively high in comparison to individuals with type 1. For example, an obese patient with type 2, presenting acutely ill, may initially require insulin doses >2 units/kg, only to fall to <0.1units/kg in weeks. Another variation in insulin therapy from type 1, is the use of insulin in combination with oral agents.

Use of insulin varies from meal boluses with rapid acting insulin analogs through enhancement of basal levels with long acting preparations. During transition periods and periods of diagnostic uncertainty with T2DM patients, it is frequently convenient to utilize intermediate and short acting or long and short acting insulin combinations identical to "conventional," or "intensive," multiple daily injection regimens used withT1DM. Young patients with T2DM, initially treated with insulin, may evolve to very low insulin requirements in weeks to months, with some patients having a "remission," in which they remain euglycemic for extended periods with no insulin replacement.

More commonly, patients initially treated with insulin, may be transitioned to therapy with oral antidiabetic agents. The approach in our clinic is to establish euglycaemia with insulin and then begin therapy with an oral agent. We usually employ metformin, at low dose, coupling initiation with a 50% reduction in the total insulin dose. If glycemic control is maintained with subsequent insulin weaning, insulin can be discontinued, and the oral agent increased.

***Primary Insulin Therapy***

In specific cases, individuals may continue insulin as primary therapy. The major concerns with this approach are the increased risk of hypoglycaemia, weight gain, the higher cost of parenteral therapy and the need for more frequent self glucose monitoring. Therapeutic insulin regimens used in adults have been extensively reviewed, [193, 194] and range from continuous subcutaneous infusion, through multiple injection regimens to twice daily intermediate or once daily long-acting insulin. Insulin preparations rarely used in children with T1DM, but commonly employed in adults with T2DM, are premixed intermediate/short acting.

In adults with long-standing T2DM, there is eventual loss of β-cell function resulting in insulin deficiency. [195] These individuals require exogenous insulin to survive and are often treated with intensive insulin regimens. In our experience, it is uncommon to see this evolution in children, unless they combine insulin resistance with positive immune markers. Even in these circumstances, control is not as fragile as in T1DM, and benefit can often be gained with the addition of an oral agent, which diminishes hepatic glucose output or reduces insulin resistance. As mentioned above, this approach has also been utilized in insulin resistant adolescents with T1DM. [186] The therapeutic changes frequently employed with the progression of type 2 diabetes in adults, with succession from lifestyle change through oral agent monotherapy and combination therapy, to simple insulin regimens to basal-bolus regimens have been described.

## Comorbid Conditions

T2DM is frequently associated with the metabolic or insulin resistance syndrome. The criteria for identification of this syndrome have been specifically defined for adults by the National Cholesterol Education Program in the adult treatment panel III (ATP III). [196] The major features comprising it and which can be extrapolated to children are: obesity, glucose intolerance or type 2 diabetes, dyslipidemia, hypertension, and the polycystic ovarian syndrome in females. A more complete list of comorbid conditions seen in individuals with type 2 diabetes is shown in Table 4. In this chapter, only hypertension and dyslipidemia will be addressed. There is a large literature dealing with each in adults. The importance of treating hypertension in individuals with T2DM was confirmed in the UKPDS. [197] This study showed clearly that the microvascular complications associated with diabetes can also be delayed or reduced by aggressively treating hypertension; similarly, the adverse cardiovascular events associated with T2DM were beneficially affected by antihypertensive therapy, [198, 199] with no significant difference in outcome with inhibitors of angiotensin converting enzyme (ACE inhibitors) or with β-blockers. We use ACE inhibitors, primarily because of concerns about hypoglycaemia with compromised counter-regulatory responses, especially in adolescents who are taking insulin or insulin secretagogues. ACE inhibitors also have beneficial effects on atherosclerosis progression and prevention. [200] Though there is little information about use of these drugs in children with T2DM, they have been used in treating many forms of hypertension in children, so there is experience and information available about safety and efficacy in this age group. [201]

Atherosclerosis and macrovascular disease is the major killer of adults with diabetes, 80% of whom die from coronary artery disease (CAD), cerebrovascular disease (CVD), or peripheral arterial disease (PAD). [202]

There is a 2-4 fold increase in risk for CAD in adults with diabetes over those in the general population. This increase equates the risk for a coronary event in those with diabetes without previous myocardial infarction (MI) to the same risk level as normoglycemic individuals with a previous MI. [202] The rates of reinfarction, congestive heart failure, and death in those with diabetes and an MI are also significantly increased over a normoglycemic population. [203] The 5 year mortality rate after an infarction is twice as high in individuals with diabetes as in those without. [204]

There is also a 2-4 fold increase in PAD with diabetes. [205] The incidence and extent of PAD correlates with the severity and duration of diabetes, [206] and it is more frequently symptomatic. [207] Diabetes increases the relative risk for developing intermittent claudication 3.5 fold in men and 8.6 fold in women. Amputation rates are also increased, with the relative risk ranging from 12.7 to 23.5, depending upon the age. [208]

Cerebrovascular disease is especially devastating in adults with diabetes, as they have a 150-400% increased risk of stroke. [209, 210, 211] The stroke risk is particularly strong in the relatively young, in whom there is a 10 fold increase over the general population, [212] Following a stroke, diabetics experience a 3-fold increase in the risk for stroke related dementia, [213] double the risk of another stroke, [214] and an increase in mortality rate. [215]

The typical dyslipidemia of T2DM consists of decreased HDL cholesterol and hypertriglyceridemia. Changes in particle size and in oxidized LDL have also been described, as has their contribution to the atherosclerotic process. In adult populations, it is estimated that individuals experience at least 7 years of asymptomatic hyperglycaemia before diabetes is diagnosed. There is evidence that the dyslipidemia described in diabetes is also present before its diagnosis. [216] In children with the metabolic syndrome and at risk for diabetes, the evolution of this dyslipidemia and its risks are not yet defined. This lack of information creates a therapeutic question, for while there is little disagreement that treatment of hyperglycaemia and hypertension is indicated in children as well as adults, treating the dyslipidemia associated with T2DM, now the standard of care in adults, is not established as standard practice and is more controversial in children. We do know that the dyslipidemia of T2DM is present in children with the disease and that glycemic management alone does not significantly improve it. [217]

Atherosclerosis is described children and young adults and the dyslipidemia associated with T2DM in adults is also present in children with the disease. [218] In children, fatty vascular streaks may develop in utero. [219] The Fate of Early Lesions in Children (FELIC) study investigated lesions in cross sections of the entire aortic arch and abdominal aorta in children from 1 to 13 years of age who died in trauma or from other causes unrelated to diabetes or hyperlipidemia. Atherosclerotic lesions ranging from fatty streaks to advanced lesions were present in all individuals examined, and the lesion size increased linearly with increasing age. [220] The Pathobiological Determinants of Atherosclerosis in Youth (PDAY) study, including individuals from 15-34 years of age, found atherosclerosis beginning in the teens and progressing to advanced lesions in young adulthood. This study also documented that the severity of atherosclerosis was influenced by the same risk factors that predict risk of coronary disease in middle-aged adults. [221] PDAY also confirmed reports from the Bogalusa Heart Study showing positive relationships between an unfavorable lipoprotein profile and the extent of atherosclerosis in the aorta and coronary arteries. [222] These observations coupled with recent information suggesting that individuals with T2DM diagnosed in childhood develop complications as early as the third decade of life, [223] give rise to increasing concern about cardiovascular complications occurring earlier with all the attendant implications.

Some have used this information to suggest that early treatment of dyslipidemia is indicated, although there are contrary arguments. [224] There are no published clinical trials of therapy of dyslipidemia in children with T2DM or the IRS, so approaches must be extrapolated from experience in adult studies and from that with children who have familial hypercholesterolemia. Guidelines for the treatment of dyslipidemia in adults are established. [225, 226]

In children, as in adults, treatment should start with diet modification and a goal of reducing LDL. Tracking studies have shown that children with hypercholesterolemia continue this pattern into adulthood. [227] The establishment of good dietary habits early in life may positively affect lifetime dietary choices. If 6 weeks with the dietary modifications do not reduce LDL below 100, and if this adult target is to be used for children, pharmacotherapy may be employed.

Resins, one class of drugs used to reduce serum cholesterol, bind to bile acids in the small intestine and prevents their reabsorption. This action initiates a chain of events leading to up-regulation of LDL receptors on liver cells and increased LDL clearance.

Fibric acids reduce lipids by increasing lipoprotein lipase activity and decreasing the production of triglycerides by the liver. [228] Gemfibrozil has been shown to reduce TG and moderately increase HDL in adults, but it has also been associated with increases in LDL. [229] Although, there are few studies of fibrates in children, a 1981study treated 17 hyperlipidemic children between the ages of 4 and 19 years with fenofibrate. [230] After 3 months of therapy, their mean total cholesterol decreased by 22% and their TG by 39%. The only reported adverse effects were modest increases in AST and ALT. A more recent study of hyperlipidemia in 12 children with the nephrotic syndrome, found that gemfibrozil reduced total cholesterol by 34%, LDL by 30%, and TG by 53% over a four month interval. [231]

Statins inhibit HMG-CoA reductase and *de novo* cholesterol production, up-regulating LDL receptors and increasing LDL clearance. In adult studies, statins have decreased LDL as much as 18-55%. Children with familial hypercholesterolemia tolerate statins well, with no inhibition of growth or development of abnormal serum chemistries. [232] Many statin preparations are available commercially, and several have been approved by the FDA for use in children with hypercholesterolemia. Atorvastatin, at a dose of 20mg/d, has been approved for children aged 10-17 years, as has pravastatin for children aged 8-18 years, with a maximum dose of 40mg/d. Simvastatin has also been approved for use in children between the ages of 10-17 years. In addition to their role in lowering cholesterol, these drugs also appear to be beneficial for prevention of arteriosclerotic vascular disease and acute cardiac events by other mechanisms, especially through an anti-inflammatory effect. [233]

Ezetimibe is the first of a new class of drugs for cholesterol lowering. It works at the intestinal brush border to selectively inhibit the absorption of cholesterol and phytosterols by as much as 54% with no effect on lipid-soluble vitamins. The response to this decrease in dietary cholesterol is a mild up-regulation of HMG-CoA reductase to produce more cholesterol. As a result, ezetimibe's effect is greatest when used in conjunction with a HMG-CoA reductase inhibitor. Ezetimibe, a relatively small pill, is taken once a day, offering easy compliance. It also has an adverse-event profile that is similar to placebo. This combination of ease of administration and safety could combine to make it an important drug for use in children.

Large studies in adult patients with diabetes have demonstrated the benefits of lipid lowering therapy in the prevention of mortality and morbidity from arterioscleotic vascular disease. It has also been demonstrated that combination therapy directed at the vascular disease is more effective than therapy directed against one or another of the underlying risk factors. [234]

The subject of dyslipidemia and T2DM in adolescents has been reviewed. [235] The chronology of the atherosclerotic process [236] suggests that intervention in the first two decades of life to prevent development or progression may differ from the therapy prescribed in older adults. For example, antiplatelet or plaque stabilization therapy may be unnecessary in a younger population without unstable plaques. Therapy for prevention of lipid accumulation, on the other hand, would still be beneficial in prevention strategies.

## Prevention of Type 2 Diabetes

Prevention of diabetes in children is yet an unexplored area. Because the rise in the frequency of T2DM has paralleled the rise in obesity, attention has been focused on trying general societal change. This has not been age specific and has not been done in controlled studies, but the efforts have targeted improving diets, encouraging increased physical activity, and a general decrease in calorie consumption.

We do know from the Diabetes Prevention Program (DPP), that intensive efforts to improve diet and exercise decreased the rate of progression of individuals from impaired glucose tolerance to diabetes from that of a control population. In this study of more than 3,000 individuals, the progression to diabetes was 11.0/100 person years in the control group compared to 4.8 in the intensive lifestyle intervention group. The frequency in the third group, given 850 mg of metformin each day was 7.8/100 patient years. [237] Very similar results have been reported from The Finnish Diabetes Prevention Study. [238]

## Conclusions

Type 2 diabetes is rapidly becoming a significant national and international health problem in children and adolescents. Early epidemiologic information suggests that the disease in children has comparable demographics and follows similar clinical patterns to those described in adults. There are certainly differences between adults and children in clinical course and in the difficulties involved in diagnosis and therapy. There is no reason to suspect that the role of insulin resistance is any less important in children. Indeed, the information discussed in this book confirms its important role. Reduction in insulin resistance is important in diabetes therapy, including therapy of hyperglycaemia and of the comorbidities associated with diabetes. It is also clear that the early information we have about prevention of T2DM strongly suggests that strategies to prevent diabetes must address improving insulin sensitivity as well as preserving β-cell function.

## References

[1] Paulson EP, Richenderfer L, Ginsberg-Fellner F: Plasma glucose, free fatty acids, and immunoreactive insulin in sixty-six obese children. *Diabetes* 17:261-269, 1968

[2] American Diabetes Association: Report of the expert committee on the diagnosis and classification of diabetes mellitus. *Diabetes Care* 21(S2):B1-B167, 1998. American Diabetes Association: Type 2 diabetes in children and adolescents. *Diabetes Care* 23:1, 2000.

[3] Savage PJ, Bennett PH, Senter GR, et al: High prevalence of diabetes in young Pima Indians. *Diabetes* 28:937, 1979.

[4] Dean HE, Mundy RLL, Moffatt M: Non-insulin-dependent diabetes mellitus in Indian children in Manitoba. *Can Med Assoc* J 147:52, 1992.

[5] Fagot-Campana A, Pettit DJ, Engelgau MM, et al: Type 2 diabetes among North American children and adolescents: an epidemiological review and a public health perspective. *J Pediatr* 136:664, 2000.

[6] Pinhas-Hamiel O, Dolan LM, Daniels SR, et al: Increased incidence of non-insulin-dependent diabetes mellitus among adolescents. *J Pediatr* 128:608-615, 1996.

[7] Scott CR, Smith JM, Cradock M, Pihoker C: Characteristics of youth-onset non-insulin-dependent-diabetes mellitus and insulin-dependent diabetes mellitus at diagnosis. *Pediatrics* 100:84, 1997.

[8] Neufeld ND, Raffal LJ, Landon C, et al: Early presentation of type 2 diabetes in Mexican-American youth. *Diabetes Care* 21:80, 1998.
[9] Glaser N, Jones KL: Non-insulin-dependent diabetes mellitus in Mexican-American children. *West J Med* 168:11, 1998.
[10] Kitagawa T, Owada M, Urakami T, Tajima N: Epidemiology of type 1 (insulin-dependent) and type 2 (non-insulin-dependent) diabetes mellitus in Japanese children. *Diabetes Res Clin Pract.* 24(Suppl):S7-S13, 1994.
[11] Braun B, Zimmermann MB, Kretchmer N, et al: Risk factors for diabetes and cardiovascular disease in young Australian aborigines. *Diabetes Care* 19, 472, 1996.
[12] Wei J-N, Sung F-C, Lin C-C, et al: National surveillance for type 2 diabetes mellitus in Taiwanese children. *JAMA* 290:1345, 2003.
[13] Kahn SE: The relative contributions of insulin resistance and β-cell dysfunction to the pathophysiology of type 2 diabetes. *Diabetologia* 46:3, 2003.
[14] Bergman RN, Finegood DT, Kahn SE: The evolution of beta-cell dysfunction and insulin resistance in type 2 diabetes. *Eur J Clin Invest* 32:35, 2002.
[15] Kahn CR: The Gordon Wilson Lecture. Lessons about the control of glucose homeostasis and the pathogenesis of diabetes from knockout mice. *Trans Am Clin Climatol Assoc* 114:125, 2003.
[16] DeFronzo RA: Pathogenesis of type 2 (non-insulin dependent) diabetes mellitus: A balanced overview. *Diabetologia* 35:389, 1992.
[17] Freychet P, Roth J, Neville DM, Jr. "Insulin receptors in the liver: specific binding of (125 I) insulin to the plasma membrane and its relation to insulin bioactivity." *Proc Natl Acad Sci USA* 68:1833-7, 1971.
[18] Ullrich A, Bell JR, Chen EY, Herrera R, Petruzzelli LM, Dull, TJ, Gray A, Coussens L, Liao YC, Tsubokawa M, et al. "Human insulin receptor and its relationship to the tyrosine kinase family of oncogenes." *Nature* 313:756-61,1985.
[19] Czech MP, "The nature and regulation of the insulin receptor: structure and function." *Ann Rev Physiol* 47:357-81, 1985.
[20] Kahn CR, White MF, "The insulin receptor and the molecular mechanism of insulin action." *J Clin Invest* 82:1151-6, 1988.
[21] White MF, Maron R, Kahn CR, "Insulin rapidly stimulates tyrosine phosphorylation of a Mr-185,000 protein in intact cells." *Nature* 318:183-6, 1985.
[22] Sun XJ, Rothenberg P, Kahn CR, Backer JM, Araki E, Wilden PA, Cahill DA, Goldstein BJ, White MF, "Structure of the insulin receptor substrate IRS-1 defines a unique signal transduction protein." *Nature* 352:73-7, 1991.
[23] Sun XJ, Wang LM, Zhang Y, Yenush L, Myers MG, Jr., Glasheen E, Lane WS, Pierce JH, White MF, "Role of IRS-2 in insulin and cytokine signaling." *Nature* 377:173-7, 1995.
[24] Lavan BE, Lane WS, Lienhard GE, "The 60-kDa phosphotyrosine protein in insulin-treated adipocytes is a new member of the insulin receptor substrate family." *J Biol Chem* 272: 11439-43, 1997.
[25] Lavan BE, Fantin VR, Chang ET, Lane WS, Keller SR, Lienhard GE, "A novel 160-kDa phosphotyrosine protein in insulin-treated embryonic kidney cells is a new member of the insulin receptor substrate family." *J Biol Chem* 272: 21403-7, 1997.
[26] White MF, "The IRS-signaling system: a network of docking proteins that mediate insulin and cytokine action." *Recent Prog Horm Res* 53, 119-38, 1998.

[27] Yenush L, Makati KJ, Smith-Hall J, Ishibashi O, Myers MG, Jr., White MF, "The pleckstrin homology domain is the principal link between the insulin receptor and IRS-1." *J Biol Chem* 271:24300-6, 1996.
[28] Eck MJ, Dhe-Paganon S, Trub T, Nolte RT, Shoelson SE, "Structure of the IRS-1 PTB domain bound to the juxtamembrane region of the insulin receptor." *Cell* 85:695-705, 1996.
[29] Virkamaki A, Ueki K, Kahn CR, "Protein-protein interaction in insulin signaling and the molecular mechanisms of insulin resistance." *J Clin Invest* 103:931-43, 1999.
[30] Alessi DR, Downes CP, "The role of PI 3-kinase in insulin action." *Biochim Biophys Acta* 1436:151-64, 1998.
[31] Alessi DR, Deak M, Casamayor, A, Caudwell FB, Morrice N, Norman DG, Gaffney P, Reese CB, MacDougall CN, Harbison D, Ashworth A, Bownes M, "3-Phosphoinositide-dependent protein kinase-1 (PDK1): structural and functional homology with the Drosophila DSTPK61 kinase." *Curr Biol* 7:776-89, 1997.
[32] Farese RV, "Insulin-sensitive phospholipid signaling systems and glucose transport. Update II." *Exp Biol Med* (Maywood) 226:283-95, 2001.
[33] Bellacosa A, Testa JR, Staal SP, Tsichlis PN, "A retroviral oncogene, akt, encoding a serine-threonine kinase containing an SH2-like region." *Science* 254:274-7, 1991.
[34] Downward J, "Mechanisms and consequences of activation of protein kinase B/Akt." *Curr Opin Cell Biol* 10: 262-7, 1998.
[35] Le Good JA, Ziegler WH, Parekh DB, Alessi DR, Cohen P, Parker PJ, "Protein kinase C isotypes controlled by phosphoinositide 3-kinase through the protein kinase PDK1." *Science* 281:2042-5, 1998.
[36] Kotani K, Ogawa W, Matsumoto M, Kitamura T, Sakaue H, Hino Y, Miyake K, Sano W, Akimoto K, Ohno S, Kasuga M, "Requirement of atypical protein kinase clambda for insulin stimulation of glucose uptake but not for Akt activation in 3T3-L1 adipocytes." *Mol Cell Biol* 18:6971-82, 1998.
[37] Ravichandran LV, Esposito DL, Chen J, Quon MJ, "Protein kinase C-zeta phosphorylates insulin receptor substrate-1 and impairs its ability to activate phosphatidylinositol 3-kinase in response to insulin." *J Biol Chem* 276:3543-9, 2001.
[38] Cross DA, Alessi DR, Cohen P, Andjelkovich M, Hemmings BA, "Inhibition of glycogen synthase kinase-3 by insulin mediated by protein kinase B." *Nature* 378:785-9, 1995.
[39] Scott PH, Brunn GJ, Kohn AD, Roth RA, Lawrence JC, Jr., "Evidence of insulin-stimulated phosphorylation and activation of the mammalian target of rapamycin mediated by a protein kinase B signaling pathway." *Proc Natl Acad Sci* USA 95:7772-7, 1998.
[40] Pause A, Belsham GJ, Gingras AC, Donze O, Lin TA, Lawrence JC, Jr., Sonenberg N, "Insulin-dependent stimulation of protein synthesis by phosphorylation of a regulator of 5'-cap function." *Nature* 371:762-7, 1994.
[41] Brady MJ, Saltiel AR, "The role of protein phosphatase-1 in insulin action." *Recent Prog Horm Res* 56:57-73, 2001.
[42] Hashimoto N, Feener EP, Zhang WR, Goldstein BJ, "Insulin receptor protein-tyrosine phosphatases. Leukocyte common antigen-related phosphatase rapidly deactivates the insulin receptor kinase by preferential dephosphorylation of the receptor regulatory domain." *J Biol Chem* 267:13811-4, 1992.

[43] Elchebly M, Cheng A, Tremblay ML, “Modulation of insulin signaling by protein tyrosine phosphatases.” *J Mol Med* 78:473-82, 2000.

[44] Rocchi S, Tartare-Deckert S, Sawka-Verhelle D, Gamha A, van Obberghen E, “Interaction of SH2-containing protein tyrosine phosphatase 2 with the insulin receptor and the insulin-like growth factor-I receptor: studies of the domains involved using the yeast two-hybrid system.” *Endocrinology* 137:4944-52, 1996.

[45] Baumann CA, Ribon V, Kanzaki M, Thurmond DC, Mora S, Shigematsu S, Bickel PE, Pessin JE, Saltiel AR, “CAP defines a second signalling pathway required for insulin-stimulated glucose transport.” *Nature* 407:202-7, 2000.

[46] Martin SS, Haruta T, Morris AJ, Klippel A, Williams LT, Olefsky JM, “Activated phosphatidylinositol 3-kinase is sufficient to mediate actin rearrangement and GLUT4 translocation in 3T3-L1 adipocytes.” *J Biol Chem* 271:17605-8, 1996.

[47] Wiese RJ, Mastick CC, Lazar DF, Saltiel AR, “Activation of mitogen-activated protein kinase and phosphatidylinositol 3'-kinase is not sufficient for the hormonal stimulation of glucose uptake, lipogenesis, or glycogen synthesis in 3T3-L1 adipocytes.” *J Biol Chem* 270: 3442-6, 1995.

[48] Avruch J, Khokhlatchev A, Kyriakis JM, Luo Z, Tzivion G, Vavvas D, Zhang XF, “Ras activation of the Raf kinase: tyrosine kinase recruitment of the MAP kinase cascade.” 2001; *Recent Prog Horm Res* 56:127-55, 2001.

[49] Pulverer BJ, Kyriakis JM, Avruch J, Nikolakaki E, Woodgett JR, “Phosphorylation of c-jun mediated by MAP kinases.” *Nature* 353:670-4, 1991.

[50] Derijard B, Hibi M, Wu IH, Barrett T, Su B, Deng T, Karin M, Davis RJ, “JNK1: a protein kinase stimulated by UV light and Ha-Ras that binds and phosphorylates the c-Jun activation domain.” *Cell* 76:1025-37, 1994.

[51] Kimball SR, Vary TC, Jefferson LS, “Regulation of protein synthesis by insulin.” *Annu Rev Physiol* 56:321-48, 1994.

[52] Given BD, Mako ME, Tager HS, Baldwin D, Markese J, Rubenstein AH, Olefsky J, Kobayashi M, Kolterman O, Poucher R, “Diabetes due to secretion of an abnormal insulin.” *N Engl J Med* 302:129-35, 1980.

[53] Olefsky JM, Saekow M, Tager H, Rubenstein AH, “Characterization of a mutant human insulin species.” *J Biol Chem* 255:6098-105, 1980.

[54] Randle PJ, Garland PB, Hales CN, Newsholme EA, “The glucose fatty-acid cycle. Its role in insulin sensitivity and the metabolic disturbances of diabetes mellitus.” *Lancet* 1:785-9, 1963.

[55] Kruszynska YT, Worrall DS, Ofrecio J, Frias JP, Macaraeg G, Olefsky JM, “Fatty acid-induced insulin resistance: decreased muscle PI3K activation but unchanged Akt phosphorylation.” *J Clin Endocrinol Metab* 87:226-34, 2002.

[56] Boden G, Chen X, Ruiz J, White JV, Rossetti L, “Mechanisms of fatty acid-induced inhibition of glucose uptake.” *J Clin Invest* 93:2438-46, 1994.

[57] Staehr P, Hother-Nielsen O, Landau BR, Chandramouli V, Holst JJ, Beck-Nielsen H, “Effects of free fatty acids per se on glucose production, gluconeogenesis, and glycogenolysis.” *Diabetes* 52:260-7, 2003.

[58] Laws A, “Free fatty acids, insulin resistance and lipoprotein metabolism.” *Curr Opin Lipidol* 7:172-7, 1996.

[59] Shimabukuro M, Zhou YT, Levi M, Unger RH, “Fatty acid-induced beta cell apoptosis: a link between obesity and diabetes.” *Proc Natl Acad Sci USA* 95:2498-502, 1998.

[60] Ruan H, Lodish HF, "Insulin resistance in adipose tissue: direct and indirect effects of tumor necrosis factor-alpha." *Cytokine Growth Factor Rev* 14:447-55, 2003.
[61] Hotamisligil GS, Arner P, Caro JF, Atkinson RL, Spiegelman BM, "Increased adipose tissue expression of tumor necrosis factor-alpha in human obesity and insulin resistance." *J Clin Invest* 95:2409-15, 1995.
[62] Hotamisligil GS, Shargill NS, Spiegelman BM, "Adipose expression of tumor necrosis factor-alpha: direct role in obesity-linked insulin resistance." *Science* 259:87-91, 1993.
[63] Lang CH, Dobrescu C, Bagby GJ, "Tumor necrosis factor impairs insulin action on peripheral glucose disposal and hepatic glucose output." *Endocrinology* 130:43-52, 1992.
[64] Hotamisligil GS, Spiegelman BM, "Tumor necrosis factor alpha: a key component of the obesity-diabetes link." *Diabetes* 43:1271-8, 1994.
[65] Hotamisligil, GS, "The role of TNFalpha and TNF receptors in obesity and insulin resistance." J Intern Med 245:621-5, 1999.
[66] Hotamisligil, GS, Peraldi P, Budavari A, Ellis R, White MF, Spiegelman BM, "IRS-1-mediated inhibition of insulin receptor tyrosine kinase activity in TNF-alpha- and obesity-induced insulin resistance." *Science* 271:665-8, 1996.
[67] Febbraio MA, Pedersen BK, "Muscle-derived interleukin-6: mechanisms for activation and possible biological roles." *Faseb J* 16:1335-47, 2002.
[68] Kanemaki T, Kitade H, Kaibori M, Sakitani K, Hiramatsu Y, Kamiyama Y, Ito S, Okumura T, "Interleukin 1beta and interleukin 6, but not tumor necrosis factor alpha, inhibit insulin-stimulated glycogen synthesis in rat hepatocytes." *Hepatology* 27:1296-303, 1998.
[69] Tsigos C, Papanicolaou DA, Kyrou I, Defensor R, Mitsiadis CS, Chrousos GP, "Dose-dependent effects of recombinant human interleukin-6 on glucose regulation." *J Clin Endocrinol Metab* 82:4167-70, 1997.
[70] Chandran M, Phillips SA, Ciaraldi T, Henry RR, "Adiponectin: more than just another fat cell hormone?" *Diabetes Care* 26:2442-50, 2003.
[71] Hotta K, Funahashi T, Arita Y, Takahashi M, Matsuda M, Okamoto Y, Iwahashi H, Kuriyama H, Ouchi N, Maeda K, Nishida M, Kihara S, Sakai N, Nakajima T, Hasegawa K, Muraguchi M, Ohmoto Y, Nakamura T, Yamashita S, Hanafusa T, Matsuzawa Y, "Plasma concentrations of a novel, adipose-specific protein, adiponectin, in type 2 diabetic patients." *Arterioscler Thromb Vasc Biol* 20:1595-9, 2000.
[72] Berg AH, Combs TP, Du X, Brownlee M, Scherer PE, "The adipocyte-secreted protein Acrp30 enhances hepatic insulin action." *Nat Med* 7:947-53, 2001.
[73] Fruebis J, Tsao TS, Javorschi S, Ebbets-Reed D, Erickson MR, Yen FT, Bihain BE, Lodish HF, "Proteolytic cleavage product of 30-kDa adipocyte complement-related protein increases fatty acid oxidation in muscle and causes weight loss in mice." *Proc Natl Acad Sci USA* 98:2005-10, 2001.
[74] Taylor SI, "Lilly Lecture: molecular mechanisms of insulin resistance. Lessons from patients with mutations in the insulin-receptor gene." *Diabetes* 41:1473-90, 1992.
[75] Okamoto H, Accili D, "In vivo mutagenesis of the insulin receptor." *J Biol Chem* 278:28359-62, 2003.
[76] Lei HH, Coresh J, Shuldiner AR, Boerwinkle E, Brancati FL, "Variants of the insulin receptor substrate-1 and fatty acid binding protein 2 genes and the risk of type 2

diabetes, obesity, and hyperinsulinemia in African-Americans: the Atherosclerosis Risk in Communities Study." *Diabetes* 48:1868-72, 1999.

[77] Yoshimura R, Araki E, Ura S, Todaka M, Tsuruzoe K, Furukawa N, Motoshima H, Yoshizato K, Kaneko K, Matsuda K, Kishikawa H, Shichiri M, "Impact of natural IRS-1 mutations on insulin signals: mutations of IRS-1 in the PTB domain and near SH2 protein binding sites result in impaired function at different steps of IRS-1 signaling." *Diabetes* 46:929-36, 1997.

[78] Terauchi Y, Tsuji Y, Satoh S, Minoura H, Murakami K, Okuno A, Inukai K, Asano T, Kaburagi Y, Ueki K, Nakajima H, Hanafusa T, Matsuzawa Y, Sekihara H, Yin Y, Barrett JC, Oda H, Ishikawa T, Akanuma Y, Komuro I, Suzuki M, Yamamura K, Kodama T, Suzuki H, Kadowaki T, et al., "Increased insulin sensitivity and hypoglycaemia in mice lacking the p85 alpha subunit of phosphoinositide 3-kinase." *Nat Genet* 21:230-5, 1999.

[79] Hunter SJ, Garvey WT, "Insulin action and insulin resistance: diseases involving defects in insulin receptors, signal transduction, and the glucose transport effector system." *Am J Med* 105:331-45, 1998.

[80] Obermaier-Kusser B, White MF, Pongratz DE, Su Z, Ermel B, Muhlbacher C, Haring HU, "A defective intramolecular autoactivation cascade may cause the reduced kinase activity of the skeletal muscle insulin receptor from patients with non-insulin-dependent diabetes mellitus." *J Biol Chem* 264:9497-504, 1989.

[81] Freidenberg GR, Henry RR, Klein HH, Reichart DR, Olefsky JM, "Decreased kinase activity of insulin receptors from adipocytes of non-insulin-dependent diabetic subjects." *J Clin Invest* 79:240-50, 1987.

[82] Smith U, Axelsen M, Carvalho E, Eliasson B, Jansson PA, Wesslau C, "Insulin signaling and action in fat cells: associations with insulin resistance and type 2 diabetes." *Ann N Y Acad Sci* 892:119-26, 1999.

[83] Kim YB, Nikoulina SE, Ciaraldi TP, Henry RR, Kahn BB, "Normal insulin-dependent activation of Akt/protein kinase B, with diminished activation of phosphoinositide 3-kinase, in muscle in type 2 diabetes." *J Clin Invest* 104:733-41, 1999.

[84] Andreelli F, Laville M, Ducluzeau PH, Vega N, Vallier P, Khalfallah Y, Riou JP, Vidal H, "Defective regulation of phosphatidylinositol-3-kinase gene expression in skeletal muscle and adipose tissue of non-insulin-dependent diabetes mellitus patients." *Diabetologia* 42:358-64, 1999.

[85] Rondinone CM, Wang LM, Lonnroth P, Wesslau C, Pierce JH, Smith U, "Insulin receptor substrate (IRS) 1 is reduced and IRS-2 is the main docking protein for phosphatidylinositol 3-kinase in adipocytes from subjects with non-insulin-dependent diabetes mellitus." *Proc Natl Acad Sci USA* 94:4171-5, 1997.

[86] Bjornholm M, Kawano Y, Lehtihet M, Zierath JR, "Insulin receptor substrate-1 phosphorylation and phosphatidylinositol 3-kinase activity in skeletal muscle from NIDDM subjects after in vivo insulin stimulation." *Diabetes* 46:524-7, 1997.

[87] Krook A, Roth RA, Jiang XJ, Zierath JR, Wallberg-Henriksson H, "Insulin receptor substrate-1 phosphorylation and phosphatidylinositol 3-kinase activity in skeletal muscle from NIDDM subjects after in vivo insulin stimulation." *Diabetes* 47:1281-6, 1998.

[88] Cusi K, Maezono K, Osman A, Pendergrass M, Patti ME, Pratipanawatr T, DeFronzo RA, Kahn CR, Mandarino LJ, "Insulin receptor substrate-1 phosphorylation and

phosphatidylinositol 3-kinase activity in skeletal muscle from NIDDM subjects after in vivo insulin stimulation." *J Clin Invest* 105:311-20, 2000.

[89] Kim YB, Kotani K, Ciaraldi TP, Henry RR, Kahn BB, "Insulin-stimulated protein kinase C lambda/zeta activity is reduced in skeletal muscle of humans with obesity and type 2 diabetes: reversal with weight reduction." *Diabetes* 52:1935-42, 2003.

[90] Carvalho E, Eliasson B, Wesslau C, Smith U, "Impaired phosphorylation and insulin-stimulated translocation to the plasma membrane of protein kinase B/Akt in adipocytes from Type II diabetic subjects." *Diabetologia* 43:1107-15, 2000.

[91] Nikoulia SE, Ciaraldi TP, Mudaliar S, Mohideen P, Carter L, Henry RR, "Potential role of glycogen synthase kinase-3 in skeletal muscle insulin resistance of type 2 diabetes." *Diabetes* 49:263-71, 2000.

[92] Thorburn AW, Gumbiner G, Bulacan F, Wallace P, Henry RR, "Intracellular glucose oxidation and glycogen synthase activity are reduced in non-insulin-dependent (type II) diabetes independent of impaired glucose uptake." *J Clin Invest* 85:522-9, 1990.

[93] Vollenweider P, Menard B, Nicod P, "Insulin resistance, defective insulin receptor substrate 2-associated phosphatidylinositol-3' kinase activation, and impaired atypical protein kinase C (zeta/lambda) activation in myotubes from obese patients with impaired glucose tolerance." *Diabetes* 51:1052-9, 2002.

[94] Pedersen O, Bak JF, Andersen PH, Lund S, Moller DE, Flier JS, Kahn BB, "Evidence against altered expression of GLUT1 or GLUT4 in skeletal muscle of patients with obesity or NIDDM." *Diabetes* 39:865-70, 1990.

[95] Garvey WT, Maianu L, Hancock JA, Golichowski AM, Baron A, "Gene expression of GLUT4 in skeletal muscle from insulin-resistant patients with obesity, IGT, GDM, and NIDDM." *Diabetes* 41:465-75, 1992.

[96] Smith U, "Gene expression of GLUT4 in skeletal muscle from insulin-resistant patients with obesity, IGT, GDM, and NIDDM." *Int J Obes Relat Metab Disord* 26:897-904, 2002.

[97] American Diabetes Association: Type 2 diabetes in children and adolescents. *Diabetes Care* 23:1, 2000.

[98] Yu L, Gianani R, Eisenbarth GS: Quantitation of gluctamic acid decarboxylase autoantibody levels in prospectively evaluated relatives of patients with type I diabetes. *Diabetes* 43:1229, 1994.

[99] National Institutes of Diabetes and Digestive and Kidney Diseases. Diabetes Statistics. Bethesda, MD: NIDDK, 1995; NIH publication no. 96-3926.

[100] The DCCT Research Group: The effect of intensive treatment of diabetes on the development and progression of long-term complications in insulin-dependent diabetes mellitus. *New Eng J Med* 329:977, 1993.

[101] National Institutes of Health. Consensus development conference on diet and exercise in non-insulin-dependent diabetes mellitus. *Diabetes Care* 10:639, 1987.

[102] American Diabetes Association. Evidence-based nutrition principles and recommendations for the treatment and prevention of diabetes and related complications. *Diabetes care 25(suppl. 1)*:S50, 2002.

[103] Diabetes Prevention Program Research Group: Reduction in the incidence of type 2 diabetes with lifestyle intervention or metformin. *New Eng J Med* 346:393, 2002.

[104] Jones KL, Arslanian S, Peterokova VA et al: Effect of metformin in pediatric patients with type 2 diabetes: A randomized controlled trial. *Diabetes Care* 25:89, 2002

[105] Dean H: Dancing with many different ghosts: Treatment of youth with type 2 diabetes. *Diabetes Care* 25: 237, 2002.
[106] Jones KL: Non-insulin dependent diabetes mellitus in children and adolescents. *Clin Pediatr* 37:103, 1998.
[107] Franz MJ, Bantle JP, Beebe CA, et al: Evidence-based nutrition principles and recommendations for the treatment and prevention of diabetes and related complications (Technical Review) *Diabetes Care* 25:S136, 2002.
[108] Rossetti L, "Glucose toxicity: the implications of hyperglycaemia in the pathophysiology of diabetes mellitus." *Clin Invest Med* 18:255-60, 1995.
[109] Pedersen O, Hother-Nielsen O, Bak J, Hjollund E, Beck-Nielsen H, "Effects of sulfonylureas on adipocyte and skeletal muscle insulin action in patients with non-insulin-dependent diabetes mellitus." *Am J Med* 90:22S-28S, 1991.
[110] Doyle ME, Egan JM, "Pharmacological agents that directly modulate insulin secretion." *Pharmacol Rev* 55:105-31, 2003.
[111] Ladriere L, Bjorkling F, Malaisse WJ, "Stimulation of insulin release in hereditarily diabetic rats by mixed molecules formed of nateglinide and a succinic acid ester." *Int J Mol Med* 5:63-5, 2000.
[112] Bailey CJ, Turner RC, "Metformin." *N Engl J Med* 334:574-9, 1996.
[113] Lalau JD, Lacroix C, Compagnon P, de Cagny B, Rigaud JP, Bleichner G, Chauveau P, Dulbecco P, Guerin C, Haegy JM, et al., "Role of metformin accumulation in metformin-associated lactic acidosis." *Diabetes Care* 18:779-84, 1995.
[114] Zhou G, Myers R, Li Y, Chen Y, Shen X, Fenyk-Melody J, Wu M, Ventre J, Doebber T, Fujii N, Musi N, Hirshman MF, Goodyear LJ, Moller DE, "Role of AMP-activated protein kinase in mechanism of metformin action." *J Clin Invest* 108:1167-74, 2001.
[115] DeFronzo RA, Barzilai N, Simonson DC, "Mechanism of metformin action in obese and lean noninsulin-dependent diabetic subjects." *J Clin Endocrinol Metab* 73:1294-301, 1991.
[116] Morel Y, Golay A, Perneger T, Lehmann T, Vadas L, Pasik C, Reaven GM, "Metformin treatment leads to an increase in basal, but not insulin-stimulated, glucose disposal in obese patients with impaired glucose tolerance." *Diabet Med* 16:650-5, 1999.
[117] Campbell LK, White JR, Campbell RK, "Acarbose: its role in the treatment of diabetes mellitus."*Ann Pharmacother* 30:1255-62, 1996.
[118] Lebovitz HE, "Postprandial hyperglycaemic state: importance and consequences." *Diabetes Res Clin Pract 40(Suppl):*S27-8, 1998.
[119] Nauck MA, Holst JJ, Willms B, Schmiegel W, "Glucagon-like peptide 1 (GLP-1) as a new therapeutic approach for type 2-diabetes." *Exp Clin Endocrinol Diabetes* 105:187-95, 1997.
[120] Buse J, "Effects of five-day dosing of synthetic extendin-4 (Ac2993) Type 2 Diabetes." *Diabetes 29(Suppl):*A100, 2000.
[121] Fineman MS, Bicsak TA, Shen LZ, Taylor K, Gaines E, Varns A, Kim D, Baron AD, "Effect on glycemic control of exenatide (synthetic exendin-4) additive to existing metformin and/or sulfonylurea treatment in patients with type 2 diabetes." *Diabetes Care* 26:2370-7, 2003.
[122] Ahren B, Simonsson E, Larsson H, Landin-Olsson M, Torgeirsson H, Jansson PA., Sandqvist M, Bavenholm P, Efendic S, Eriksson JW, Dickinson S, Holmes D,

"Inhibition of dipeptidyl peptidase IV improves metabolic control over a 4-week study period in type 2 diabetes." *Diabetes Care* 25:869-75, 2002.

[123] Weyer C, Maggs, DG, Young AA, Kolterman OG, "Amylin replacement with pramlintide as an adjunct to insulin therapy in type 1 and type 2 diabetes mellitus: a physiological approach toward improved metabolic control." *Curr Pharm Des* 7:1353-73, 2001.

[124] Hollander PA, Levy P, Fineman MS, Maggs DG, Shen LZ, Strobel SA, Weyer C, Kolterman OG, "Pramlintide as an adjunct to insulin therapy improves long-term glycemic and weight control in patients with type 2 diabetes: a 1-year randomized controlled trial." *Diabetes Care* 26:784-90, 2003.

[125] Saltiel AR, Olefsky JM, "Thiazolidinediones in the treatment of insulin resistance and type II diabetes." *Diabetes* 45:1661-9, 1996.

[126] Spiegelman BM, "PPAR-gamma: adipogenic regulator and thiazolidinedione receptor." *Diabetes* 47:507-14, 1998.

[127] Young PW, Cawthorne MA, Coyle PJ, Holder JC, Holman GD, Kozka IJ, Kirkham D, M, Lister CA, Smith SA, "Repeat treatment of obese mice with BRL 49653, a new potent insulin sensitizer, enhances insulin action in white adipocytes. Association with increased insulin binding and cell-surface GLUT4 as measured by photoaffinity labeling." *Diabetes* 44:1087-92, 1995.

[128] Maeda N, Takahashi M, Funahashi T, Kihara S, Nishizawa H, Kishida K, Nagaretani H, Matsuda M, Komuro R, Ouchi N, Kuriyama H, Hotta K, Nakamura T, Shimomura I, Matsuzawa Y, "PPARgamma ligands increase expression and plasma concentrations of adiponectin, an adipose-derived protein." *Diabetes* 50:2094-9, 2001.

[129] Szalkowski D, White-Carrington S, Berger J, Zhang B, "Antidiabetic thiazolidinediones block the inhibitory effect of tumor necrosis factor-alpha on differentiation, insulin-stimulated glucose uptake, and gene expression in 3T3-L1 cells." *Endocrinology* 136:1474-81, 1995.

[130] Miyazaki Y, Mahankali A, Matsuda M, Mahankali S, Hardies J, Cusi K, Mandarino LJ, DeFronzo RA, "Metabolic effects of visceral fat accumulation in type 2 diabetes." *J Clin Endocrinol Metab* 87:2784-91, 2002.

[131] Burant CF, Sreenan S, Hirano K, Tai TA, Lohmiller J, Lukens J, Davidson NO, Ross S Graves RA, "Troglitazone action is independent of adipose tissue." *J Clin Invest* 100:2900-8, 1997.

[132] Park KS, Ciaraldi TP, Lindgren K, Abrams-Carter L, Mudaliar S, Nikoulina SE, Tufari, SR, Veerkamp JH, Vidal-Puig A, Henry RR, "Troglitazone effects on gene expression in human skeletal muscle of type II diabetes involve up-regulation of peroxisome. *J Clin Endocrin Metab* 83:2830-5, 1998.

[133] Park KS, Ciaraldi TP, Abrams-Carter L, Mudaliar S, Nikoulina SE, Henry RR., "Troglitazone regulation of glucose metabolism in human skeletal muscle cultures from obese type II diabetic subjects." *J Clin Endocrinol Metab* 83:1636-43, 1998.

[134] Martens FM, Visseren FL, Lemay J, de Koning EJ, Rabelink TJ, "Metabolic and additional vascular effects of thiazolidinediones." *Drugs* 62:1463-80, 2002

[135] Zhang B, Salituro G, Szalkowski D, Li Z, Zhang Y, Royo I, Vilella D, Diez MT, Pelaez, F, Ruby C, Kendall RL, Mao X, Griffin P, Calaycay J, Zierath JR, Heck JV, Smith RG, Moller DE, "Discovery of a small molecule insulin mimetic with antidiabetic activity in mice." *Science* 284:974-7, 1999.

[136] Li M, Youngren J F, Manchem VP, Kozlowski M, Zhang BB, Maddux BA, Goldfine ID, "Small molecule insulin receptor activators potentiate insulin action in insulin-resistant cells." *Diabetes* 50:2323-8, 2001.

[137] Manchem VP, Goldfine ID, Kohanski RA, Cristobal CP, Lum RT, Schow SR, Shi S, Spevak WR, Laborde E, Toavs DK, Villar HO, Wick MM, Kozlowski MR, "Novel small molecule that directly sensitizes the insulin receptor in vitro and in vivo." *Diabetes* 50:824-30, 2001.

[138] Elchebly M, Payette P, Michaliszyn E, Cromlish W, Collins S, Loy AL, Normandin D, Cheng A, Himms-Hagen J, Chan CC, Ramachandran C, Gresser MJ, Tremblay ML, Kennedy BP, "Increased insulin sensitivity and obesity resistance in mice lacking the protein tyrosine phosphatase-1B gene." *Science* 283:1544-8, 1999.

[139] Cline GW, Johnson K, Regittnig W, Perret P, Tozzo E, Xiao L, Damico C, Shulman GI, "Effects of a novel glycogen synthase kinase-3 inhibitor on insulin-stimulated glucose metabolism in Zucker diabetic fatty (fa/fa) rats." *Diabetes* 51:2903-10, 2002.

[140] Nikoulina SE, Ciaraldi TP, Mudaliar S, Carter L, Johnson K, Henry RR, "Inhibition of glycogen synthase kinase 3 improves insulin action and glucose metabolism in human skeletal muscle." *Diabetes* 51:2190-8, 2002.

[141] Martinez A, Castro A, Dorronsoro I, Alonso M, "Glycogen synthase kinase 3 (GSK-3) inhibitors as new promising drugs for diabetes, neurodegeneration, cancer, and inflammation." *Med Res Rev* 22:373-84, 2002.

[142] Gerich JE: Oral hypoglycemic agents. *N Engl J Med* 321:1231, 1989.

[143] Turner RC, Cull CA, Frighi V, et al: Glycemic control with diet, sulfonylurea, metformin, or insulin in patients with type 2 diabetes mellitus. *JAMA* 281:2005, 1999.

[144] Chang AM, Halter JB: Aging and insulin secretion. *Am J Physiol Endocrinol Metab* 284:E7-12, 2003.

[145] Heine RJ: Role of sulfonylureas in non-insulin-dependent diabetes mellitus: Part II. "The cons." *Horm Metab Res* 28:522,1996.

[146] Riddle MC, McDaniel PA, Tive LA: Glipizide-GITS does not increase the hypoglycemic effect of mild exercise during fasting in NIDDM. *Diabetes Care* 20:992, 1997.

[147] Dills DG, Schneider J: The glimepride/glyburide research group: Clinical evaluation f Glimepiride versus glyburide in NIDDM in a double-blind comparative study. *Hor Metab Res* 28:426, 1996.

[148] University Group Diabetes Program: A study of the effects of hypoglyemic agents on vascular complications in patients with adult-onset diabetes: Mortality results. *Diabetes* 19:785, 1970.

[149] Malaisse WJ. Mechanism of action of a new class of insulin secretagogues. *Exp Clin Endocrinol Diabetes* 107 (Suppl 4):140, 1999.

[150] Hu S, Wang S, Fanelli B, et al. Pancreatic beta-cell K(ATP) channel activity and membrane-binding studies with nateglinide: a comparison with sulfonylureas and repaglinide. *J Pharmacol Exp Ther* 293: 444, 2000.

[151] Damsbo P, Clauson P, Marbury TC, et al. A double-blind randomized comparison of meal-related glycemic control by repaglinide and glyburide in well controlled type 2 diabetic patients. *Diabetes Care* 22:789, 1999.

[152] Jovanovic L, Dailey G III, Huang WC, et al. Repaglinide in type 2 diabetes: a 24 week, fixed-dose efficacy and safety study. *J Clin Pharmacol* 40: 49, 2000..

[153] Keilson L, Mather S, Walter YJ, et al: Synergistic effects of nateglinide and meal administration on insulin secretion in patients with type 2 diabetes mellitus. *J Clin Endocrinol Metab* 85: 1081, 2000.
[154] Marre M, Gall LV, Usadel K, et al.: Nateglinide improves glycemic control when added to metformin monotherapy: results of a randomized trial with type 2 diabetes patients. *Dia Obesity and Metab 4*: 177, 2002.
[155] Bailey CJ: Biguanides and NIDDM. *Diabetes Care* 15:755, 1992.
[156] Lalau JD, Race JM: Lactic acidosis in metformin therapy: searching for a link with metformin in reports of 'metformin-associated lactic acidosis'. *Diabetes Obes Metab* 3:195, 2001.
[157] Spiller HA, Weber JA, Winter ML et al: Multicenter case series of pediatric metformin ingestion. *Ann Pharmacother* 34:1385, 2000.
[158] Fantus IG, Brosseau R: Mecahnism of action of metformin: insulin receptor and postreceptor effects in vitro and in vivo. *J Clin Endocrinol Metab* 63:898, 1986.
[159] Cusi K, DeFronzo RA: Metformin: a review of its metabolic effects. *Diabetes Rev* 6:89, 1998.
[160] Davidson MB, Peters AL: An overview of metformin in the treatment of type 2 diabetes mellitus. *Am J Med* 102:99, 1997.
[161] American Diabetes Association: Type 2 diabetes in children and adolescents (consensus statement). *Diabetes Care* 23:381, 2000.
[162] Bastyr EJ, Stuart CA, Brodows RG, et al.: Therapy focused on lowering postprandial glucose, not fasting glucose, may be superior for lowering HbA1C. *Diabetes Care* 23:1236, 2000.
[163] Lebovitz HE: α-Glucosidase inhibitors as agents in the treatment of diabetes. *Diab Rev 6:*132, 1998.
[164] Hollander P: Safety profile of acarbose, an α-glucosidase inhibitor. *Drugs 44(suppl 2):*47, 1992.
[165] Hoffman J, Spengler M: Efficacy of 24-week monotherapy with acarbose, metformin or placebo in dietary treated NIDDM patients: the Essen-II study. *Am J Med* 103:483, 1997.
[166] Hara T, Nakamura J, Koh N, et al: An importance of carbohydrate ingestion for the expression of the effect of an α-glucosidase inhibitor in NIDDM. *Diabetes Care* 19:642, 1996.
[167] Saltiel AF, Olefsky JM: Thiazolidinediones in the treatment of isuilin resistance and type II diabetes. *Diabetes* 45:1661, 1996.
[168] Olefsky JM: Treatment of insulin resistance with peroxisome proliferators-activated receptors. *J Clin Invest* 106:467, 2000.
[169] Fonseca VA, Valiquett TR, Huang SM, et al: Troglitazone monotherapy improves glycemi control in patients with type 2 diabetes mellitus: a randomized, controlled study. *J Clin Endo Metab* 83:3169, 1998.
[170] Horton ES, Whitehouse F, Ghazzi MN, et al: Troglitazone in combination with sulfonylurea restores glycemic control in patients with type 2 diabetes. *Diabetes Care* 21:1462, 1998.
[171] Schwartz S, Raskin P, Fonseca V, et al: Effect of troglitazone in insulin-treated patients with type II diabetes mellitus. *N Engl J Med* 338:861, 1998.

[172] Fonseca V, Foyt HL, Shen K, Whitcomb RW: Long-term effects of troglitazone: open-label extension studies in type 2 diabetes patients. *Diabetes Care* 23:354, 2000.

[173] Gitlin N, Julie NL, Spurr CL, et al: Two cases of severe clinical and histologic hepatotoxicity associated with troglitazone. *Ann Int Med* 129:36, 1998.

[174] Aronoff S, Rosenblatt S, Braithwaite S, et al, for the Pioglitazone 001 Study Group. Pioglitazone hydrochloride monotherapy improves glycemic control in the treatment of patients with type 2 diabetes: A 6-month randomized placebo-controlled dose-response study. *Diabetes Care* 23:1605, 2000.

[175] Lebovitz HE, Dole JF, Patwardhan R, et al: Rosiglitazone monotherapy is effective in patients with type 2 diabetes. *J Clin Endocrinol Metab* 86:280, 2001.

[176] Parulkar AA, Pendergrass ML, Grnada-Ayala R, et al: Nonhypoglycemic effects of thiazolidinediones. *Ann Intern Med* 135:307, 2001.

[177] Braunstein S: Cardiovascular disease and benefits of thiazolidinediones. *Postgrad Med* Spec No:45-52, 2003.

[178] Plutzky J, Viberti G, Haffner S: Atherosclerosis in type 2 diabetes mellitus and insulin resistance: mechanistic links and therapeutic targets. *J Diabetes Complications* 16:401, 2002.

[179] Patel J, Anderson RJ, Rappaport EB: Rosiglitazone monotherapy imporves glycaemic control in patients with type 2 diabetes: A twelve-week, randomized, placebo-controlled study. *Diabetes Obes Metab.* 1:165, 1999.

[180] Wolffenbuttel BH, Gomis R, SquatritoS, et al: Addition of low-dose rosiglitazone to sulphonylurea therapy improves glycaemic control in type 2 diabetic patients. *Diabetic Med* 17:40, 2000.

[181] Fonseca V, Rosenstock J, Patwardhan R, Salzman A: Effect of metformin and rosiglitazone combination therapy in patients with type 2 diabetes mellitus: a randomized controlled trial. *JAMA* 283:1695, 2000.

[182] Raskin P, Rendell M, Riddle MC, et al: A randomized trial of rosiglitazone therapy in patients with inadequately controlled insulin-treated type 2 diabetes. *Diabetes Care* 24:1226, 2001.

[183] Lebovitz HE, Kreider M, Freed MI: Evaluation of liver function in type 2 diabetic patients during clinical trials: Evidence that rosiglitazone does not cause hepatic dysfunction. *Diabetes Care* 25:815, 2002.

[184] Scheen AJ: Hepatotoxicity with thiazolidinediones: is it a class effect? *Drug Saf* 24:873, 2001.

[185] Tolman KG, Chandramouli J: Hepatotoxicity of the thiazolidinediones. *Clin Liv Dis* 7:369, 2003.

[186] Hamilton J, Cummings E, Zdravkovic et al: Metformin as an adjunct therapy in adolescents with type 1 diabetes and insulin resistance. *Diabetes Care* 26:138, 2003.

[187] DeFronzo RA: Pharmacologic therapy for type 2 diabetes mellitus. *Ann Intern Med* 131:281, 1999.

[188] Feinglos MN, Bethel MA: Oral agent therapy in the treatment of type 2 diabetes. *Diabetes Care 22(Suppl. 3):*C61, 1999.

[189] Buse J: Combining insulin and oral agents. *Am J Med 17(Suppl 6a):*23S, 2000.

[190] Jones KL, Haghi M: Type 2 diabetes mellitus in children and adolescents. *The Endocrinologist* 10:389, 2000.

[191] DeFronzo RA, Matsuda M, Barrett EJ: Diabetic ketoacidosis: a combined metabolic-nephrologic approach to therapy. *Diabetes Rev* 2:209, 1994.

[192] Reaven GM: Role of insulin resistance in human diabetes. *Diabetes* 37:1595,1988.

[193] Koivisto VA: Insulin therapy in type 2 diabetes. *Diabetes Care 16(Suppl. 3):*29, 1993.

[194] Ahmann AJ, Riddle MC, "Insulin therapy in type 2 diabetes mellitus." pp. 113-125. In: *Insulin Therapy*, ed. By Leahy JL and Cefalu WT. Marcel Dekker Inc. New York, New York. 2002.

[195] Kahn SE: The importance of β-cell failure in the development and progression of type 2 diabetes. *J Clin Endo Metab* 86:4047, 2001.

[196] Executive summary of the third report of the national cholesterol education program (NCEP) expert panel on detection, evaluation, and treatment of high blood cholesterol in adults (adult treatment panel III). *JAMA* 285:2846, 2001.

[197] Adler AI, Stratton IM, Neil HA, et al: Association of systolic blood pressure with macrovascular and microvascular complications of type 2 diabetes (UKPDS 36): prospective observational study. *BMJ* 321:412, 2000.

[198] UKPDS 39: UK Prospective Diabetes Study Group. Efficacy of atenolol and captopril in reducing risk of macrovascular and microvascular complications in type 2 diabetes. *BMJ* 317:713, 1998.

[199] UKPDS 38: Tight blood pressure control and risk of macrovascular and microvascular complications in type 2 diabetes. *BMJ* 318:29, 1999.

[200] Jacoby DS, Rader DJ: Renin-angitensin system and atherothrombotic disease: from genes to treatment. *Arch Intern Med* 163:1155, 2003.

[201] Flynn JT: Pharmacologic management of childhood hypertension: Current status, future challenges. *Am J Hypertension* 15:30S, 2002.

[202] Haffner SM, Lehto S, Ronnemaa T, et al. Mortality from coronary heart disease in subjects with type 2 diabetes and in nondiabetic subjects with and without prior myocardial infarction. *N Engl J Med* 339: 229, 1998.

[203] Malmberg K, Yusuf S, Gerstein HC, et al. Impact of diabetes on long-term prognosis in patients with unstable angina and non-Q-wave myocardial infarction : results of the OASIS (Organization to Assess Strategies for Ischemic Syndromes) Registry. *Circulation* 102:1014, 2000.

[204] Herlitz J, Karlson BW, Lindqvist J, et al: Rate and mode of death during five years of follow-up among patients with acute chest pain with and without a history of diabetes mellitus. *Diabet Med.* 15:308,1998.

[205] Newman AB, Siscovick DS, Manolio TA, et al. Ankle-arm index as a marker of atherosclerosis in the Cardiovascular Health Study. *Circulation.* 88P:837, 1993.

[206] Jude EB, Oyibo So, Chalmers N, Boulton AJ. Peripheral arterial disease in diabetic and nondiabetic patients. *Diabetes Care* 24:1433, 2001.

[207] Uusitupa MI, Niskanen LK, Siitonen O, et al: 5 year incidence of atherosclerotic vascular disease in relation to general risk factors, insulin level, and abnormalities in lipoprotein composition in non-insulin dependent diabetic and nondiabetetic subjects. *Circulation.* 82:27, 1990.

[208] Diabetes-related amputations of lower extremities in the Medicare population – Minnesota, 1993-1995. *MMWR Morb Mortal Wkly Rep.* 47:649, 1998.

[209] Jamrozik K, Broadhurst RJ, Forbes S, et al. Predictors of death and vascular events in the elderly. *Stroke.* 31:863, 2000.

[210] Folsom AR, Rasmussen ML, Chambless LE, et al. Prospective associations of fasting insulin, body fat distribution, and diabetes with risk of ischemic stroke. *Diabetes Care.* 22:1077, 1999.
[211] Kuusisto J, Mykkanen L, Pyorala K, et al: Non-insulin dependent diabetes and its metabolic control are important predictors of stroke in elderly subjects. *Stroke.* 25:1157, 1994.
[212] Jorgensen H, Nakayama H, Raaschou HO, et al. Stroke in patients with diabetes: The Copenhagen Stroke Study. *Stroke.* 25:1977, 1994.
[213] Luchsinger JA, Tang MX, Stern Y, et al. Diabetes mellitus and risk of Alzheimer's disease and dementia with stroke in a multiethnic cohort. *Am J Epidemiol.* 154:635, 2001.
[214] Hankey GJ, Jamrozik K, Broadhurst RJ, et al. Long term risk of first recurrent stroke in the Perth Community Stroke Study. *Stroke.* 29:2491, 1998.
[215] Tuomilehto J, Rastenyte D, Jousilahti P, et al. Diabetes mellitus as a risk factor for death from stroke. *Stroke* 27:210, 1996.
[216] Haffner SM, Stern MP, Hazuda HP, et al: Cardiovascular risk factors in confirmed prediabetic individuals: does the clock for coronary heart disease start ticking before the onset of clinical diabetes? *JAMA* 263:2893, 1990.
[217] Apedo MT, Sowers JR, Banerji MA : Cardiovascular disease in adolescents with type 2 diabetes mellitus. *J Pediatr Endocrinol Metab. Suppl 1*:519, 2002.
[218] Taha D: Hyperlipidemia in children with type 2 diabetes mellitus. *J Pediatr Endo Metab* 15:505, 2002.
[219] Palinski W, Napoli C.: Pathophysiological events during pregnancy influence the development of atherosclerosis in humans. *Trends Cardiovasc Med* 9:205-14, 1999.
[220] Napoli C, Glass CK, Witztum JL, et al: Influence of maternal hypercholesterolemia during pregnancy on the progression of early atherosclerotic lesions in childhood: Fate of Early Lesions in Children (FELIC) study. *Lancet* 354:1234, 1999.
[221] Zeiske A, Malcom G, Strong J. Natural History and Risk Factors of Atherosclerosis in children and Youth : The PDAY study. *Pediatr Pathol Mol Med.* 21:213, 2002.
[222] Berenson GS, Wattingney WA, Tracy RE, et al. Atherosclerosis of the aorta and coronary arteries and cardiovascular risk factors in persons aged 6 to 30 years and studied at necropsy (The Bogalusa Heart Study). *Am J Cardiol* 70:851, 1992.
[223] Dean H, Flett B: Natural history of type 2 diabetes diagnosed in childhood: Long term follow-up in young adult years. *Diabetes* 51:A24, 2002.
[224] Newman TB, Garber AM, Holtzman NA, et al: Problems with the report of the Expert Panel on Blood Cholesterol Levels in Children and Adolescents. *Arch Pediatr Adolesc Med* 149:241, 1995.
[225] Haffner SM: Management of dyslipidemia in adults with diabetes (Technical Review). *Diabetes Care* 21:160, 1998.
[226] American Diabetes Association: Management of dyslipidemia in adults with diabetes. *Diabetes Care* 25:S74, 2002.
[227] National Cholesterol Education Program: Report of the Expert Panel on Blood Cholesterol Levels in Children and Adolescents. *Pediatrics* 89:3S 525-584.
[228] Kesaniemi YA, Grundy SM: Influence of gemfibrozil and clofibrate on metabolism of cholesterol and plasma triglycerides in man. *JAMA* 251:2241, 1984 .

[229] Vinik AI, Colwell JA: Hyperlipidemia in Diabetes investigator Study . *Diabetes Care* 16:37, 1993.
[230] Steinmetz J, Morin C, Panek E, et al: Biological variations in hyperlipidemic children and adolescents treated with fenofibrate. *Clin Chim Act* 112:43, 1981.
[231] Buyukcelip M, Anarat A, Bayazit AK, et al: The effects of gemfibrozil in hyperlipidemia in children with persistent nephrotic syndrome. *Turk J Pediatr* 44:40, 2002.
[232] Stein EA, Illingworth DR, Kwiterovich PO, et al. Efficacy and safety of lovastatin in adolescent males with heterozygous familial hypercholesterolemia: a randomized controlled trial. *JAMA*. 281:137, 1999.
[233] Weitz-Schmidt G; Statins as anti-inflammatory agents. *Trends Pharmacol Sci* 23:482, 2002.
[234] Gaede P, Vedel P, Larsen N, et al: Multifactorial intervention and cardiovascular disease in patients with type 2 diabetes. *N Engl J Med* 348:383, 2003.
[235] Jones KL, Dewan A: Type 2 diabetes in adolescence: lipid and cardiovascular risk factors. *Curr Diab Rep* 3:255, 2003.
[236] Glass CK, Witztum JL: Atherosclerosis. The road ahead. *Cell* 104:503, 2001.
[237] Knowler WC, Barrett-Connor E, Fowler SE, et al: Reduction in the incidence of type 2 diabetes with lifestyle intervention or metformin. *N Engl J Med* 346:393, 2002.
[238] Lindstrom J, Erikson JG, Valle TT, et al: Prevention of diabetes mellitus in subjects with impaired glucose tolerance in the finnish diabetes prevention study: results from a randomized clinical trial. *J Am Soc Nephrol 14 (Suppl 2):*S108, 2003.

In: Insulin Resistance in Children and Adolescents ISBN 1-59454-215-5
Editors: D. Daneman and J. Hamilton, pp. 163-178 ©2005 Nova Science Publishers, Inc.

*Chapter 7*

# PREMATURE ADRENARCHE, POLYCYSTIC OVARY SYNDROME (PCOS) AND INSULIN RESISTANCE

***Joan Di Martino-Nardi* and Mireya H. Garcia***

Department of Pediatrics, Division of Pediatric Endocrinology,
Albert Einstein College of Medicine and the Children's Hospital
at Montefiore Medical Center, Bronx, New York

## INTRODUCTION

Polycystic Ovary Syndrome (PCOS) is a syndrome of chronic androgen excess characterized by hirsutism, acne, menstrual irregularities and/or infertility [1]. Hyperinsulinism and insulin resistance are strongly implicated in the etiology of PCOS, and women with PCOS are at increased risk for the complications of the metabolic syndrome.

Polycystic Ovary Syndrome had been described as "...the most common cause of hyperandrogenemia presenting *at or after the onset of puberty*..." [2]. However, more recently, it has been noted that "*...some patients present in mid childhood with premature adrenarche, particularly exaggerated adrenarche, true sexual precocity, overgrowth ..., or obesity....*" [3].

Over the past 10 years, the occurrence of obesity in the pediatric and adult population has increased substantially, with approximately 15% of prepubertal and pubertal children meeting the criteria for obesity [4]. Obesity is an important cause of insulin resistance and the complications of the metabolic syndrome are becoming more common in pediatrics. For example, over the past 10-15 years, the occurrence of type 2 diabetes mellitus in the pediatric population has increased dramatically. Approximately 8-45% of teens with new onset diabetes mellitus have the type 2 variant, with higher occurrences in those centers caring for minority youths [5].

---

* Send correspondence to: Joan DiMartino-Nardi, M.D., Division of Pediatric Endocrinology, Montefiore Medical Center, 111 East 210$^{th}$ Street, Bronx, NY 10467; Tel. (718) 920-4664; Fax (718) 405-5609; email: jdimartino2@aol.com. This study was supported by a generous grant from the Genentech Foundation for Growth and Development.

Type 2 diabetes mellitus is not the only complication of obesity observed in our young patients. Insulin resistance and marked hyperandrogenism have been shown to occur in prepubertal minority group girls (African-American and Caribbean Hispanic) with premature adrenarche [6]. Hence, in these young girls, the modest hyperandrogenism characteristic of premature adrenarche may be a forerunner of adult disease.

## ADRENARCHE

The term "adrenarche" refers to the maturation of the zona reticularis the adrenal glands, and is characterized by the gradual rise in androgen production that occurs normally between 6-8 years of age [7]. In particular, increases in dehydroepiandrosterone (DHEA) and dehydroepiandrosterone sulfate (DHEA-S>50mcg/dl) occur. Clinically, normal adrenarche can result in small but significant increases in growth velocity, and in the appearance of sexual hair growth (pubic hair or pubarche, and axillary hair), acne, and axillary odor after the age of 8 years in girls, and after the age of 9 years in boys. Both ACTH (adrenocorticotropic hormone), and CRH (corticotropin-releasing hormone), as well as insulin and insulin-like growth factors, have been implicated in the control of adrenarche but are not believed to be the sole regulators. Changes in nutritional status with increases in BMI (body mass index), may also have a role in adrenarche [8]. Gonadarche (maturation of the hypothalamic/pituitary/gonadal axis) and adrenarche are independent events controlled by separate mechanisms [9].

## PREMATURE ADRENARCHE

Premature adrenarche refers to the early maturation of the zona reticularis with resultant early appearance of pubic hair (pubarche) in girls before the age of 8 years, and in boys before the age of 9 years [10,11]. Axillary hair, apocrine odor, and acne may or may not be present. Clitoromegaly and penile enlargement are absent, and breast and testicular size remain prepubertal. Small increases in growth velocity and modest advances in bone maturation (within 2 SDs) can also be observed [10,11]. However, the times of initiation of gonadarche and menarche are compatible to population data [10]. Adult heights tend to be above midparental heights. The early appearance of sexual hair growth may herald early puberty or may be the first sign of clinically significant hyperandrogenism derived from a virilizing tumor or an enzymatic defect of steroidogenesis. ACTH testing (Cortrosyn 0.25mg IV with adrenal androgens measured at 0 and 60 minutes) can be performed to distinguish premature adrenarche from an enzymatic defect of steroidogenesis or an adrenal virilizing tumor.

### Premature Adrenarche: A Risk Factor for Adult Disease

Previously, premature adrenarche was thought to be a benign condition. However, recent studies indicate that certain girls with premature adrenarche may be at risk of developing functional ovarian hyperandrogenism, polycystic ovarian syndrome, and the complications of insulin resistance.

The specific etiology of the ovarian and adrenal hyperandrogenism in adolescent and adult woman with PCOS remains elusive. Several factors have been implicated, including hyperinsulinism, alterations of growth factors (IGF-1 and IGF-binding proteins), dysregulation of the hypothalamic-pituitary-ovarian unit, and enzymatic defects of steroidogenesis [12-17].

***Exaggerated Adrenarche***

As noted previously, girls with benign premature adrenarche have been reported to have androgens in the range found in normal children in the early stages of puberty. [7] Although most girls with premature adrenarche have modestly elevated androgens, many *prepubertal* African-American and Caribbean Hispanic girls evaluated have ACTH stimulated levels of 17-hydroxy-pregnenolone (17OHPreg) significantly higher than those reported for *pubertal* children of mixed ethnic background. [18-22] ACTH testing in 72 African-American and Caribbean Hispanic girls with premature adrenarche was compared with those reported for normal girls in early puberty (Figure 1) [25]. Twenty-eight percent were found to have significantly elevated stimulated 17OHPreg levels >2SD units above the mean for normal early pubertal children. The ACTH stimulated ratio of 17OHPreg/17OHProgesterone (17OHProg) also was elevated in 18% of the girls and showed a modest correlation with body mass index. Hyperresponsiveness of ACTH stimulated 17OHPreg has also been described in women with hirsutism or PCOS [23,24]. This similar finding in many African-American and Caribbean Hispanic girls with premature adrenarche suggests that the hyperandrogenism in these girls may be an early presentation of persistent adrenal and ovarian hyperandrogenism.

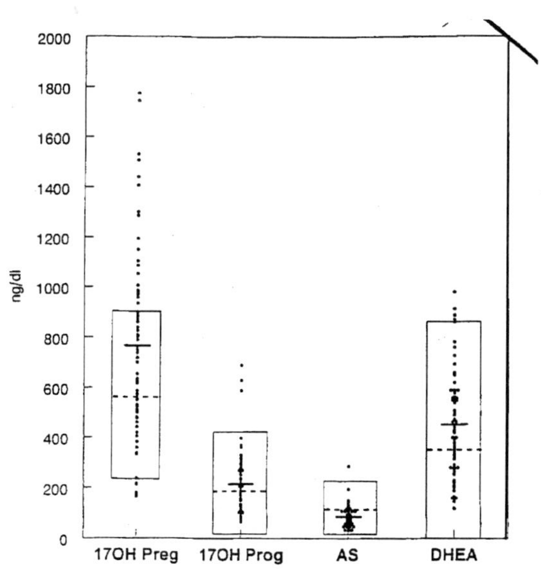


Figure 1. The 60 minute ACTH-stimulated levels of 17 α-hydroxypregnenolone, 17 α-hydoxyprogesterone, DHEA, and androstenedione in prepubertal girls with premature adrenarche. Boxes indicate the 60-minute ACTH-stimulated hormonal data (mean ± 2 SD units) in normal early pubertal girls (Tanner stages II and III). Reprinted with permission from S. Banerjee et. al. *Pediatrics* 1998;102(3) URL: ttp://www.pediatrics. org/cgi/content/full/102/3/c36.

In previous studies of girls of mixed ethnic backgrounds, the exaggerated androgen responsiveness to ACTH stimulation found in 3-13% of girls, was believed to be secondary to a mild defect of the 3β-hydroxysteroid dehydrogenase enzyme (3β-HSD). This pattern of steroid response to ACTH has also been described in women with hirsutism or PCOS who were also designated as having a mild deficiency of 3β-HSD [26-28]. However, studies of the gene encoding this enzyme have not detected an abnormality in either girls with premature adrenarche or women with PCOS with this degree of hyperandrogenism [29,30]. A defect in the gene encoding this particular enzyme was only detected in those patients with delta-5 steroids greater than 10 SD above normal levels. Although a specific etiology is yet to be identified, the hyperandrogenism in a subset of girls with premature adrenarche may persist into adolescence or adulthood and predispose them to hirsutism, acne, menstrual irregularities, polycystic ovarian syndrome, and infertility.

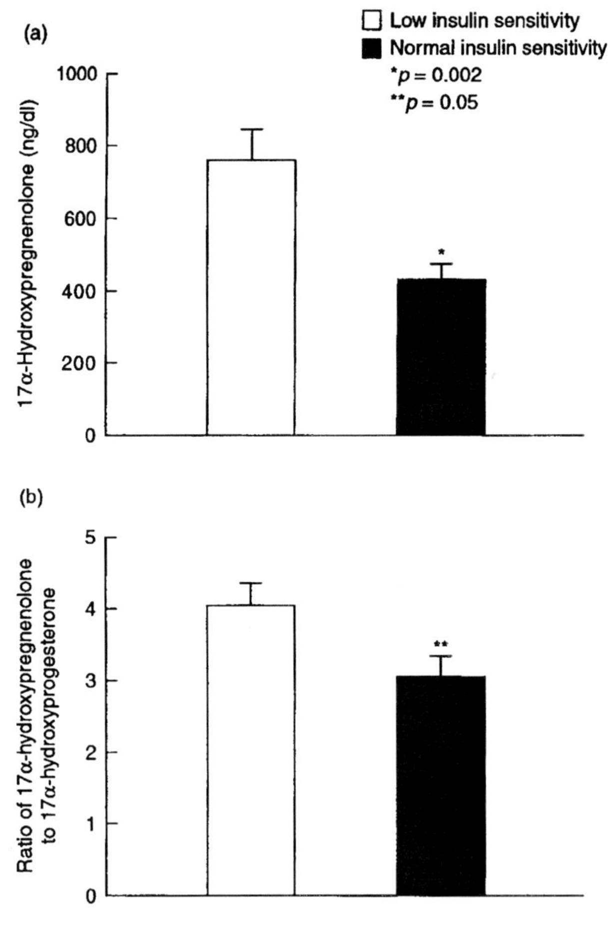


Figure 2. (a) ACTH-stimulated 17α-hydroxypregnenolone level and (b) ratio of 17α-hydroxypregnenolone:17α-hydoxyprogesterone in prepubertal girls with premature adrenarche and either low or normal insulin sensitivity. Reduced insulin sensitivity is associated with a higher 17α-hydroxypregnenolone response and a higher ratio of 17α-hydroxypregnenolone:17α-hydroxyprogesterone. Reprinted with permission from J. DiMartino-Nardi. *Acta Paediatr Suppl* 1999;433:67-72.

***Premature Adrenarche, Acanthosis Nigricans, Insulin Resistance and Alteration of Growth Factors***

Insulin has been shown to directly and indirectly stimulate ovarian and adrenal steroidogenesis; and, IGF-I has also been shown to stimulate adrenal steroidogenesis in vitro [31-34 ]. IGF-I circulates bound to several proteins. By reducing levels of IGFBP-1, insulin potentially increases the bioavailability of IGF-I. Hyperinsulinism further enhances IGF-I induced steroidogenesis by increasing IGF-I production by the liver.

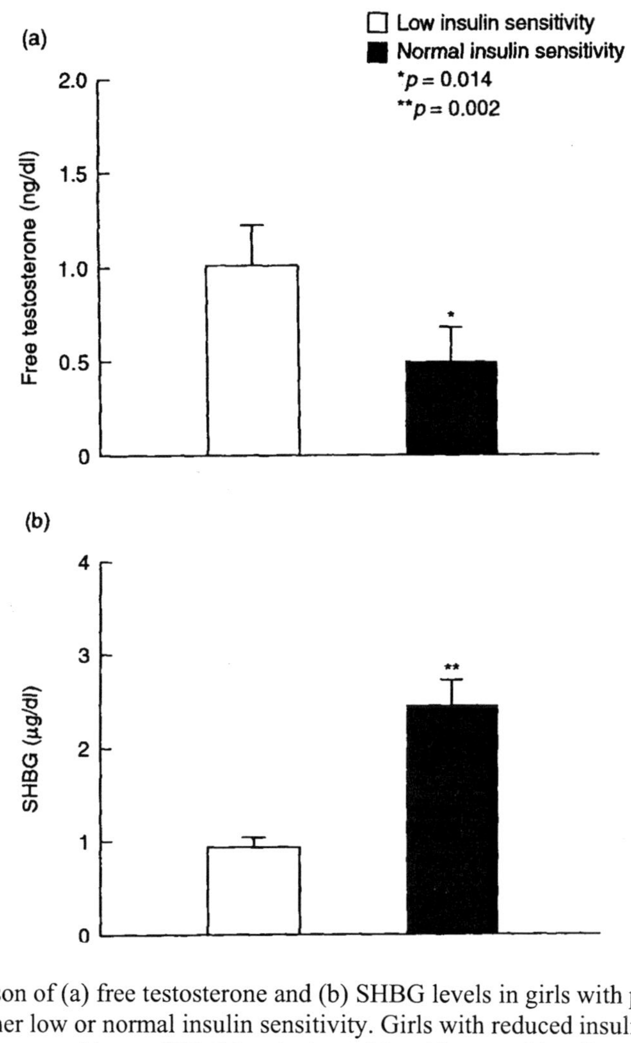


Figure 3. Comparison of (a) free testosterone and (b) SHBG levels in girls with premature adrenarche and either low or normal insulin sensitivity. Girls with reduced insulin sensitivity had higher free testosterone and lower SHBG levels than girls with normal insulin sensitivity. Reprinted with permission from J. DiMartino-Nardi. *Acta Paediatr Suppl* 1999;433:67-72.

The first report linking premature adrenarche and insulin resistance was that of 12 prepubertal African-American and Caribbean Hispanic girls with premature adrenarche. [35] Seven of the 12 girls studied had acanthosis nigricans and hyperinsulinism stemming from reduced insulin sensitivity as determined by the frequently sampled intravenous glucose tolerance test (FSIVGTT). These findings were of particular concern as Caribbean Hispanic women in general are at increased risk of developing polycystic ovarian syndrome, and African-Americans are at increased risk of developing the complications of hyperinsulinism.

As insulin and altered levels of growth factors have been implicated in the severe hyperandrogenism of PCOS, the role of insulin resistance in the hyperandrogenism in premature adrenarche was further assessed in 35 prepubertal minority group (African American and Caribbean Hispanic) girls with premature adrenarche [6]. These young girls with a mean age of 6.8 years underwent the FSIVGTT to assess insulin sensitivity ($S_I$) and 60 minute ACTH testing. Those girls with significantly reduced insulin sensitivity more than 2 SD below the mean for prepubertal girls also had significantly higher ACTH-stimulated levels of 17OHPreg and ratios of 17OHPreg/17OHProg than the girls with normal insulin sensitivity. Those girls with premature adrenarche and reduced insulin sensitivity also had reduced IGFBP-1 levels, higher levels of IGF-I, and higher ACTH-stimulated levels of 17OHPreg and a higher ratio of 17-OHPreg/17-OHProg (Figures 2,3) [36 ]. Higher basal free testosterone and lower SHBG (sex hormone binding globulin) levels also occurred in the more insulin resistant girls. These findings supported the hypothesis that insulin and IGF-I may have a role in the hyperandrogenism of premature adrenarche, just as they do in the more severe hyperandrogenism of PCOS. This is also consistent with the in vitro finding that both insulin and IGF-I augment ACTH-dependent adrenal steroidogenesis in human adrenal cell culture.

***Fasting Glucose: Insulin Ratio and Insulin Sensitivity***

Calculation of insulin sensitivity using the FSIVGTT is labor intensive. Recently, the fasting glucose: insulin ratio has been proposed as a useful screening test for insulin resistance in adult women with PCOS [37]. The glucose: insulin ratio has been compared to the insulin sensitivity determined by the FSIVGTT in girls with premature adrenarche to determine whether the ratio is a useful screening test for insulin resistance in these patients as well. [38]

Insulin sensitivity (SI) correlated significantly with the glucose: insulin ratio ($r=0.76$; $p=0.001$), fasting insulin levels ($r=-0.75$, $p<0.001$), and IGFBP-1 ($r=0.59$; $p=0.005$). No significant correlation was found with fasting glucose levels. Stepwise regression analysis with $S_I$ as the dependent variable, showed that the fasting glucose: insulin ratio was significantly predictive of $S_I$ ($p=0.002$). When viewed as a screening test for insulin resistance in girls with premature adrenarche, setting a value of the fasting glucose (ng/dL): insulin (μU/mL) ratio of less than 7 as abnormal and an $S_I$ less than $5.7\ 10^{-4}$ x $\text{min.}^{-1}$ x $\mu U^{-1}$ x $ml^{-1}$ as evidence of insulin resistance, (normal prepubertal $S_I > 5.7\ 10^{-4}$ x $min^{-1}$ x $\mu U^{-1}$ x $ml^{-1}$), the sensitivity of the fasting glucose: insulin ratio was 86.6%, and the specificity was 88.9%.(Figure 4) [9].

Furthermore, when the girls were divided into two groups based on their glucose: insulin ratio, the girls who were more insulin resistant (glucose: insulin <7) had higher ACTH stimulated levels of 17 OHPreg, free testosterone and lower sex hormone binding globulin (SHBG) levels. Fasting insulin levels were higher and IGFBP-1 levels were lower in the girls with the glucose: insulin ratio <7. Hence, a fasting glucose: insulin ratio < 7 is useful for identifying insulin resistance in Caribbean Hispanic and African-American prepubertal girls with premature adrenarche. This ratio may be a simple screening test that will help to identify the subset of girls with premature adrenarche who may have an increased risk of developing later complications of hyperinsulinemia.

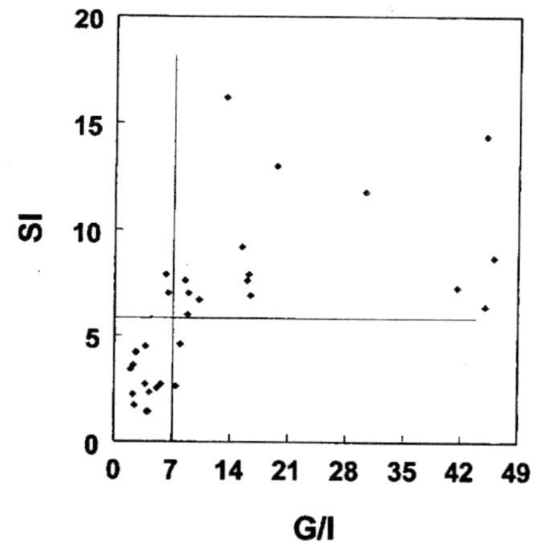


Figure 4. Regression plot of fasting glucose to insulin (G/I) ratio to insulin sensitivity ($S_I$ $10^{-4}$ x $min^{-1}$ x $\mu U^{-1}$ x $mL^{-1}$) as determined by FSIVGTT in prepubertal Caribbean Hispanic and African American girls with premature adrenarche. Reprinted with permission from P. Vuguin et. al. J *Clin Endocrinol Metab* 2001;86:4618-4621.

***Pre and Post Pubertal Findings in Premature Adrenarche***

Caribbean Hispanic and African-American subjects, in general, are at increased risk of obesity and the complications of hyperinsulinism stemming from insulin resistance. Of concern is that nearly 50% of the 35 prepubertal African-American and Caribbean Hispanic girls with premature adrenarche studied as young as 5 years of age had a significant decrease in their insulin sensitivity as assessed by the FSIVGTT [6]. These young girls were also noted to have levels of HDL cholesterol that were significantly lower than those measured in their insulin sensitive peers. Furthermore, the pattern of hyperandrogenism as well as the lower levels of SHBG and higher levels of free testosterone in these very young insulin resistant girls were similar to the observations reported in adult women with PCOS. These findings suggest that careful follow-up of African-American and Caribbean Hispanic girls is indicated.

Hyperinsulinemia (as assessed by mean serum insulin calculated after an oral glucose tolerance test) has also been reported in lean girls from Europe with premature adrenarche before and during pubertal development [39]. In postpubertal girls with a history of premature adrenarche, hyperinsulinemia was directly related to the degree of ovarian hyperandrogenism (assessed by the GnRH challenge test) [40]. Studies of 60-first degree relatives belonging to nine families with two affected adolescents have shown an increased prevalence of both type 2 diabetes mellitus and impaired glucose tolerance [41]. Throughout puberty, serum triglycerides have been found to be higher in those girls with premature adrenarche when compared with a Tanner stage- and age-matched control population. [42]

In adult women with PCOS, the administration of the GnRH-agonist, nafarelin, elicits pituitary-gonadal responses that are similar to those found in normal men and different from the response elicited in normal women [43]. Ibanez *et al.* assessed the ovarian response to challenge with the GnRH-agonist leuprolide acetate in 35 adolescents a with history of premature adrenarche who were at least 3 years beyond menarche [44]. Sixteen had clinical evidence of hyperandrogenism (hirsutism and oligomenorrhea) and had elevated baseline testosterone and/or androstenedione levels. Forty-five percent of the girls tested had a response to GnRH agonist challenge suggestive of functional ovarian hyperandrogenism.

Furthermore, this pattern of ovarian androgen hyperresponsiveness began early in puberty; became most evident during mid and late puberty, and was characterized by higher basal, peak, and incremental responses of most steroid precursors to GnRH agonist testing [45]. In addition, levels of DHEA-S and androstenedione at the time of initial evaluation of premature adrenarche correlated positively with GnRH stimulated levels of 17-OHProgesterone, done postpubertally [44].

In preliminary studies of adolescent girls whose premature adrenarche had been evaluated previously, those adolescent girls who returned with symptoms of hyperandrogenism (hirsutism, acne, menstrual irregularities) had significantly higher BMI, waist/hip ratio, ACTH stimulated androgens, and a higher mean insulin level during the OGTT than did their peers without symptoms of hyperandrogenism [46]. Those adolescent girls who returned with symptoms of hyperandrogenism also had higher ACTH stimulated androgens at the time of their initial evaluation of premature adrenarche.

Reevaluation of adrenal function in postpubertal girls from Europe with a history of premature adrenarche has also shown an increased incidence of idiopathic functional adrenal hyperandrogenism with an exaggerated DHEA, 17-OHPreg, and androstenedione response to ACTH stimulation [7].

***Relationship of Birth Weight, BMI and Insulin Sensitivity***

Children born small for gestational age have been reported to have insulin resistance and premature adrenarche [47]. It has been hypothesized that the hyperandrogenism and hyperinsulinism of premature adrenarche may have common origins in early gestation and are the result of reduced fetal weight. Recently, Ibáñez *et al.* reported that prenatal growth restriction is most pronounced in those girls with premature adrenarche, hyperinsulinism and ovarian hyperandrogenism during adolescence [47]. Ibáñez *et al.* hypothesized that perhaps the fetal undernutrition may modulate adrenarche as well as insulin sensitivity.

The association of birth weight and BMI with insulin sensitivity has also been evaluated in 22 African-American and 30 Caribbean-Hispanic patients with premature adrenarche [48]. The birth weights of these 52 prepubertal, full-term girls with premature adrenarche were compared with 970 ethnically matched controls (Cazano C., personal communication). The level of insulin sensitivity, calculated from the FSIVGTT, was available for 25 of the 52 patients.

The mean birth weight of the 52 girls with premature adrenarche was significantly lower than the birth weights of the normal controls. Furthermore, in the group of Caribbean-Hispanic patients, the birth weights of the patients with reduced insulin sensitivity was less than that of those girls with normal insulin sensitivity and of the control population. Only 6 African-American girls underwent the FSIVGTT, so a comparison of birth weight and insulin sensitivity could not be obtained.

In contrast, in Ghizzoni's study of 38 girls from Italy with premature adrenarche, birth weight did not differ from that of normal controls [49]. Also, in a study by Léger [50], hyperandrogenism was not detected in a large cohort (n=130) of women from France born small for gestational age.

Hence, the occurrence of premature adrenarche in many minority group girls may represent an early clinical manifestation of the insulin resistance syndrome. As many factors contribute to the development of insulin resistance, (i.e. obesity, genetics, birth weight, disturbed lipid metabolism), all of these may contribute to the development of premature adrenarche as well.

### Premature Adrenarche in Boys

Adrenarche in boys has not been shown to be associated with the cluster of abnormalities and reduced fetal growth as noted in girls [51].

## Polycystic Ovarian Syndrome and Insulin Resistance

The association of hirsutism, amenorrhea and enlarged multicystic ovaries was first described in 1935 by Stein and Leventhal [52]. It is now recognized as polycystic ovarian syndrome (PCOS), characterized by chronic anovulation and hyperandrogenism in the absence of hypothalamo-pituitary dysfunction, and ovarian or adrenal disease. Common hormonal derangements include hyperinsulinism, increased LH, with an increased LH:FSH ratio, normal or elevated estradiol levels and decreased SHBG. The radiographic evidence of "polycystic ovaries" need not be present. Other features include obesity, acne and acanthosis nigricans. Signs of androgen excess (seborrhea, acne, hirsutism, alopecia) are evident, although some women may not develop them due to ethnic differences in androgen sensitive target tissues [53]. The relationship between insulin resistance and PCOS has been suggested [54]. Studies have demonstrated improvement in PCOS related symptoms with the use of insulin sensitizing medications (such as Metformin) [55].

This relationship can very well explain the high risk of impaired glucose tolerance (IGT) and most likely Type 2 diabetes mellitus (T2DM) in this population.

### Pathogenesis of Insulin Resistance in Adolescents with PCOS

The etiology of insulin resistance in PCOS is not completely understood. Insulin resistance has been attributed to form part of this syndrome, although it may not be proven in all women with PCOS. Studies have demonstrated disturbances in insulin sensitivity in non-obese PCOS women [56]. The presence of obesity may exacerbate the manifestation of insulin resistance, although a decrease in weight in some cases does not improve the hyperinsulinism observed in PCOS. [57] The human ovary expresses receptors for insulin and insulin-like-growth factor I (IGF-I); this characteristic may explain why hyperinsulinism may contribute to the excess ovarian androgen production seen in PCOS. [58] Studies aimed at reducing hyperandrogenemia have failed to improve insulin sensitivity, leaning towards the hypothesis of hyperinsulinism as the basic metabolic derangement in polycystic ovarian syndrome [59].

### Insulin Sensitivity in PCOS

Hyperinsulinemia reflects peripheral insulin resistance in women with PCOS, an entity well recognized for more than 20 years. Dunaif *et al.* found that obese PCOS women (mean age 27 years), had increased glucose levels during an oral glucose tolerance test (OGTT) when compared to controls. Twenty percent of this cohort had an impaired glucose tolerance (IGT) or frank Type 2 diabetes mellitus [60]. Legro and colleagues later demonstrated an increased risk for IGT and Type 2 diabetes in a cohort of white non-hispanic, Caribbean Hispanic and African American obese and non-obese women with PCOS, when compared to controls matched by age, weight and ethnicity. It was noted that although PCOS along with age and obesity places these women at greater risk for IGT and diabetes, it can also occur in young non-obese PCOS women as well [61].

Insulin sensitivity and secretion in young adolescents has been investigated by Lewy *et al.* [62] In this cohort, young obese adolescent girls, with mean age of 12 years, and with childhood onset of PCOS, were compared to obese but nonhyperandrogenic girls. Hyperinsulinemic-euglycemic clamps to measure insulin sensitivity, and hyperglycemic clamps to determine insulin secretion were performed in both groups. PCOS girls had a 50% reduction in peripheral tissue insulin sensitivity and compensatory hyperinsulinism when compared to obese nonhyperandrogenic controls, placing them at an increased risk for T2DM. Despite the increased insulin production in the PCOS group, hepatic glucose production was similar in both groups, validating the existence of hepatic insulin resistance as well.

## Role of Insulin Resistance and ß-cell Dysfunction in PCOS

The involvement of insulin resistance and pancreatic insulin secretion in the pathogenesis of glucose intolerance in obese PCOS adolescents was recently evaluated [63]. Clamp studies performed in this population (mean age of 13 years), revealed no difference in fasting insulin and glucose levels between PCOS subjects with impaired glucose tolerance, compared to PCOS patients with normal glucose tolerance (NGT). However, hepatic glucose production was higher in the IGT group. Insulin-stimulated glucose disposal and insulin sensitivity were similar between the 2 groups. First phase insulin was lower in the IGT group, but no difference was noted in the second phase insulin concentration for both groups. These findings underscore the significance of insulin resistance and compensated abnormal insulin secretion in obese adolescents with PCOS, leading to the early development of impaired glucose tolerance, and increasing the risk for T2DM as ß-cell function deteriorates.

## Prevalence of Insulin Resistance and Glucose Intolerance

The prevalence of glucose intolerance and type 2 diabetes in adults with PCOS is estimated to be between 30-40%. A recent study showed this to be true for both lean and obese adolescents with PCOS. [64] A cohort of 27 adolescents with PCOS (ages 13.9-19.1 years), of white non- hispanic, Hispanic, and African American ethnic backgrounds, underwent an OGTT to determine the prevalence of IGT and DM. Thirty-three percent of the subjects had an abnormal glucose tolerance test. There was no significant difference with regards to ethnicity between the groups with normal and abnormal results. Although fasting plasma glucose has been suggested as a screening tool to detect glucose intolerance in PCOS subjects, a fasting plasma glucose was a poor predictor of abnormal glucose tolerance. The 2-hour glucose sample was better in detecting glucose intolerance in this high risk population.

## Metformin Therapy in PCOS and Impaired Glucose Tolerance

Metformin treatment has been shown to be beneficial without significant side effects in a group of fifteen obese adolescents with PCOS treated for three months. Arslanian and colleagues demonstrated a post-treatment increase in glucose disposal as well as a decrease in 2- hour plasma glucose in these subjects, and an improvement in glucose intolerance in eight subjects. Menstrual cycles improved in 40% of the cases studied. Furthermore, there was a decrease in androgen levels in response to ACTH stimulation. ACTH stimulated levels of androstenedione, 17OHProg and 17OHPreg levels were lower post treatment, supporting the role of insulin-sensitizing therapy in decreasing adrenal and ovarian hyperandrogenism in PCOS. Metformin was helpful in ameliorating insulin resistance, decreasing fasting insulin and improving glucose tolerance [65]. Ibáñez and co-workers used a combination of flutamide (an antiandrogen) and metformin in 30 non-obese teenage girls, (age range 13.6-18.6 years), with PCOS. After 9 months of treatment a significant decrease of body fat and increased lean body mass was observed. Ovulation rate increased as well. Similar findings have been noted with metformin monotherapy, but to a lesser effect. Androgen levels decreased in addition to the improvement of hirsutism [66]. Recently, Ibáñez completed a 12 month prevention study of low birth weight, lean adolescents with a history of precocious pubarche, at risk for PCOS, and demonstrated amelioration of signs of hyperinsulinism and hyperandrogensim with metformin therapy compared to untreated controls [67]. Further prospective observation will be required to determine if the metformin actually prevents PCOS in this at-risk cohort.

These studies further imply the significance of hyperinsulinism as the culprit of the ensuing hyperandrogenism evident in PCOS.

# CONCLUSION

Although premature adrenarche has been thought to be a benign normal variant of puberty, studies of minority group girls from the United States and European girls from Italy and Spain indicate that for certain girls, premature adrenarche represents an early clinical presentation of the insulin resistance syndrome. Furthermore, studies of young girls with premature adrenarche provide the opportunity to elucidate the early mechanisms involved in the development of PCOS. Hyperinsulinism stemming from insulin resistance and premature adrenarche may have a common underlying pathogenic mechanism or perhaps the hyperinsulinism itself stimulates both ovarian and adrenal steroidogenesis with resultant ovarian and adrenal hyperandrogenism. Perhaps the early identification of these patients will permit early therapy, such as lifestyle changes, including dietary and activity intervention, and, possibly the use of insulin sensitizing therapy. Normalization of hyperandrogenism, hirsutism, hyperinsulinism, and ovulation in PCOS teens with an insulin sensitizer, such as metformin, underlines the importance of insulin resistance, with compensated hyperinsulinism as the common denominator in PCOS. Obesity plays an important role, but insulin resistance may be present in the absence of increased body weight. With glucose intolerance as a prelude to type 2 diabetes mellitus, adolescents with PCOS are at an increased risk for many other associated metabolic co-morbidities. The health ramifications implied strongly support the need for future studies to discern the usefulness of insulin sensitizers in this at-risk young population.

## References


[1] Dunaif A. Insulin resistance and the polycystic ovary syndrome: mechanism and implications for pathogenesis. *Endocr Rev* 1997;18:774-800.

[2] Rosenfield RL. The ovary and female sexual maturation. In: *Sperling M. Pediatric Endocrinology:* W.B. Saunders 1996: 329-385.

[3] Rosenfield RL. Puberty in the female and its disorders. In: *Sperling M. Pediatric Endocrinology:* W.B. Saunders 2002: 455-518.

[4] NCHS, CDC: Prevalence of overweight among children and adolescents. United States, 1999 [Internet]. Available from *www.cdc.gov/nchs/ products/pubs/pubd/ hestats/ over99fig1.htm.*

[5] Rosenbloom AL, Joe JR, Young RS, Winter WE. Emerging epidemic of type 2 diabetes in youth. *Diabetes Care* 1999;22:345-354.

[6] Vuguin P, Linder B, Rosenfeld RG, Saenger P, DiMartino-Nardi J. The role of insulin sensitivity, insulin-like growth factor and insulin-like growth factor binding proteins 1 and 3 in the hyperandrogenism of African-American and Caribbean Hispanic girls with premature adrenarche. *JCEM* 1999;84:2037-2042.

[7] Ibáñez L, DiMartino-Nardi J, Potau N, Saenger P. Premature adrenarche–normal variant or forerunner of adult disease. Endrocrine Reviews 2000;21: 671-696.

[8] Remer T, Marz F. Role of nutritional status in the regulation of adrenarche. *J Clin Endocrinol Metab* 1999;84:3936-3944.

[9] Sklar CA, Kaplan SI, Grumbach MM. Evidence of dissociation between adrenarche and gonadarche:studies in patients with idiopathic precocious puberty, gonadal dysgenesis, isolated gonadotropin deficiency, and constitutionally delayed growth and development. *J Clin Endocrinol Metab* 1980;51:548-556.

[10] Ibáñez L, Virdis R, Potau N, Zampolli M, Ghizzoni L, Albisu MA, Carrascosa A, Bernasconi S, Vicens-Calvet E. Natural history of premature pubarche: an auxological study. *J Clin Endocrinol Metab* 1992;74:254-257.

[11] Pere A, Voutilainen R, Perheentupa A, Peter M. Follow-up of growth and steroids in premature adrenarche. *Eur J Pediatr* 1995;154:346-352.

[12] Giudice L. The insulin like growth factor system in normal and abnormal human ovarian follicle development. *Am J Med* 1995:1A485-1A535.

[13] Voutilainen R, Franks S, Mason H, Martikainen H. Expression of insulin like growth factor (IGF) IGF-binding protein and IGF-receptor messenger ribonucleic acids in normal and polycystic ovaries. *J Clin Endocrinol Metab* 1996;81:1003-1008.

[14] Rosenfield RL. Evidence that idiopathic functional adrenal hyperandrogenism is caused by dysregulation of adrenal steroidogenesis and that hyerinsulinemia may be involved. Editorial. *J Clin Endocrinol Metab* 1996;81:878-880.

[15] Nestler JE, Clore JN, Blackard WG. The central role of obesity (hyperinsulinemia) in the pathogenesis of polycystic ovary syndrome. Am J Obs Gyn 1989;161:1095-2097.

[16] Ibáñez L, Potau N, Zampolli M et al. Hyperinsulinemia in postpubertal girls with a history of premature pubarche and functional ovarian hyperandrogenism. *J Clin Endocrinol Metab* 1996;81:1237-1243.

[17] Apter D, Butzow T, Laughlin GA, Yen SSC. Accelerated 24-hour luteinizing hormone pulsatile activity in adolescent girls with ovarian hyperandrogenism: relevance to the development phase of polycystic ovarian syndrome. *J Clin Endocrinol Metab* 1994;79:119-125.

[18] Temeck JW, Pang S, Nelson C, New MI. Genetic defects of steroidogenesis in premature pubarche. *J Clin Endocrinol Metab* 1987;64:609-617.

[19] Morris AH, Reiter EO, Geffner ME, Lippe BM, Itami RM, Mayes DM. Absence of nonclassical congenital adrenal hyperplasia in patients with precocious adrenarche. *J Clin Endocrinol Metab* 1989;69:709-715.

[20] Hawkins LA, Chasalow FI, Blethen SL. The role of adrenocorticotrophin testing in evaluating girls with premature adrenarche and hirsutism/oligomenorrhea. *J Clin Endocrinol Metab* 1992;64:248-253.

[21] Siegel SF, Finegold DN, Urban MD, McVie R, Lee PA. Premature adrenarche: etiological heterogeneity. *J Clin Endocrinol Metab* 1992; 74:239-247.

[22] Oberfield SE, Mayes DM, Levine LS. Adrenal steroidogenic function in a Black and Hispanic population with precocious pubarche. *J Clin Endocrinol Metab* 1990;70:76-82.

[23] Lachelin GCL, Barnett M, Hopper BR, Brink G, Yen SSC. Adrenal function in normal women and women with the polycystic ovarian syndrome. *J Clin Endocrinol Metab* 1979;49:892-898.

[24] McKenna TJ, Miller RB, Liddle GW. Plasma pregnenolone and 17-OH Pregnenolone in patients with adrenal tumors, ACTH excess or iodiopathic hirsutism. *J Clin Endocrinol Metab* 1977;44:231-236.

[25] Banerjee S, Raghavan S, Wasserman EJ, Linder B, Saenger P, DiMartino-Nardi J. Hormonal findings in African-American and Caribbean Hispanic Girls with Premature Adrenarche: Implications for Polycystic Ovarian Syndrome. Pediatrics 1998;102(3) URL: *http://www.pediatrics.org/cgi/content/full/102/3/c36.*

[26] Lucky AW, Rosenfield RL, McGuire J, Rudy S, Helke J. Adrenal androgen hyper-responsiveness to adrenocorticotropin in women with acne and/or hirsutism: adrenal enzyme defects and exaggerated adrenarche. *J Clin Endocrinol Metab* 1986;62:840-848.

[27] Lobo RA, Goebelsmann U. Evidence for reduced 3-β-ol-hydroxysteroid dehydrogenase activity in some hirsute women thought to have polycystic ovary syndrome. *J Clin Endocrinol Metab* 1981;53:394-400.

[28] Pang S, Lerner AJ, Stoner E, et al. Late-onset adrenal steroid 3β-hydroxysteroid dehydrogenase deficiency. A cause of hirsutism in pubertal post pubertal women. *J Clin Endocrinol Metab* 1985;60:428-439.

[29] Chang YT, Zhang L, Alkaddour HS, et al. Absence of molecular defect in the type II 3β-HSD gene in premature pubarche children and hirsute female patients with moderately decreased adrenal 3β-HSD activity. *Pediatr Res* 1995;37:820-824.

[30] Sakkal-Alkaddour H, Zhang L, Yang X, et al. Studies of 3β-hydroxysteroid dehydrogenase genes in infants and children manifesting premature pubarche and

increased adrenocorticotropin stimulated delta 5-steroid levels. *J Clin Endocrinol Metab* 1996;81:3961-3965.

[31] Bianchi P, Toscano V, Monaco G, Marano G, Lubrano C, Sciarra F. Effects of ACTH, insulin and insulin like growth factor I on guinea pig adrenal fasciculata-glomerulosa cells [Abstract]. *J Endocrinol Invest* 1993;16:88.

[32] Hernandez ER, Resnick CE, Holtzclaw WD, Payne D, Adashi E. Insulin as a regulator of androgen biosynthesis by cultured rat ovarian cells: cellular mechanism(s) underlying physiological and pharmacological hormonal actions. *Endocrinology* 1988;122:2034-2043.

[33] Barbieri RL, Makris A, Randall RW, Daniels G, Kistner RW, Ryan KJ. Insulin stimulates androgen accumulations in incubations of ovarian stroma obtained from woman with hyperandrogenism. *J Clin Endocrinol Metab* 1986;62:904-910.

[34] Poretsky L, Kalin MF. The gonadotropic functions of insulin. Endocr Rev 1987;8:132-141.

[35] Oppenheimer E, Linder B, DiMartino-Nardi J. Decreased insulin sensitivity in prepubertal girls with premature adrenarche and acanthosis nigricans. *J Clin Endocrinol Metab* 1995;80:614-618.

[36] DiMartino-Nardi J. Premature adrenarche: findings in prepubertal African-American and Caribbean-Hispanic girls. *Acta Paediatr Suppl* 1999;433:67-72.

[37] Legro RS, Finegood DT, Dunaif A. A fasting glucose to insulin ratio is a useful measure of insulin sensitivity in women with polycystic ovary syndrome. *J Clin Endocrinol Metab* 1998;83:2964-2968.

[38] Vuguin P, Saenger P, DiMartino-Nardi J. Fasting glucose insulin ratio: a useful measure of insulin resistance in girls with premature adrenarche. *J Clin Endocrinol Metab* 2001;86:4618-4621.

[39] Ibáñez L, Potau N, Zampolli M, Rique S, Saenger P, Carrascosa A. Hyperinsulinemia and decreased insulin-like growth factor binding protein-1 are common features in prepubertal and postpubertal girls with a history of premature pubarche. *J Clin Endocrinol Metab* 1997;82:2283-2288

[40] Ibáñez L, Potau N, Zampolli M, Prat N, Virdis R, Vicens-Calvet E, Carrascosa A. Hyperinsulinemia in postpubertal girls with a history of premature pubarche and functional ovarian hyperandrogenism.. *J Clin Endocrinol Metab* 1996;81:1237-1243.

[41] Ibáñez L, Castell C, Tesserras R, Potau N. Increased prevalence of unknown type 2 diabetes mellitus and impaired glucose tolerance in first-degree relatives of girls with a history of precocious pubarche. *Clin Endocrinol* 1999;51:395-401.

[42] Ibáñez L, Potau N, Chacon P, Pascual C, Carrascosa A. Hyperinsulinemia, dyslipidemia and cardiovascular risk in girls with a history of premature pubarche. *Diabetologia* 1998;41:1057-1063.

[43] Barnes RB, Rosenfield RL, Burnstein S. Ehrmann DA. Pituitary-ovarian responses to nafarelin testing in the polycystic ovary syndrome. *N Engl J Med* 1989;320:559-565.

[44] Ibáñez L, Potau N, Virdis R, Zampolli M, Terzi C, Gussinyé M, Carrascosa A, Vicens-Calvet E. Postpubertal outcome in girls diagnosed of premature pubarche during childhood: increase frequency of functional ovarian hyperandrogenism. *J Clin Endocrinol Metab* 1993;76:1599-1603.

[45] Ibáñez L, Potau N, Sample M, Street ME, Carrascosa A. Girls diagnosed with premature pubarche show an exaggerated ovarian androgen synthesis from the early

stages of puberty: evidence from gonadotropin-releasing hormone agonist testing. *Fertil Steril* 1997;67:849-855.

[46] DiMartino-Nardi J. Pre- and postpubertal findings in premature adrenarche. *J Ped Endocrinol Metab* 2000;13:1265-1269.

[47] Ibáñez L, Potau N, Francois I, de Zegher F. Precocious pubarche, hyperinsulinism and ovaria*n hyperandrogenism in girls: relation to reduced fetal growth.* J Clin Endocrinol Metab 1998;83:3558-3562.

[48] Grinstein GP, Vuguin P, Saenger P, DiMartino-Nardi J. The relationship between birth weight (BW), body mass index (BMI) and insulin sensitivity ($S_I$) in prepubertal Caribbean Hispanic (CH) and Black African-American (BAA) girls with premature adrenarche. *Pediatric Research* 1999; 45:89A.

[49] Ghizzoni L, Milani S. The natural history of premature adrenarche. *J Pediatr Endocrinol Metab* 2000;13:1247-1251.

[50] Jaquet D, Léger J, Chevenne D, Czernichow P, Levy-Marchal C. Intrauterine growth retardation predisposes to insulin resistance but not to hyperandrogenism in young women. *J Clin Endocrinol Metab* 1999;84:3945-3949.

[51] Potau N, Ibáñez L, Sanchez-Ufarte C, Rique S, de Zegher F. Pronounced adrenarche and precocious pubarche in boys. *Horm Res* 1999;51:238-241.

[52] Stein I, Leventh*al* M. Amenorrhea associated with bilateral polycystic ovaries. *Am J Obstet Gynecol* 1935;29:181-191.

[53] Carmina E, Koyama T, Chang L, Stanczyk FZ, Lobo RA. Does ethnicity influence the prevalence of adrenal hyperandrogenism and insulin resistance in polycystic ovary syndrome. *Am J Obstet Gynecol* 1992;167:1807-1812.

[54] Burghen GA, Givens JR, Kitabchi AE. Correlation of hyperandrogenism with hyperinsulinism in polycystic ovarian disease. *J Clin Endocrinol Metab* 1980;50:113-116.

[55] Lord JM, Flight IH, Norman RJ. Metformin in polycystic ovary syndrome: systematic review and meta-analysis. *Bmj.* Oct 25 2003;327(7421):951-953.

[56] Dunaif A, Segal KR, Futterweit W, Dobrjansky A. Profound peripheral *insulin resistance independent of obesity, in polycystic ovary syndrome. Diabetes* 1989;38:1165-1174.

[57] Robinson S, Chan SP, Spacey S, Anyaoku V, Johnston DG, Franks S. Postprandial thermogenesis is reduced in polycystic ovary syndrome and is associated with increased insulin resistance. *Clin Endocrinol* 1992;36:537-543.

[58] Franks S, Gilling-Smith C, Watson H, Willis D. Insulin action in the normal and polycystic ovary. *Endocrinol Metab Clin North Am* 1999;28:361-378.

[59] Diamanti-Kandarakis E, Mitrakou A, Hennes MMI, Platanissiotis D, Kaklas N, Spina J, Georgiadou E, Hoffmann RG, Kissebah AH, Raptis S. *Insulin sensitivity and antiandrogenic therapy in women with polycystic ovary syndrome* 1995;44:525-531.

[60] Dunaif A, Graf M, Mandeli J, Laumas V, Dobrjansky A. Characterization of groups of hyperandrogenic women with acanthosis nigricans, impaired glucose tolerance an/or hyperinsulinemia. *J Clin Endocrinol Metab* 1987;65:499-507.

[61] Legro RS, Kunselman AR, Dodson WC, Dunaif A. Prevalence and predictors of risk for type 2 diabetes mellitus and impaired glucose tolerance in polycystic ovary syndrome: A prospective, controlled study in 254 affected women. *J Clin Endocrinol Metab* 1999;84:402-408.

[62] Lewy V, Danadian K, Witchel SF, Arslanian SA. Early metabolic abnormalities in adolescent girls with polycystic ovarian syndrome. *J Pediatr* 2001;138:38-44.
[63] Arslanian SA, Lewy V, Danadian K. Glucose intolerance in obese adolescents with polycystic ovary syndrome: Role of insulin resistance and ß-cell dysfunction and risk of cardiovascular disease. *J Clin Endocrinol Metab* 2001;86:66-71.
[64] Palmert MR, Gordon CM, Kartashov AI, Legro RS, Emans SJ, Dunaif A. Screening for abnormal glucose tolerance in adolescents with polycystic ovary syndrome. *J Clin Endocrinol Metab* 2002;87:1017-1023.
[65] Arslanian SA, Lewy V, Danadian K, Saad R. Metformin therapy in obese adolescents with polycystic ovary syndrome and impaired glucose tolerance: amelioration of exaggerated adrenal response to adrenocorticotropin with reduction of insulinemia/insulin resistance. *J Clin Endocrinol Metab* 2002;87:1555-1559.
[66] Ibáñez L, Ong K, Ferrer A, Amin R, Dunger D. Low dose flutamide-metformin therapy reverses insulin resistance and reduces fat mass in nonobese adolescents with ovarian hyperandrogenism. *J Clin Endocrinol Metab* 2002;88:2600-2606.
[67] Ibanez L, Ferrer A, Ong K, Amin R, Dunger D, de Zegher F. Insulin sensitization early after menarche prevents progression from precocious pubarche to polycystic ovary syndrome. *J Pediatr.* Jan 2004;144(1):23-29.)

In: Insulin Resistance in Children and Adolescents ISBN 1-59454-215-5
Editors: D. Daneman and J. Hamilton, pp. 179-208 ©2005 Nova Science Publishers, Inc.

*Chapter 8*

# INSULIN RESISTANCE IN TYPE 1 DIABETES AND OTHER CONDITIONS

***Judith Simoneau-Roy, Denis Daneman and Jill Hamilton***
University of Toronto

## INTRODUCTION

Insulin resistance (IR) can be defined as a subnormal glucose response to endogenous or exogenous insulin. It is most often considered in relation to common disease states associated with obesity, such as type 2 diabetes, hypertension, polycystic ovarian syndrome and the metabolic syndrome and primarily affecting adults. However, IR has been increasingly identified as an integral component a wide spectrum of disorders affecting children, and, more particularly adolescents (see chapters 5,6,7). In this chapter, we highlight the evidence for insulin resistance in other specific medical conditions affecting youth, namely type 1 diabetes, cystic fibrosis, survivors of childhood cancer thalassemia major and genetic and acquired syndromes of insulin resistance, including lipodystrophic syndromes. We discuss the pathophysiology, clinical manifestations and treatment of insulin resistance in these populations, with specific emphasis on the pediatric literature.

## TYPE 1 DIABETES

Insulin resistance in type 1 diabetes was first described over 30 years ago in patients who required increasing doses of insulin to control their glucose levels. At that time, insulin resistance was believed to be secondary to anti-insulin antibodies against animal-derived insulin [1]. Although this phenomenon is now almost nonexistent with the use of both highly purified animal and recombinant human insulin, a number of other factors contribute to IR in type 1 diabetes, many of which are relevant during adolescence. Specifically, IR in type 1 diabetes has been noted at disease onset, with episodes of diabetic ketoacidosis (DKA), during adolescence (see Chapter 4), and during periods of poor metabolic control. The increasing prevalence of obesity in youth may be another contributing factor to IR in this age group.

## Onset of Type 1 Diabetes: Insulin Resistance and the Honeymoon Period

Following insulin treatment, acidosis corrects, hormonal status returns to a non-stress level, and utilization of alternate substrates such as FFA and ketones are minimal. In addition, as serum glucose levels are normalized or near-normalized, there is a lessening of glucose toxicity at the level of the β-cell resulting in improved residual endogenous insulin secretion. As a consequence, in the early weeks after diagnosis of type 1 diabetes, many patients exhibit a period of metabolic stability associated with decreased insulin requirement, called the remission or "honeymoon" period [2]. The "honeymoon" period is usually characterized by insulin dose requirements below 0.5 units/kg/day in the face of near normal glucose and HbA1c levels, and is known to last for periods of weeks to months. Older teens and adults tend to have a longer lasting remission period than do younger children [3, 4].

For many years, the remission period was presumed to be due to recovery of residual insulin secretion with reversal of the glucose toxicity present at diagnosis. However, residual insulin secretion alone has been unable to account for all of the metabolic changes during this period [3]. Yki-Jarvinen et al prospectively studied the natural course of insulin sensitivity in adults with newly diagnosed type 1 diabetes using the insulin clamp technique. Two weeks following the diagnosis of diabetes, when pH, free fatty acid and counterregulatory hormone levels had normalized, there remained a 32% lower rate of glucose uptake in individuals with type 1 diabetes, compared to controls. This indicates persistence of a significant degree of IR shortly after diagnosis [4]. Basal hepatic glucose production was also 56% higher in individuals with type 1 diabetes than in controls, but hepatic glucose output was completely and normally suppressed during euglycemic hyperinsulinemic clamps, indicating normal hepatic insulin sensitivity. Thus, the increased IR in the first few months following diagnosis is predominantly due to defective glucose uptake in peripheral tissues such as skeletal muscle [5].

In longer term studies, Yki-Jarvinen and her colleagues demonstrated significant improvement in insulin sensitivity such that it approached levels of nondiabetic controls [5]. Those patients who no longer required exogenous insulin therapy during the honeymoon period demonstrated 40% greater insulin sensitivity than those requiring exogenous insulin. Fasting C-peptide was not found to be related to the degree of clinical remission. Other studies examining insulin secretion during the honeymoon also do not demonstrate a relationship between HbA1c, fasting and stimulated C-peptide levels and insulin dose, thus indirectly supporting an important role for changes in insulin sensitivity/resistance in expression of the honeymoon period [2, 3]. Clamp studies done in adults with type 1 diabetes one year after diagnosis show that insulin sensitivity deteriorates as the remission period reaches its completion and is approximately 40% lower than controls, with a wide inter-individual range. In one study, the degree of insulin resistance was positively correlated with HbA1c, insulin dose and relative body weight [4]. Clearly, factors other than endogenous insulin secretion contribute to insulin sensitivity and to the degree of clinical remission and length of the honeymoon period. Specifically, effective diabetes management with achievement of near normoglycaemia may improve insulin sensitivity and prolong the presence of residual insulin secretion [6, 7].

## Diabetic Ketoacidosis (DKA)

Resistance to insulin had been demonstrated in patients during diabetic ketoacidosis (DKA) as early as 1963 [8]. In the 1980's, Barrett et al compared insulin action (6 U/hr after 6-10 U bolus) in 15 adults with DKA to 6 normal volunteers made hyperglycemic with a combined glucose and somatostatin infusion. In those with DKA, the fractional glucose turnover and t ½ of the fall in plasma glucose was reduced 10 fold compared to controls, and the mean glucose clearance was 8% of controls. They concluded that marked IR is present in virtually all individuals with DKA (Figure 1) [9].

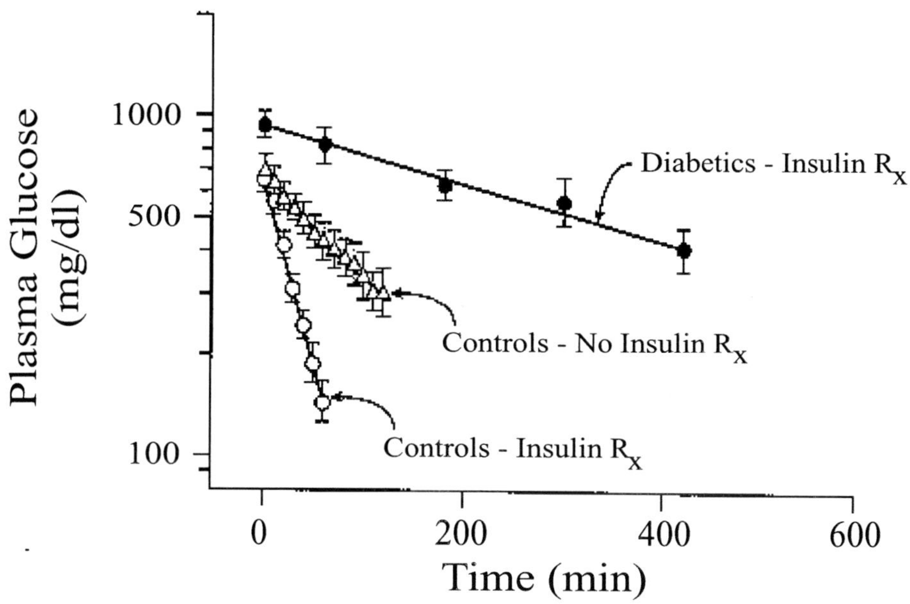


Figure 1: Time course of decline in plasma glucose in the ketoacidotic diabetic subjects (N=15) and in normal volunteers (N=6) after insulin treatment, and in normal volunteers not receiving exogenous insulin. [9] Copyright © 1982 American Diabetes Association from *Diabetes*, Vol. 31, 1982. Reprinted with permission from The American Diabetes Association

The etiology of IR during DKA is complex and multifactorial. Insulin deficiency, coupled with increased levels of the counterregulatory stress hormones, cortisol, growth hormone (GH), glucagon and catecholamines, leads to a state promoting glycogenolysis, gluconeogenesis, lipolysis and ketogenesis, while decreasing glucose utilization and glucose removal [10, 11]. At the same time, the increasing levels of alternative fuel substrates, particularly free fatty acids (FFA) and ketones, further inhibit insulin-mediated glucose utilization in peripheral tissues. To evaluate this, Ginsberg and colleagues measured insulin sensitivity in 9 patients newly diagnosed with type 1 diabetes while in DKA, and revaluated them again 2 - 7 weeks following diagnosis. They demonstrated that GH, cortisol and FFA were increased at diagnosis and then declined following initiation of insulin therapy, and that cortisol and FFA significantly correlated with the degree of IR [12].

Free fatty acids inhibit glucose metabolism via several mechanisms. They are transported intra-cellularly and undergo β-oxidation by the mitochondria. Accumulation of FFA results in increased acetyl-CoA and citrate generated from the Krebs cycle. These in turn inhibit important enzymes necessary for glycolysis. Accumulation of intermediary glucose metabolites such as glucose-6-phosphate then exacerbates the defect in glycolysis by impairing glucose transport [13]. (Figure 2) Human physiologic studies using intralipid infusions have confirmed in vivo that FFAs act as peripheral antagonists of insulin action, primarily through inhibition of glucose oxidation [14-16].

Finally, hyperglycaemia itself is also known to interfere with glucose disposal directly and indirectly by various mechanisms: (i) effects on the pancreatic β-cell ("glucose toxicity") through induction of oxidative stress and free radicals leading to both down regulation of insulin synthesis and secretion as well as beta cell apoptosis, and (ii) direct inhibition of glucose transport in skeletal muscle [17-19].

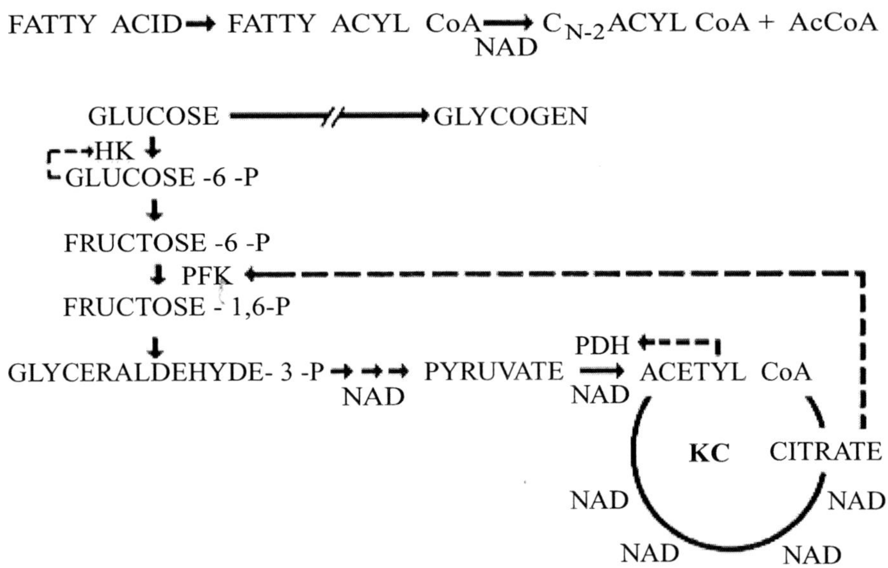


Figure 2: Randle cycle. Enhanced free fatty acid oxidation depletes NAD stores, leading to an inhibition of the Krebs cycle (KC) and a resultant increase in intracellular citrate abd acetyl-CoA concentrations. Accumulation of acetyl-CoA and citrate leads to the inhibition of pyruvate dehydrogenase (PDH) and phosphofructokinase (PFK), respectively. Build up of glucose-6-P inhibits hexokinase, leading to an inhibition of glucose transport into cell. The decrease in glucose transport, in combination with an inhibition effect of fatty acetyl-CoA on glycogen synthase, results in diminished glycogen formation. Dashed lines represent sites of inhibition of glucose metabolism (13). 

## Puberty

Puberty is a period of considerable hormonal and psychological change, which is coupled with a significant deterioration in insulin sensitivity (see also Chapter 4). Nondiabetic youth respond to the increase in IR by increasing endogenous insulin secretion. Resultant hyperinsulinemia is very effective in maintaining euglycaemia, since nondiabetic adolescents do not exhibit hyperglycaemia during puberty [20-22]. IR peaks in mid-puberty and then declines in early adulthood, and is more pronounced in girls than boys [23]. In nondiabetic youth, the IR of puberty is likely an adaptive response in that it relates more particularly to glucose homeostasis than to defects in either fat or protein deposition. The ensuing hyperinsulinemia may lead to enhanced fat and protein deposition essential to the pubertal growth spurt [24].

Amiel and colleagues compared the results of euglycemic insulin-clamp studies in adults and prepubertal and pubertal children with and without type 1 diabetes. In nondiabetic pubertal children, insulin-stimulated glucose metabolism was significantly reduced compared with that of prepubertal children and adults, despite comparable hyperinsulinemia. Similarly, the response to insulin was 25-30% lower in the diabetic pubertal children than in the diabetic prepubertal children and adults. At each stage of development, insulin sensitivity was decreased by 33-42% in the children with diabetes. In all the groups of children studied, the response to insulin was inversely correlated with the mean 24-hour levels of growth hormone. Among the diabetic children, the glycosylated hemoglobin levels were substantially higher in the pubertal children than in the prepubertal children although the daily insulin doses tended to be higher [21]. Arslanian also demonstrated a 43% decrease of insulin-mediated glucose utilization rate in adolescent girls compared to boys with diabetes, after matching for age, pubertal status, BMI and HbA1c [25]. Unlike in nondiabetic youth, the IR of puberty may be maladaptive in the teen with type 1 diabetes in that the higher insulin dosages required to maintain good metabolic control may lead to excess weight gain and its physical and psychological consequences [26].

The normal physiologic pubertal increase in IR, exaggerated in type 1 diabetes, may be an important factor contributing to the deterioration in metabolic control that often occurs during adolescence. Typically, adolescents with type 1 diabetes experience higher HbA1c levels despite increased daily insulin requirements. In a large cross-sectional study of 2873 children in 18 countries, HbA1c increased to a mean maximum of 9-9.5% during puberty, coincident with an increased daily insulin dosage, and the effect was most marked in adolescent females [27]. Similarly, the adolescent subgroup in the Diabetes Control and Complications Trial (DCCT) had an average 1% higher HbA1c with increased weight gain compared to adults, in both conventional and intensive treatment groups, despite a higher insulin dose requirement (1.0 u/kg/day versus 0.6 U/kg/day in the adult cohort) [28].

Several physiologic factors may account for the increased insulin resistance in pubertal youth with type 1 diabetes. Sex steroids are not generally believed to play a major role, as levels are higher during adult life, coincident with improving insulin sensitivity following completion of puberty [21, 23]. However, growth hormone (GH) is a known counterregulatory hormone, and both baseline and peak GH levels increase steadily during puberty and are temporally related to the nadir of insulin sensitivity [29]. GH secretion is also higher in teens with type 1 diabetes compared to their non-diabetic peers at each stage of development [21, 30, 31]. Furthermore, plasma GH levels during clamp studies were 129%

higher in girls than in boys, supporting GH as the major factor contributing to the difference in other insulin sensitivity during puberty between girls and boys, with and without diabetes [25].

The etiology of the exaggerated GH secretion in type 1 diabetes, may relate to lower insulin-like growth factor-1 (IGF-1) and GH binding protein (GHBP) levels documented in adolescents with type 1 diabetes, compared to healthy nondiabetic controls [21, 32-34]. This finding, highly specific to type 1 diabetes, has been hypothesized to be due to the lack of effect of intra-hepatic insulin regulation of the GH-IGF-1 axis. Insulin delivered portally normally increases GHBP synthesis. GHBP serve a dual function as carrier proteins of GH and also as receptor subunits for GH binding [32]. Subcutaneous insulin bypasses the portal circulation, thus decreasing the intra-hepatic insulin effect on GHBP synthesis and leading to decreased GH action. Consequently, production of IGF-1 diminishes, with loss of normal negative feedback of the IGF-1/GH axis to the hypothalamus [35]. This leads to an exaggerated GH level and contributes to peripheral IR [33, 34]. Also, some studies have shown that both GH and insulin are required for hepatic IGF-1 synthesis, so that lost of portal delivery of insulin may directly reduce IGF-1 synthesis, again contributing to increased GH secretion seen in type 1 diabetes [36].

In support of this hypothesis, several studies have demonstrated an inverse relationship between insulin sensitivity and IGF-1 level in adolescents [21, 31, 37, 38]. Adult studies where insulin was administered intra-peritoneally have shown improvement in hepatic GH resistance and a reversible increase in GHBP, IGF-1 and IGFBP-3 [39].

Thus, alterations in the GH/IGF-1 axis, both in term of spontaneous hypersecretion of GH and lower IGF-1 levels, seem to be the most plausible reason to understand the mechanism of decreased insulin sensitivity during puberty in patients with type 1 diabetes.

## Poor Metabolic Control

Chronic hyperglycaemia or 'glucose toxicity' can lead to insulin resistance as described in the section on diabetic ketoacidosis [40]. Yki-Jarvinen et al demonstrated in subjects with type 1 diabetes that insulin action significantly decreased after a period of time of 24 hours of sustained hyperglycaemia compared to the euglycemic state [41]. Moreover, restoration of euglycaemia in poorly controlled patients with type 1 diabetes improves glucose uptake in muscle [42]. Poor metabolic control is linked to elevated free fatty acids in both type 1 and type 2 diabetes, which also exacerbates IR [43-45]. Dyslipidemia in youth with type 1 diabetes correlates with increased HbA1c [46, 47].

Intensive insulin therapy with achievement of near normoglycaemia can lead to restoration of insulin sensitivity [48]. This improvement in insulin sensitivity is associated with improved metabolic control and may account for the decreasing insulin dose requirements noted clinically in many of these patients.

## Treatment of Insulin Resistance in Type 1 Diabetes

During adolescence, the patient, family and multidisciplinary diabetes team must adopt a dynamic approach to the diabetes regimen as puberty is not only a time of insulin resistance but also one of rapid physical and psychological growth. Appropriate insulin therapy, either by intermittent injection or continuous subcutaneous infusion, remains the cornerstone of treatment for type 1 diabetes. However, some of the oral hypoglycaemic agents used to treat type 2 diabetes might be useful adjunctive therapy for individuals with IR. The major benefit of improved insulin action may be facilitation of improved metabolic control.

### *Metformin*

The biguanide metformin acts primarily to decrease hepatic production of glucose with modest improvement of peripheral insulin sensitivity [49]. The combination of metformin and insulin has been evaluated in children and adolescents with type 1 diabetes in a few studies, including two randomized controlled trials [50-53].

We conducted a double-blinded, placebo-controlled trial to examine the efficacy of metformin in 27 poorly controlled adolescents with type 1 diabetes and high insulin dose requirements (HbA1c >8<11%; insulin dose > 1unit/kg/day) [51]. Using metformin in doses of 25-30 mg/kg/day up to a maximum of 2000 mg/day, we found a significant reduction in HbA1c (mean decrease of 0.6%) and insulin dose (mean decrease of 0.14 u/kg/day) over a 3-month period, without an associated increase in BMI. There was no difference in severe hypoglycaemia or in gastrointestinal side effects between the two groups. This combination of a reduction in insulin dose/kg and lower HbA1c without weight gain provides strong clinical evidence of enhanced insulin action. Insulin sensitivity was measured by the Minimal Model of Bergman using the frequently sampled intravenous glucose tolerance test: there was a trend towards improving insulin sensitivity in the metformin-treated group, but this did not reach statistical significance, likely because of the wide range of results and difficulties in Minimal Model analysis in individuals treated with exogenous insulin.

Särnblad et al. reported similar results in a double-blinded, placebo-controlled trial of 26 adolescents with type 1 diabetes [50]. After 3 months, a reduction of HbA1c of 0.9% was achieved in the metformin group compared to 0.3% in the placebo group. They found no change in either BMI or insulin dose. Two other smaller uncontrolled studies have shown similar improvement in HbA1c with metformin adjunctive treatment [52, 53]. Studies involving hyperinsulinemic euglycemic clamp have shown improvement in glucose utilisation in those treated with metformin [50, 52]. The theoretical risk of lactic acidosis in ketosis-prone individuals requires that close supervision of teens with type 1 diabetes be maintained when metformin is combined with insulin in an attempt to achieve optimal clinical outcomes.

### *Thiazolidinediones (TZD's)*

Thiazolidinediones are a relatively new class of insulin-sensitizing agents and their use has not been evaluated in type 1 diabetes. These drugs have been extensively studied in adults with type 2 diabetes and demonstrate amelioration of IR, improvement of hyperglycaemia and reduction of hyperinsulinaemia [54]. Given their more significant impact on peripheral insulin sensitivity, one would expect that TZDs would be more effective than metformin in reducing insulin dose and improving metabolic control when used as adjunctive therapy in individuals with type 1 diabetes. Studies of the efficacy of new TZD's in adolescents with type 1 diabetes are currently underway.

***Acarbose***

Acarbose, an α-glucosidase inhibitor, delays carbohydrate digestion by competitive enzyme inhibition. This drug was also evaluate as adjunctive therapy to insulin in adults with type 1 diabetes. Despite its modest positive effect in decreasing HbA1c and post-prandial blood sugar, its use is limited by the high prevalence of gastrointestinal side effects [55-57].

***Insulin-like Growth Factor-1 (IGF-1)***

A few studies have evaluated the use of IGF-l as an adjunctive agent in type 1 diabetes because of its potential hypoglycaemic and anabolic properties. The rationale for the use of recombinant human IGF-1 (rhIGF-1) in individuals with type 1 diabetes stems from the demonstration of dysregulation of the GH/IGF-1 axis, with low serum levels of IGF-1 and exaggerated secretion of growth hormone (GH). One study used isotope techniques during an hyperinsulinemic clamp in adults to demonstrate that IGF-1 administration resulted in increased insulin-mediated glucose uptake [58]. Another study evaluated daily IGF-1 injection in adolescents with type 1 diabetes, with the aim of restoring IGF-1 levels to normal. After a single dose of 40 μg/kg at night, mean GH nocturnal secretion decreased (19.4 +/- 4.0 compared with 33.6 +/- 5.8 mU/l; p = 0.01 ) and insulin requirements to maintain euglyceamia improved significantly (0.25 +/- 0.02 compared with 0.31 +/- 0.04 mU.kg-1.min-1; p = 0.03) [59].

Acerini et al treated 53 adolescents with type 1 diabetes with 40 μg/kg of rhIGF-1 for 24 weeks in a randomized placebo controlled trial [36]. The median reduction in HbA1c was 0.6% after 12 weeks of treatment but this improvement was not sustained and disappeared completely by the end of the 24 week trial. The authors presumed that this was the result of poor compliance with IGF-1 injections.

One potential disadvantage of this treatment is that IGF-1 exhibits mitogenic activity which may accelerate retinopathy and nephropathy [60]. The largest treatment study, done in 223 individuals aged 11-66 years, demonstrated worrisome adverse events of edema and acceleration of retinopathy in the groups treated with higher doses [61]. This may negate the potential benefits of the small reduction in long-term risk of micro-vascular complications accomplished by improving metabolic control [61, 62].

***Pirenzipine***

Pirenzipine is an oral anticholinergic drug which inhibits the GH response to GHRH in individuals with type 1 diabetes [63]. Halldin et al have performed detailed physiologic studies in 11 adolescents with hyperinsulinemic euglycemic clamps before and after 3 weeks therapy with pirenzipine [64]. HbA1c fell by 0.9%, with improved insulin sensitivity by clamp measurement, but there was no significant differences in pattern of GH secretion assessed by 24 hour serum sampling, IGF-1 levels or IGFBP-1 levels. Thus, the improvement in metabolic control may be a study effect and not via changes in GH secretion affecting insulin sensitivity. Placebo-controlled studies are needed to assess potential role of anticholinergic agents such as pirenzipine in the management of teens with type 1 diabetes.

In summary, adjunctive therapy to treat the IR associated with type 1 diabetes in adolescents is of potential benefit, but there remains a paucity of well-controlled studies. Metformin is the best studied and does appear to be both safe and modestly effective in the short-term. As the prevalence of childhood obesity continues to rise, teens with type 1 diabetes may exhibit an increasing number of features of IR and the metabolic syndrome.

Thus, judicious use of insulin-sensitizing agents along with insulin may be of benefit to an increasingly greater number of youth with type 1 diabetes, specifically during the period of enhanced IR of puberty.

## CYSTIC FIBROSIS

Cystic fibrosis (CF), an autosomal recessive disease affecting 1 in 2000-2500 children, results from mutation in the chloride channel, which leads to hyperviscosity of ductular secretion and progressive damage to many organs, particularly the lungs and pancreas. The disease is characterized by chronic pulmonary infection and various degrees of endocrine pancreatic insufficiency leading to malabsorption and malnutrition. Most patients with the common mutation associated with CF, namely Δ508, have evidence of pancreatic exocrine insufficiency at a very young age [65]. As life expectancy has improved to a mean of about 30 years in many centres [66-69], pancreatic endocrine dysfunction has been recognized increasingly and associated with negative health outcomes [66, 70, 71]. Cystic fibrosis-related diabetes (CFRD) may be insidious in onset, with most patients being asymptomatic for many years before the disease is recognized. The natural history of CRFD is quite variable, and is influenced by a host of factors such as nutrition, chronic pulmonary activity and acute lung infections, use of glucocorticoids, the presence of associated glucagon deficiency, malabsorption and liver dysfunction [72].

In a five year prospective study of 191 patients with CF over 2 years of age, Lanng et al found an increase in CFRD from 11 to 24%, with an annual incidence averaging 3.8% [73]. They employed oral glucose tolerance testing to define CFRD and found it superior to either fasting glucose or HbA1c measurements in this group. Of note, in those over 10 years of age, the prevalence of CFRD increased from 16 to 34% and in those over 20 years of age from 25 to 53%. The prevalence of impaired glucose tolerance remained stable except in the older age group in which it decreased from 32 to 9% as full blown CFRD steadily increased. In a recent report from our institution, Solomon et al studied 94 patients aged 9-18 years using the OGTT [74]. They found impaired glucose tolerance in 17% and CFRD in 4.3%. Abnormal glucose tolerance was associated exclusively with severe mutations in the CF gene and exocrine pancreatic insufficiency. Moreover, a large questionnaire survey done in CF clinics of North America and Europe reported a prevalence of 5-6% of CFRD in the paediatric population [75, 76].

CFRD is thought to arise from the loss of pancreatic islet cell mass with resulting insulin and glucagon deficiency. This occurs secondary to progressive fibrosis and destruction of the pancreatic islets [77]. The first phase insulin secretion is impaired in both IGT and CFRD, insulin response to OGTT is delayed and the maximal insulin peak diminished [78-82]. However, the role of peripheral IR in the pathogenesis of CFRD remains unclear.

Studies of the contribution of IR to the onset and expression of abnormal glucose homeostasis in CF have yielded conflicting and inconclusive results [80, 83-88]. For example, Hardin et al studied 18 CF patients (8 with normal glucose tolerance, 5 with IGT and 5 with CFRD) and 20 lean controls using a 3-step hyperinsulinemic-euglycemic clamp: all CF groups were insulin resistant compared to controls, with the lowest insulin sensitivity found in the group with IGT [86]. Of note, there was a striking correlation between IR and poor clinical status (r=0.85). Similarly, Holl and colleagues studied 71 CF subjects and 59 controls using OGTT [87]. They found that CF patients with IGT or CFRD did not have reduced insulin secretion, but did show evidence of increased glucose to insulin ratios indicating IR. They concluded that IR likely contributes to the hyperlgycemia in these subjects. Conversely, Yung [88] and Lombardo [89] and colleagues were unable to demonstrate a role for IR in abnormal glucose metabolism in 68 and 14 CF patients respectively, using OGTT and calculated measures of insulin sensitivity.

The differences in the studies above may relate in part to different techniques used to detect IR and to differences in age, lung functional and nutritional status in those studied. The hyperinsulinemic-euglycemic clamp technique may be a more sophisticated and accurate measure of IR than either that derived from an OGTT or from fasting insulin and glucose measurements (e.g. HOMA-IR).

The mechanism of IR in subjects with CFRD has been also been investigated. One possible explanation for the peripheral insulin resistance seen in these subjects may be via "glucose toxicity," whereby chronic hyperglycaemia leads to a deterioration in insulin action [83, 86]. One study found both raised TNF-α levels in the circulation and impaired GLUT-4 translocation in muscle biopsies in CF compared to control subjects. Both correlated with impaired glucose disposal rates calculated from clamp studies [90]. Hardin et al have also suggested that CF subjects have several defects in substrate utilization, including de novo lipogenesis and elevated hepatic glucose production which may also contribute to the abnormalities in glucose homeostasis [91].

In conclusion, it appears that IR is a frequent finding in those with CFRD, but its role in the pathophysiology of abnormal glucose metabolism in CF remains to be proven. Future longitudinal studies are needed both to determine the relative contributions of insulin deficiency and IR to the pathogenesis of glucose intolerance and diabetes in these patients. Furthermore, a more in depth analysis of the factors contributing to IR, both hepatic and peripheral is warranted. Finally, given its anabolic actions and its theoretical ability to provide relative β-cell rest, it is timely to study the effects of early and aggressive insulin therapy on nutritional status, pulmonary function and diabetes prevention in CF.

## SURVIVORS OF CHILDHOOD CANCER

With improvements in cancer treatment, more children are surviving to adulthood and are exposed to long-term effects of cancer therapies. Recent studies have confirmed an in overall excess mortality rate in adults who were treated for childhood cancers (up to 10.8 fold, CI 10.3-11.2), with a 5 to 12.5 increase in mortality from cardiovascular disease, which is the most frequent cause of death after cancer (original or recurrent disease) [92-95].

Risk factors for development of obesity, IR and cardiovascular disease in patients treated for cancer, are not limited to, but may include damage to the hypothalamic-pituitary axis from tumour, surgery or radiation, leading to hormone deficiencies and dysregulation of appetite/energy homeostasis, decreased physical activity with chronic illness or disability, and cytotoxic effects of medications such as chemotherapy and steroids on body composition and energy metabolism [96-101]. Growth hormone deficiency (GHD) is by far the most common endocrine abnormality in childhood survivors, especially after cranial irradiation [102]. GHD has been well documented to lead to IR in adults and to improve with GH replacement [103,

104]. Most of the paediatric literature to date has explored issues related to development of obesity and the metabolic syndrome.

## Obesity

It is now well recognized that survivors of various childhood malignancies have an increased prevalence of obesity (Table 1). In particular, studies that have examined survivors of acute lymphoblastic leukemia (ALL) found an increased risk for obesity in the initial years after therapy and at time of final height [105-107]. Didi and co-workers found that the two main factors associated with increase in BMI z score were the younger age at diagnosis of ALL and female gender, whereas, the development of obesity was not associated with treatment with cranial irradiation or GH deficiency. In contrast, Sklar and his colleagues have analysed data from the Childhood Cancer Survivor Study (CCSS) which show that cranial radiation therapy was a major independent predictor of obesity [106, 107]. CCSS, the biggest retrospective study of ALL childhood survivors, revealed an Odds Ratio (OR) for obesity of 2.59 (95% CI, 1.88-3.55) for females who received cranial irradiation > 20 Gy, and an OR of 1.86 (95% CI, 1.33-2.57) for men. The greatest risk was among females with ALL diagnosed before 4 years of age, treated with a combination of chemotherapy and cranial radiation > 20 Gy (OR 3.8; 95% CI 2.34-5.99). Interestingly, later diagnosis (older than 15 years) and treatment with chemotherapy alone or in combination with lower dose of cranial irradiation (<20 Gy) were not associated with an increased risk of developing obesity [107].

Data from patients with treated brain tumors are also quite concerning. A recent retrospective analysis of 156 children who survived a brain tumor for more than 5 years after treatment were evaluated for risk factors of obesity [96]. Lustig identified hypothalamic damage, due to the tumor location, surgery or radiation therapy, as the primary risk factor for the development of obesity. In particular, patients diagnosed at younger age (less than 6 years) and those who received more than 51 Gy of cranial radiation in the hypothalamic region were at greater risk. After stratification by tumor histology, they found that patients with craniopharyngioma were the most vulnerable to increases in BMI after treatment. Other cohort studies have also shown hypothalamic obesity in 35 to 60% after a craniopharyngioma therapy, putting these patients at very high risk for future development of IR and its consequences [108-110].

## Metabolic Syndrome in Cancer Survivors

While many studies focus on the prevalence of obesity in childhood cancer survivors, very few have examined its consequences. The largest cross-sectional study reporting features of the metabolic syndrome was done in 50 young adult survivors (23 females, mean age at follow-up 18.3 years) of non-brain tumor childhood cancer (28 acute lymphoblastic leukemia 7 lymphoma, 7 Wilms tumor and 8 other cancers) treated with different combinations of chemotherapy and irradiation. They found that one third of young survivors met the criteria of obesity (> 120% ideal body weight) compared to 10% of controls, and that most survivors had a pro-atherogenic lipid profile, consisting of low HDL and low HDL/Total cholesterol ratio. Fasting glucose and insulin levels were also higher in patients than in controls (4.7 ± 0.5

vs. 4.0 ± 0.5 mmol/L and 102 ± 43 vs. 78 ± 31 pmol/L). Sixteen percent of all survivors had the combination of obesity, hyperinsulinemia and low HDL, whereas none of the 50 age-matched controls exhibited this pattern [111]. Similarly, another study that assessed the cardiovascular risk factors in 26 young adults survivors of childhood ALL found 62% with at least one, and 30% with two or more, risk factors for cardiovascular disease (obesity, hypertension, dyslipidemia, elevated fasting glucose, elevated fasting insulin). Morever, patients who received cranial irradiation were heavier and had a more atherogenic profile (higher TG and VLDL), although intimal-medial thickness was not significantly different between the groups [112]. Lastly, Taskinen et al compared glucose and lipids metabolism in 23 long-term survivors of bone-marrow transplantation in childhood (8 ALL, 4 severe aplastic anemia and 11 other conditions) to 13 patients in remission from leukemia, and 23 age and sex matched healthy controls. They found that only the patients who had undergone bone marrow transplant exhibited significantly more features of the metabolic syndrome than the other groups, including increased IR measured by HOMA, impaired glucose tolerance, type 2 diabetes, abdominal obesity and hypertriglyceridemia [113].

Finally, only one study has explored features of the metabolic syndrome after childhood craniopharyngioma, a tumor often associated with hypothalamic obesity. Fifteen patients (7 to 19 years of age) were evaluated for insulin sensitivity using a 40 minute IV glucose tolerance test, fasting lipid profile and body composition, and compared to 9 age, sex, BMI and pubertal stage-matched controls. Craniopharyngioma patients had increased truncal fat (by DEXA), higher triglycerides levels and lower HDL levels, but were not found to have increased IR [114]. These results are somewhat contradictory to other reports of increased fasting and secreted insulin in children with hypothalamic obesity, which is hypothesized to be due to increased vagally-mediated stimulated insulin secretion following hypothalamic damage, and has been shown to be improved with octreotide, a drug which decreases insulin sensitivity [96, 115, 116]. Further studies are required to identify both risk factors for development of the metabolic syndrome in these populations, and the mechanisms by which these abnormalities occur.

## Thalassemia Major

Thalassemias are congenital haemolytic anemias resulting from impaired synthesis of one or more globin chains (the $\alpha$ and $\beta$ chains). Individuals with $\beta$-thalassemia major (TM) require monthly blood transfusions and chelation therapy to minimize iron overload [117, 118]. Chronic iron deposition can lead to cardiac and hepatic dysfunction, as well as many endocrine abnormalities, including diabetes [119].

Secondary hemochromatosis was recognized as a cause of diabetes mellitus in children with thalassemia major in the early 1970's [120, 121]. Data from Europe suggests that the prevalence of diabetes in children with thalassemia major is approximately 5%, and of impaired glucose tolerance more than 25% [122]. Direct iron-induced damage to pancreatic $\beta$-cell and impairment of insulin secretion was initially thought to be the sole pathophysiologic disturbance leading to diabetes [119, 120, 123, 124]. However, Meckel et al, using the euglycemic clamp, demonstrated 30% decreased insulin sensitivity (Si) in 12 children with thalassemia (4 pre-pubertal and 8 pubertal) compared to controls, suggesting that IR may contribute to the development of diabetes in $\beta$-thalassemia [125].

**Table 1: Obesity in ALL Childhood Survivors**

| Authors | Year | Study population | N (%F) | Age (yr) | Obesity Definition | Prevalence of Obesity | Risk Factors for Obesity |
|---|---|---|---|---|---|---|---|
| Didi [105] | 1995 | ALL | 114 (55%F) | 16.2 [13.3-20.6] | BMI > $85^{th}$ %ile | 46.5 % | Younger age at Dx, female gender |
| Sklar [106] | 2000 | ALL | 126 (53% F) | 18.3 ± 0.2 | BMI > $85^{th}$ %ile | 30.2% | Cranial irradiation |
| Oeffinger [107] | 2003 | ALL compared to siblings | 1765 (49%F) | 24.1 ± 4.9 | BMI > 30 $kg/m^2$ | 17% v/s 12 % in siblings | Younger age at Dx, female gender, cranial irradiation |

**Table 2: Genetic Defects of Insulin Action**

| Genetics Defect | Mode of Inheritance and Gene involve | Clinical Features |
|---|---|---|
| ***Insulin Receptor Pathway:*** | | |
| • Donohue Syndrome (Leprechaunism) | AR, IR mutation | IUGR and postnatal growth retardation, severe insulin resistance, "leprechaun" facies, lipoatrophy, mild hirsutism; very high insulin level, fatal in the first year of life |
| • Rabson-Mendenhall Syndrome | IR mutation | Childhood presentation of insulin resistance, dental and nail dysplasia, pineal hyperplasia; most develop severe DKA |
| • Type A Syndrome-Acanthosis | 10-15% IR mutation | Development of insulin resistance at puberty, hyperandrogenism, acanthosis, risk of glucose intolerance, no obesity, no lipoatrophy, no insulin receptor antibodies |
| ***Fat Cell and Lipid Metabolism Pathway*: *Inherited Lipodystrophies*** | | |
| Congenital, Generalized | | |
| • Berardinelli-Seip Syndrome | AR | Extreme lack of adipose tissue from birth, accelerated growth and acromegaloid features, acanthosis, hepatomegaly; lack of visceral, intra-muscular and bone marrow fat |
| Type 1 (BSCL1) | 9q34, AGPAT2 gene | BSCL1:spare mechanical adipose tissues (joints, orbits, scalp, palms, soles…) |
| Type 2 (BSCL2) | 11q13, Seipin gene | BSCL2: mild mental retardation, hypertrophic cardiomyopathy; distinctive lack of mechanical adipose tissues |
| • Variants: AREYLD* and SHORT** syndromes | AR, Gene unknown | Generalized lipodystrophies and dysmorphisms |

**Table 2: Genetic Defects of Insulin Action (continued)**

| Genetics Defect | Mode of Inheritance and Gene involve | Clinical Features |
|---|---|---|
| Familial Partial Localized | | |
| • Dunnigan Syndrome (FPLD) | AD, 1q21-22, LMNA gene; Lamin A/C proteins | Progressive symmetric lipoatrophy of arms, legs and trunk at puberty, spare face, neck and labia majora; normal stores of intermuscular, intra-abdominal, intrathoracic and bone marrow fat |
| • Kobberling's Syndrome (FPL) | X-linked or AD, mutation in PPAR-γ gene | Loss of subcutaneous fat from extremities, variable loss in the face |

AD: Autosomal Dominant
AR: Autosomal Recessive
IR: Insulin Receptor
*Acrorenal field defect, Ectodermal dysplasia and lipoatrophic diabetes
**Short stature, Hyperextensibility of joints, Ocular depression, Rieger anomaly (defects of iris and cornea) and Teething delay

Adapted from Garg A, *NEJM* 350;1220-34;2004 and Ten S. *JCEM* 89;2526-2539;2004

Subsequently, other investigators, using FSIGT in nondiabetic children and young adults with β-thalassemia, have confirmed that Si is 40-50% lower than age, BMI and pubertal-matched healthy controls [126, 127] . In one study of 7 nondiabetic adolescents with β-thalassemia (14 ± 1 years, BMI 19 ± 1, Tanner stage 2-4) Si was inversely correlated with iron overload (r= -.707 P= 0.006). Hepatic insulin extraction was also found to be lower in the hyperinsulinemic patients than in normo-insulinemic patients and controls (49% vs. 73 % vs. 77%), and was also inversely correlated with iron overload [127]. A study of 10 thalassemic patients (age 21.7 ± 1.2 yrs, BMI 19.7 ± 0.6) also demonstrated reduced hepatic insulin extraction compared to 10 healthy controls [126]. Most, but not all, other investigators have reported a negative correlation between Si and markers of iron overload (hepatic iron stores, serum ferritin or transfusion number) [125, 128-130]. Taken together, these data suggest that the liver may be susceptible to insult from iron accumulation, and that hepatic IR is the primary cause of hyperinsulinemia in these patients with β-thalassemia.

Recently, Cario et al assessed insulin sensitivity and β-cell secretion by using OGTT in a larger study of young adults with β-thalassemia major with varying degrees of glucose tolerance. Thalassemic patients were found to have higher fasting and integrated glucose levels compared to controls, even in those with normal glucose tolerance (NGT). Patients with impaired glucose tolerance (IGT) had highest, but delayed levels of insulin in response to an OGTT, and patients with diabetes had lower insulin levels. As a group, thalassemic patients showed significantly lower insulin secretion capacity. No correlation of insulin secretion with serum ferritin or hepatic iron concentration was found. There was, however, a negative correlation between C-peptide/insulin ratio, which reflects insulin extraction, and age, a surrogate parameter for iron overload in thalassemia. Fasting insulin sensitivity indices ($ISI_{HOMA}$ and $ISI_{Quicki}$) revealed decreased insulin sensitivity in both IGT and diabetic patients, but not in NGT patients compared to controls [131].

In summary, the development of secondary diabetes in β-thalassemia major appears to result from a combination of hepatic IR with progressive deterioration of the pancreatic beta cell function presumably due to iron overload in vulnerable tissues. The contribution of inflammation, which is associated with IR, and markers of IR such as C-reactive peptide and tumor necrosis alpha remains to be explored.

## Genetic and Acquired Insulin Resistance Syndromes

The ADA etiologic classification of diabetes mellitus includes type 1, type 2 and other conditions associated with abnormality of glucose metabolism, such as diabetes associated with genetic defects of β-cell function (MODY) or genetic defects of insulin action, endocrinopathies, drug and chemical-induced diabetes, and some rare genetic syndromes associated with diabetes [132]. Here we focus on the genetic and acquired defects which have been associated with IR and briefly discuss medications used in children that can lead to impaired insulin action and diabetes.

## Genetic Defects in Insulin Action and Inherited Lipodystrophies

Donohue and Rabson-Mendenhall syndromes are rare pediatric conditions of severe IR caused by different insulin receptor mutations [133-137]. They present during infancy and childhood with hyperinsulinemia, fasting hypoglycaemia and post-prandial hyperglycaemia. They can be distinguished from each other by their facial features and their natural history, Donohue Syndrome being more severe at presentation and generally lethal in the first year of life. Patients with Type A Syndrome-Acanthosis present with signs of insulin resistance at puberty and share characteristics similar to women with lean PCOS. This inherited syndrome is more frequent in blacks with 10-15% of those tested having mutations in the insulin receptor. The absence of insulin receptor auto-antibodies and the lack of association with auto-immune diseases, such as alopecia, vitiligo, arthritis and nephritis distinguishes Type A syndrome from Type B Syndrome, an uncommon form of acquired IR due to antibodies directed at the insulin receptor [138].

Lipodystrophies are clinically heterogeneous disorders characterized by an unusual amount and distribution of fat tissue, atrophy of subcutaneous fat, and clinical and biochemical features of insulin resistance including acanthosis nigricans, hyperandrogenism, PCOS in females, glucose intolerance, hypertriglyceridemia and hepatic steatosis. They are primarily secondary to lipid metabolism pathway defects (e.g. AGPAT) or mutations in genes important for adipocyte formation (e.g. PPAR-γ) or maintenance (e.g. LMNA) [139, 140]. They can be subdivided into broad categories; genetic (congenital), and acquired, and generalized or partial lipodystrophies. The age of onset of presentation can vary from infancy to puberty to adulthood, depending on the mutation involved. Generally, the metabolic consequences of the disorders correlate with the degree of loss of fat [140].

The clinical presentation and molecular knowledge of the most frequent genetic defects in insulin action seen in the pediatric population are summarized in Table 2.

## Acquired Lipodystrophies

Acquired lipodystrophies are more common in the general population than inherited lipodystrophies. With the exception of HIV-associated lipodystrophy, most acquired lipodystrophies present during childhood. They can be classified as acquired generalized lipodystrophy (AGL, Lawrence syndrome), acquired partial lipodystrophy (APL, Barraquer-Simons syndrome), lipodystrophy in HIV infected patients (LD-HIV) and localized lipodystrophies.

Lawrence syndrome, the acquired generalized form, is believed to occur following immune-mediated loss of adipocytes [140]. It has been reported in 80 patients, affecting primarily white females, and begins in childhood and adolescence [141]. An episode of panniculitis occurs in one quarter of the patients before the development of this lipodystrophy, while another quarter have an associated autoimmune condition, such as dermatomyositis, juvenile rheumatoid arthritis, Sjogren's syndrome, chronic active hepatitis or Hashimoto thyroiditis. The fat loss affects the face, arms and legs primarily. Some patients have a loss of subcutaneous fat from the palms and soles, as in type 2 congenital generalized lipodystrophy (BSCL2), but unlike most of the inherited generalized forms, there is preservation of bone marrow fat. Acanthosis nigricans and hepatic steatosis have been reported to develop during childhood, along with extreme insulin resistance, diabetes, hypertriglyceridemia and low levels of leptin and adiponectin [142, 143].

Barraquer-Simons syndrome, is an acquired partial lipodystrophy which is related to low levels of serum C3 and presence of an autoantibody, C3 nephritic factor [144, 145]. The C3 nephritic factor is believed to activate the complement pathway, leading to consumption of C3 and lysis of adipocytes [146]. Barraquer-Simons syndrome has been described in 250 patients, demonstrates a male preponderance, and results in loss of fat primarily in face, neck and upper body with sparing of hips and legs [140]. IR and metabolic abnormalities are less frequent than in all the other lipodystrophies, but later development of membranoproliferative glomerulonephritis, systemic lupus erythematosus and juvenile dermatomyositis has been reported [147-149].

Lastly, lipodystrophy in HIV infected patients (LD-HIV) occurs in approximately 50% of adult patients treated with protease inhibitors (PIs) for more than a year. The mechanism of PI-induced lipodystrophy is thought to be related to alteration in PPAR-γ and sterol regulatory element-binding protein-1 (SREBP-1) expression; important factors for adipogenesis [140, 150]. In adults, fat loss occurs primarily in the face and extremities, leaving a cushingoid phenotype with double chin, buffalo hump and abdominal obesity. Dyslipidemia, fasting and postprandial hyperinsulinemia are common, but development of diabetes is infrequent [151]. In children, LD-HIV has been reported less frequently ( 6-18%) and the degree of metabolic abnormalities seem to be restricted to elevation of total, LDL cholesterol and triglycerides [152-156].

## Drug -Induced Diabetes

A large number of medications can interfere with the glucose metabolism, either by direct toxicity to the pancreatic β-cells (e.g. cyclosporine and tacrolimus), by interfering with insulin release (e.g. thiazides and phenytoin) or by inducing insulin resistance (e.g. glucocorticoids, growth hormone) [157].

Glucocorticoids are the most common drugs known to impair glucose metabolism. Their diabetogenic effects are related to a combination of increased gluconeogenesis and decreased peripheral glucose uptake in muscle and adipose tissues [158, 159]. IR is thought to occur both at receptor and post-receptor levels [160, 161], and there is an increased risk of hyperglycaemia and secondary diabetes with higher dose and systemic use in susceptible patients [157]. Most studies of glucocorticoid-induced diabetes in children are reported in the renal transplant literature, and pathophysiologic studies examining IR in children treated with steroids are absent. The reported incidence of steroid-induced diabetes is lower than found in adults (3-7% compared to > 20%) [162-165]. Risk factors for development of steroid-induced diabetes include: a family history of type 2 diabetes, African-American ethnicity and concomitant use of tacrolimus [162, 163].

L-asparaginase, often used in combination with prednisone in children with leukemia, has also been recognized to induce diabetes; and some youth have even presented in diabetic ketoacidosis [166]. Hyperglycaemia affects about 10% of children during their remission induction therapy, and the timing often follows the first dose of L-asparaginase. Older age (over 10 years), presence of obesity, family history of diabetes mellitus and Down syndrome were reported to be the main risk factors associated with L-asparaginase-induced diabetes

[167]. Hyperglycaemia normalizes in most children after cessation of the medication, although transient therapy with insulin may be required [166, 167]. One putative mechanism for the transient diabetes seen with this drug may be decreased insulin synthesis secondary to depletion of endogenous L-asparagine [166]. Individuals treated with L-asparaginase demonstrate lower serum insulin and higher glucagon levels [168].

Lastly, several medications which are used to treat central nervous system disorders in children and youth are known to increase weight gain and predispose to insulin resistance. The most commonly used include valproate and the atypical antipsychotics, clozapine and olanzapine [169-176]. In one study, 58% of children treated with valproate experienced weight gain with 14% increasing to above the 85$^{th}$ percentile for age and gender [170]. Other studies in children and adults demonstrate both increased weight gain and increase fasting insulin levels with valproate therapy [169, 171]. There have also been recent concerns about the occurrence of diabetes and weight gain among children and adolescents treated with atypical antipsychotic (AAP) medications. While there are no published data on the prevalence of obesity in children associated with these medications, clozapine and olanzapine have been reported to cause increased appetite and substantial weight gain in children treated for various psychiatric conditions [172-176]. The development of new-onset diabetes in non-obese adults suggest also mechanisms unrelated to weight gain [177]. For unknown reasons, schizophrenia itself is also associated with an increased risk on diabetes in adults, even in untreated patients, and the use of AAP increases further the risk [178, 179]. The relationship between abnormal glucose metabolism and AAP is stronger for clozapine and olanzapine [173], and studies have shown that hyperglycaemia is not dose-dependent, improves with discontinuation of these drugs, and recurs on reintroduction of the medication [178, 179].The exact mechanisms of insulin resistance induced by AAP are not fully understood, but identified risk factors include presence of schizophrenia, baseline overweight or weight gain during treatment, African-American ethnicity and family or personal history of diabetes [179, 180]. Thus it appears that youth most at-risk for development of type 2 diabetes, may also be vulnerable to the effects of these drugs.

## CONCLUSION

Insulin resistance may be associated with various conditions commonly encountered in the pediatric age group, including type 1 diabetes, β-thalassemia major and cystic fibrosis. It may also be an unintended consequence of therapy of childhood diseases, including cancer, numerous conditions requiring steroid therapy, and in those receiving medications acting on the central nervous system which influence weight gain. There are also rare conditions, such as the lipodystrophies, associated with insulin resistance that present primarily during childhood. There is very little in the literature in regards to treatment or prevention of insulin resistance in these conditions, and further research is warranted, given the known long-term morbidity associated with insulin resistance and its associated metabolic complications.

## References

[1] Kahn CR, Rosenthal AS. Immunologic reactions to insulin: insulin allergy, insulin resistance, and the autoimmune insulin syndrome. *Diabetes Care* 1979;2(3):283-95.

[2] Madsbad S, Krarup T, Regeur L, Faber OK, Binder C. Insulin secretory reserve in insulin dependent patients at time of diagnosis and the first 180 days of insulin treatment. *Acta Endocrinol* (Copenh) 1980;95(3):359-63.

[3] Sochett EB, Daneman D, Clarson C, Ehrlich RM. Factors affecting and patterns of residual insulin secretion during the first year of type 1 (insulin-dependent) diabetes mellitus in children. *Diabetologia* 1987;30(7):453-9.

[4] Yki-Jarvinen H, Koivisto VA. Natural course of insulin resistance in type I diabetes. *N Engl J Med* 1986;315(4):224-30.

[5] Yki-Jarvinen H, Koivisto VA. Insulin sensitivity in newly diagnosed type 1 diabetics after ketoacidosis and after three months of insulin therapy. J Clin Endocrinol Metab 1984;59(3):371-8.

[6] Simonson DC, Tamborlane WV, Sherwin RS, Smith JD, DeFronzo RA. Improved insulin sensitivity in patients with type I diabetes mellitus after CSII. *Diabetes* 1985;34 Suppl 3:80-6.

[7] Effect of intensive therapy on residual beta-cell function in patients with type 1 diabetes in the diabetes control and complications trial. A randomized, controlled trial. The Diabetes Control and Complications Trial Research Group. *Ann Intern Med* 1998;128(7):517-23.

[8] Walker BG, Phear DN, Martin FI, Baird CW. Inhibition of Insulin by Acidosis. *Lancet* 1963;186:964-5.

[9] Barrett EJ, DeFronzo RA, Bevilacqua S, Ferrannini E. Insulin resistance in diabetic ketoacidosis. *Diabetes* 1982;31(10):923-8.

[10] Krane EJ. Diabetic ketoacidosis. Biochemistry, physiology, treatment, and prevention. *Pediatr Clin North Am* 1987;34(4):935-60.

[11] Schade DS, Eaton RP. The temporal relationship between endogenously secreted stress hormones and metabolic decompensation in diabetic man. *J Clin Endocrinol Metab* 1980;50(1):131-6.

[12] Ginsberg HN. Investigation of insulin resistance during diabetic ketoacidosis: role of counterregulatory substances and effect of insulin therapy. *Metabolism* 1977;26(10):1135-46.

[13] DeFronzo RA, Bonadonna RC, Ferrannini E. Pathogenesis of NIDDM. A balanced overview. *Diabetes Care* 1992;15(3):318-68.

[14] Randle PJ, Garland PB, Hales CN, Newsholme EA. The glucose fatty-acid cycle. Its role in insulin sensitivity and the metabolic disturbances of diabetes mellitus. *Lancet* 1963;1:785-9.

[15] Lee KU, Lee HK, Koh CS, Min HK. Artificial induction of intravascular lipolysis by lipid-heparin infusion leads to insulin resistance in man. *Diabetologia* 1988;31(5):285-90.

[16] Jensen CB, Storgaard H, Holst JJ, Dela F, Madsbad S, Vaag AA. Insulin secretion and cellular glucose metabolism after prolonged low-grade intralipid infusion in young men. *J Clin Endocrinol Metab* 2003;88(6):2775-83.

[17] Zierath JR, Kawano Y. The effect of hyperglycaemia on glucose disposal and insulin signal transduction in skeletal muscle. *Best Pract Res Clin Endocrinol Metab* 2003;17(3):385-98.
[18] Wu L, Nicholson W, Knobel SM, et al. Oxidative stress is a mediator of glucose toxicity in insulin-secreting pancreatic islet cell lines. *J Biol Chem* 2004;279(13):12126-34.
[19] Kajimoto Y, Kaneto H. Role of oxidative stress in pancreatic beta-cell dysfunction. *Ann N Y Acad Sci* 2004;1011:168-76.
[20] Caprio S, Plewe G, Diamond MP, et al. Increased insulin secretion in puberty: a compensatory response to reductions in insulin sensitivity. *J Pediatr* 1989;114(6):963-7.
[21] Amiel SA, Sherwin RS, Simonson DC, Lauritano AA, Tamborlane WV. Impaired insulin action in puberty. A contributing factor to poor glycemic control in adolescents with diabetes. *N Engl J Med* 1986;315(4):215-9.
[22] Amiel SA, Caprio S, Sherwin RS, Plewe G, Haymond MW, Tamborlane WV. Insulin resistance of puberty: a defect restricted to peripheral glucose metabolism. *J Clin Endocrinol Metab* 1991;72(2):277-82.
[23] Moran A, Jacobs DR, Jr., Steinberger J, et al. Insulin resistance during puberty: results from clamp studies in 357 children. *Diabetes* 1999;48(10):2039-44.
[24] Caprio S. Insulin: the other anabolic hormone of puberty. *Acta Paediatr Suppl* 1999;88(433):84-7.
[25] Arslanian SA, Heil BV, Becker DJ, Drash AL. Sexual dimorphism in insulin sensitivity in adolescents with insulin-dependent diabetes mellitus. *J Clin Endocrinol Metab* 1991;72(4):920-6.
[26] Hamilton J, Daneman D. Deteriorating diabetes control during adolescence: physiological or psychosocial? *J Pediatr Endocrinol Metab* 2002;15(2):115-26.
[27] Mortensen HB, Hougaard P. Comparison of metabolic control in a cross-sectional study of 2,873 children and adolescents with IDDM from 18 countries. The Hvidore Study Group on Childhood Diabetes. *Diabetes Care* 1997;20(5):714-20.
[28] Effect of intensive diabetes treatment on the development and progression of long-term complications in adolescents with insulin-dependent diabetes mellitus: Diabetes Control and Complications Trial. Diabetes Control and Complications Trial Research Group. *J Pediatr* 1994;125(2):177-88.
[29] Luna AM, Wilson DM, Wibbelsman CJ, et al. Somatomedins in adolescence: a cross-sectional study of the effect of puberty on plasma insulin-like growth factor I and II levels. *J Clin Endocrinol Metab* 1983;57(2):268-71.
[30] Edge JA, Dunger DB, Matthews DR, Gilbert JP, Smith CP. Increased overnight growth hormone concentrations in diabetic compared with normal adolescents. *J Clin Endocrinol Metab* 1990;71(5):1356-62.
[31] Tapanainen P, Kaar ML, Leppaluoto J, Huttunen NP, Knip M. Normal stimulated growth hormone secretion but low peripheral levels of insulin-like growth factor I in prepubertal children with insulin-dependent diabetes mellitus. *Acta Paediatr* 1995;84(6):646-50.
[32] Munoz MT, Barrios V, Pozo J, Argente J. Insulin-like growth factor I, its binding proteins 1 and 3, and growth hormone-binding protein in children and adolescents with

insulin-dependent diabetes mellitus: clinical implications. *Pediatr Res* 1996;39(6):992-8.

[33] Clayton KL, Holly JM, Carlsson LM, et al. Loss of the normal relationships between growth hormone, growth hormone-binding protein and insulin-like growth factor-I in adolescents with insulin-dependent diabetes mellitus. *Clin Endocrinol (Oxf)* 1994;41(4):517-24.

[34] Bereket A, Lang CH, Wilson TA. Alterations in the growth hormone-insulin-like growth factor axis in insulin dependent diabetes mellitus. *Horm Metab Res* 1999;31(2-3):172-81.

[35] Connors MH. Growth in the diabetic child. *Pediatr Clin North Am* 1997;44(2):301-6.

[36] Acerini CL, Patton CM, Savage MO, Kernell A, Westphal O, Dunger DB. Randomised placebo-controlled trial of human recombinant insulin-like growth factor I plus intensive insulin therapy in adolescents with insulin-dependent diabetes mellitus. *Lancet* 1997;350(9086):1199-204.

[37] Travers SH, Jeffers BW, Bloch CA, Hill JO, Eckel RH. Gender and Tanner stage differences in body composition and insulin sensitivity in early pubertal children. J *Clin Endocrinol Metab* 1995;80(1):172-8.

[38] Bloch CA, Clemons P, Sperling MA. Puberty decreases insulin sensitivity. *J Pediatr* 1987;110(3):481-7.

[39] Hanaire-Broutin H, Sallerin-Caute B, Poncet MF, et al. Effect of intraperitoneal insulin delivery on growth hormone binding protein, insulin-like growth factor (IGF)-I, and IGF-binding protein-3 in IDDM. *Diabetologia* 1996;39(12):1498-504.

[40] Reaven GM, Sageman WS, Swenson RS. Development of insulin resistance in normal dogs following alloxan-induced insulin deficiency. *Diabetologia* 1977;13(5):459-62.

[41] Yki-Jarvinen H. Acute and chronic effects of hyperglycaemia on glucose metabolism. *Diabetologia* 1990;33(10):579-85.

[42] Yki-Jarvinen H, Helve E, Koivisto VA. Hyperglycaemia decreases glucose uptake in type I diabetes. *Diabetes* 1987;36(8):892-6.

[43] Caprio S, Amiel S, Tamborlane WV, Gelfand RA, Sherwin RS. Defective free-fatty acid and oxidative glucose metabolism in IDDM during hypoglycaemia. Influence of glycemic control. *Diabetes* 1990;39(2):134-41.

[44] Hawkins M, Tonelli J, Kishore P, et al. Contribution of elevated free fatty acid levels to the lack of glucose effectiveness in type 2 diabetes. *Diabetes* 2003;52(11):2748-58.

[45] Staehr P, Hother-Nielsen O, Landau BR, Chandramouli V, Holst JJ, Beck-Nielsen H. Effects of free fatty acids per se on glucose production, gluconeogenesis, and glycogenolysis. *Diabetes* 2003;52(2):260-7.

[46] Azad K, Parkin JM, Court S, Laker MF, Alberti KG. Circulating lipids and glycaemic control in insulin dependent diabetic children. *Arch Dis Child* 1994;71(2):108-13.

[47] Wiltshire EJ, Hirte C, Couper JJ. Dietary fats do not contribute to hyperlipidemia in children and adolescents with type 1 diabetes. *Diabetes Care* 2003;26(5):1356-61.

[48] Tamborlane WV, Hintz RL, Bergman M, Genel M, Felig P, Sherwin RS. Insulin-infusion-pump treatment of diabetes: influence of improved metabolic control on plasma somatomedin levels. *N Engl J Med* 1981;305(6):303-7.

[49] Daniel JR, Hagmeyer KO. Metformin and insulin: is there a role for combination therapy? *Ann Pharmacother* 1997;31(4):474-80.

[50] Sarnblad S, Kroon M, Aman J. Metformin as additional therapy in adolescents with poorly controlled type 1 diabetes: randomised placebo-controlled trial with aspects on insulin sensitivity. *Eur J Endocrinol* 2003;149(4):323-9.
[51] Hamilton J, Cummings E, Zdravkovic V, Finegood D, Daneman D. Metformin as an adjunct therapy in adolescents with type 1 diabetes and insulin resistance: a randomized controlled trial. *Diabetes Care* 2003;26(1):138-43.
[52] Lacigova S, Rusavy Z, Jankovec Z, Kyselova P. [Metformin in the treatment of type 1 diabetics--a placebo controlled study]. *Cas Lek Cesk* 2001;140(10):302-6.
[53] Gomez R, Mokhashi MH, Rao J, et al. Metformin adjunctive therapy with insulin improves glycemic control in patients with type 1 diabetes mellitus: a pilot study. *J Pediatr Endocrinol Metab* 2002;15(8):1147-51.
[54] Hauner H. The mode of action of thiazolidinediones. *Diabetes Metab Res Rev* 2002;18 Suppl 2:S10-5.
[55] Sels JP, Verdonk HE, Wolffenbuttel BH. Effects of acarbose (Glucobay) in persons with type 1 diabetes: a multicentre study. *Diabetes Res Clin Pract* 1998;41(2):139-45.
[56] Hollander P, Pi-Sunyer X, Coniff RF. Acarbose in the treatment of type I diabetes. *Diabetes Care* 1997;20(3):248-53.
[57] Riccardi G, Giacco R, Parillo M, et al. Efficacy and safety of acarbose in the treatment of Type 1 diabetes mellitus: a placebo-controlled, double-blind, multicentre study. *Diabet Med* 1999;16(3):228-32.
[58] Carroll PV, Christ ER, Umpleby AM, et al. IGF-I treatment in adults with type 1 diabetes: effects on glucose and protein metabolism in the fasting state and during a hyperinsulinemic-euglycemic amino acid clamp. *Diabetes* 2000;49(5):789-96.
[59] Cheetham TD, Jones J, Taylor AM, Holly J, Matthews DR, Dunger DB. The effects of recombinant insulin-like growth factor I administration on growth hormone levels and insulin requirements in adolescents with type 1 (insulin-dependent) diabetes mellitus. *Diabetologia* 1993;36(7):678-81.
[60] Flyvbjerg A. Role of growth hormone, insulin-like growth factors (IGFs) and IGF-binding proteins in the renal complications of diabetes. *Kidney Int Suppl* 1997;60:S12-9.
[61] Thrailkill KM, Quattrin T, Baker L, Kuntze JE, Compton PG, Martha PM, Jr. Cotherapy with recombinant human insulin-like growth factor I and insulin improves glycemic control in type 1 diabetes. RhIGF-I in IDDM Study Group. *Diabetes Care* 1999;22(4):585-92.
[62] Hyer SL, Sharp PS, Brooks RA, Burrin JM, Kohner EM. Serum IGF-1 concentration in diabetic retinopathy. *Diabet Med* 1988;5(4):356-60.
[63] Krassowski J, Rogala H, Jeske W, Zgliczynski S. [Inhibition of growth hormone (GH) response to GHRH in diabetes mellitus type 1 after blockade of the cholinergic system with pirenzepine*]. Pol Arch Med Wewn* 1992;88(1):25-9.
[64] Halldin MU, Brismar K, Tuvemo T, Gustafsson J. Insulin sensitivity and lipolysis in adolescent girls with poorly controlled type 1 diabetes: effect of anticholinergic treatment. *Clin Endocrinol (Oxf)* 2002;57(6):735-43.
[65] Lanng S, Schwartz M, Thorsteinsson B, Koch C. Endocrine and exocrine pancreatic function and the delta F508 mutation in cystic fibrosis. *Clin Genet* 1991;40(5):345-8.
[66] Finkelstein SM, Wielinski CL, Elliott GR, et al. Diabetes mellitus associated with cystic fibrosis. *J Pediatr* 1988;112(3):373-7.

[67] Reisman J, Corey M, Canny G, Levison H. Diabetes mellitus in patients with cystic fibrosis: effect on survival. *Pediatrics* 1990;86(3):374-7.

[68] Elborn JS, Shale DJ, Britton JR. Cystic fibrosis: current survival and population estimates to the year 2000. *Thorax* 1991;46(12):881-5.

[69] FitzSimmons SC. The changing epidemiology of cystic fibrosis. *J Pediatr* 1993;122(1):1-9.

[70] Lanng S, Thorsteinsson B, Nerup J, Koch C. Influence of the development of diabetes mellitus on clinical status in patients with cystic fibrosis. *Eur J Pediatr* 1992;151(9):684-7.

[71] Lanng S, Thorsteinsson B, Nerup J, Koch C. Diabetes mellitus in cystic fibrosis: effect of insulin therapy on lung function and infections. *Acta Paediatr* 1994;83(8):849-53.

[72] Hardin DS, Moran A. Diabetes mellitus in cystic fibrosis. *Endocrinol Metab Clin North Am* 1999;28(4):787-800, ix.

[73] Lanng S, Hansen A, Thorsteinsson B, Nerup J, Koch C. Glucose tolerance in patients with cystic fibrosis: five year prospective study. *Bmj* 1995;311(7006):655-9.

[74] Solomon MP, Wilson DC, Corey M, et al. Glucose intolerance in children with cystic fibrosis. *J Pediatr* 2003;142(2):128-32.

[75] Cystic Fibrosis Foundation. Cystic Fibrosis Foundation National Patient Registry: 1997 *Annual Data Report*. Bethesda; 1998.

[76] Rosenecker J, Eichler I, Kuhn L, Harms HK, von der Hardt H. Genetic determination of diabetes mellitus in patients with cystic fibrosis. Multicenter Cystic Fibrosis Study Group. *J Pediatr* 1995;127(3):441-3.

[77] Lohr M, Goertchen P, Nizze H, et al. Cystic fibrosis associated islet changes may provide a basis for diabetes. An immunocytochemical and morphometrical study. *Virchows Arch A Pathol Anat Histopathol* 1989;414(2):179-85.

[78] Cucinotta D, Conti Nibali S, Arrigo T, et al. Beta cell function, peripheral sensitivity to insulin and islet cell autoimmunity in cystic fibrosis patients with normal glucose tolerance. *Horm Res* 1990;34(1):33-8.

[79] Lanng S, Thorsteinsson B, Roder ME, et al. Pancreas and gut hormone responses to oral glucose and intravenous glucagon in cystic fibrosis patients with normal, impaired, and diabetic glucose tolerance. *Acta Endocrinol (Copenh)* 1993;128(3):207-14.

[80] Austin A, Kalhan SC, Orenstein D, Nixon P, Arslanian S. Roles of insulin resistance and beta-cell dysfunction in the pathogenesis of glucose intolerance in cystic fibrosis. *J Clin Endocrinol Metab* 1994;79(1):80-5.

[81] Lippe BM, Sperling MA, Dooley RR. Pancreatic alpha and beta cell functions in cystic fibrosis. *J Pediatr* 1977;90(5):751-5.

[82] Moran A, Diem P, Klein DJ, Levitt MD, Robertson RP. Pancreatic endocrine function in cystic fibrosis. *J Pediatr* 1991;118(5):715-23.

[83] Moran A, Pyzdrowski KL, Weinreb J, et al. Insulin sensitivity in cystic fibrosis. *Diabetes* 1994;43(8):1020-6.

[84] Holl RW, Heinze E, Wolf A, Rank M, Teller WM. Reduced pancreatic insulin release and reduced peripheral insulin sensitivity contribute to hyperglycaemia in cystic fibrosis. *Eur J Pediatr* 1995;154(5):356-61.

[85] Lanng S, Thorsteinsson B, Roder ME, Nerup J, Koch C. Insulin sensitivity and insulin clearance in cystic fibrosis patients with normal and diabetic glucose tolerance. *Clin Endocrinol (Oxf)* 1994;41(2):217-23.

[86] Hardin DS, LeBlanc A, Lukenbough S, Seilheimer DK. Insulin resistance is associated with decreased clinical status in cystic fibrosis. *J Pediatr* 1997;130(6):948-56.
[87] Holl RW, Wolf A, Thon A, et al. Insulin resistance with altered secretory kinetics and reduced proinsulin in cystic fibrosis patients. *J Pediatr* Gastroenterol Nutr 1997;25(2):188-93.
[88] Yung B, Noormohamed FH, Kemp M, Hooper J, Lant AF, Hodson ME. Cystic fibrosis-related diabetes: the role of peripheral insulin resistance and beta-cell dysfunction. *Diabet Med* 2002;19(3):221-6.
[89] Lombardo F, De Luca F, Rosano M, et al. Natural history of glucose tolerance, beta-cell function and peripheral insulin sensitivity in cystic fibrosis patients with fasting euglycaemia. *Eur J Endocrinol* 2003;149(1):53-9.
[90] Hardin DS, Leblanc A, Marshall G, Seilheimer DK. Mechanisms of insulin resistance in cystic fibrosis. *Am J Physiol Endocrinol Metab* 2001;281(5):E1022-8.
[91] Hardin DS, LeBlanc A, Para L, Seilheimer DK. Hepatic insulin resistance and defects in substrate utilization in cystic fibrosis. *Diabetes* 1999;48(5):1082-7.
[92] Green DM, Hyland A, Chung CS, Zevon MA, Hall BC. Cancer and cardiac mortality among 15-year survivors of cancer diagnosed during childhood or adolescence. *J Clin Oncol* 1999;17(10):3207-15.
[93] Mertens AC, Yasui Y, Neglia JP, et al. Late mortality experience in five-year survivors of childhood and adolescent cancer: the Childhood Cancer Survivor Study. *J Clin Oncol* 2001;19(13):3163-72.
[94] Robertson CM, Hawkins MM, Kingston JE. Late deaths and survival after childhood cancer: implications for cure. *Bmj* 1994;309(6948):162-6.
[95] Hawkins MM, Kingston JE, Kinnier Wilson LM. Late deaths after treatment for childhood cancer. *Arch Dis Child* 1990;65(12):1356-63.
[96] Lustig RH, Post SR, Srivannaboon K, et al. Risk factors for the development of obesity in children surviving brain tumors. *J Clin Endocrinol Metab* 2003;88(2):611-6.
[97] Pinto G, Bussieres L, Recasens C, Souberbielle JC, Zerah M, Brauner R. Hormonal factors influencing weight and growth pattern in craniopharyngioma. *Horm Res* 2000;53(4):163-9.
[98] Goorin AM, Borow KM, Goldman A, et al. Congestive heart failure due to adriamycin cardiotoxicity: its natural history in children. *Cancer* 1981;47(12):2810-6.
[99] Gottdiener JS, Appelbaum FR, Ferrans VJ, Deisseroth A, Ziegler J. Cardiotoxicity associated with high-dose cyclophosphamide therapy. *Arch Intern Med* 1981;141(6):758-63.
[100] Harz KJ, Muller HL, Waldeck E, Pudel V, Roth C. Obesity in patients with craniopharyngioma: assessment of food intake and movement counts indicating physical activity. *J Clin Endocrinol Metab* 2003;88(11):5227-31.
[101] Sainsbury CP, Newcombe RG, Hughes IA. Weight gain and height velocity during prolonged first remission from acute lymphoblastic leukaemia. *Arch Dis Child* 1985;60(9):832-6.
[102] Shalet SM. Endocrine consequences of treatment of malignant disease. *Arch Dis Child* 1989;64(11):1635-41.
[103] Johansson JO, Fowelin J, Landin K, Lager I, Bengtsson BA. Growth hormone-deficient adults are insulin-resistant. *Metabolism* 1995;44(9):1126-9.

[104] Hwu CM, Kwok CF, Lai TY, et al. Growth hormone (GH) replacement reduces total body fat and normalizes insulin sensitivity in GH-deficient adults: a report of one-year clinical experience. *J Clin Endocrinol Metab* 1997;82(10):3285-92.

[105] Didi M, Didcock E, Davies HA, Ogilvy-Stuart AL, Wales JK, Shalet SM. High incidence of obesity in young adults after treatment of acute lymphoblastic leukemia in childhood. *J Pediatr* 1995;127(1):63-7.

[106] Sklar CA, Mertens AC, Walter A, et al. Changes in body mass index and prevalence of overweight in survivors of childhood acute lymphoblastic leukemia: role of cranial irradiation. *Med Pediatr Oncol* 2000;35(2):91-5.

[107] Oeffinger KC, Mertens AC, Sklar CA, et al. Obesity in adult survivors of childhood acute lymphoblastic leukemia: a report from the Childhood Cancer Survivor Study. *J Clin Oncol* 2003;21(7):1359-65.

[108] Curtis J, Daneman D, Hoffman HJ, Ehrlich RM. The endocrine outcome after surgical removal of craniopharyngiomas. *Pediatr Neurosurg* 1994;21 Suppl 1:24-7.

[109] Muller HL, Bueb K, Bartels U, et al. Obesity after childhood craniopharyngioma--German multicenter study on pre-operative risk factors and quality of life. *Klin Padiatr* 2001;213(4):244-9.

[110] Long-term outcomes for surgically resected craniopharyngiomas. *Neurosurgery* 2000;46(2):291-302; discussion -5.

[111] Talvensaari KK, Lanning M, Tapanainen P, Knip M. Long-term survivors of childhood cancer have an increased risk of manifesting the metabolic syndrome. J *Clin Endocrinol Metab* 1996;81(8):3051-5.

[112] Oeffinger KC, Buchanan GR, Eshelman DA, et al. Cardiovascular risk factors in young adult survivors of childhood acute lymphoblastic leukemia. *J Pediatr Hematol Oncol* 2001;23(7):424-30.

[113] Taskinen M, Saarinen-Pihkala UM, Hovi L, Lipsanen-Nyman M. Impaired glucose tolerance and dyslipidaemia as late effects after bone-marrow transplantation in childhood. *Lancet* 2000;356(9234):993-7.

[114] Srinivasan S, Ogle GD, Garnett SP, Briody JN, Lee JW, Cowell CT. Features of the metabolic syndrome after childhood craniopharyngioma. *J Clin Endocrinol Metab* 2004;89(1):81-6.

[115] Blatniczky L, Kautzky L, Peter F. Insulin metabolism in hypothalamic obesity. Exp *Clin Endocrinol* 1990;96(1):83-9.

[116] Lustig RH, Rose SR, Burghen GA, et al. Hypothalamic obesity caused by cranial insult in children: altered glucose and insulin dynamics and reversal by a somatostatin agonist. *J Pediatr* 1999;135(2 Pt 1):162-8.

[117] Necheles TF, Chung S, Sabbah R, Whitten D. Intensive transfusion therapy in thalassemia major: an eight-year follow-up. *Ann N Y Acad Sci* 1974;232(0):179-85.

[118] Weiner M, Karpatkin M, Hart D, et al. Cooley anemia: high transfusion regimen and chelation therapy, results, and perspective. *J Pediatr* 1978;92(4):653-8.

[119] McIntosh N. Endocrinopathy in thalassaemia major. *Arch Dis Child* 1976;51(3):195-201.

[120] Lassman MN, Genel M, Wise JK, Hendler R, Felig P. Carbohydrate homeostasis and pancreatic islet cell funtion in thalassemia. *Ann Intern Med* 1974;80(1):65-9.

[121] Flynn DM, Fairney A, Jackson D, Clayton BE. Hormonal changes in thalassaemia major. *Arch Dis Child* 1976;51(11):828-36.

[122] Multicentre study on prevalence of endocrine complications in thalassaemia major. Italian Working Group on Endocrine Complications in Non-endocrine Diseases. *Clin Endocrinol (Oxf)* 1995;42(6):581-6.
[123] Zuppinger K, Molinari B, Hirt A, et al. Increased risk of diabetes mellitus in beta-thalassemia major due to iron overload. *Helv Paediatr Acta* 1979;34(3):197-207.
[124] Saudek CD, Hemm RM, Peterson CM. Abnormal glucose tolerance in beta-thalassemia major. *Metabolism* 1977;26(1):43-52.
[125] Merkel PA, Simonson DC, Amiel SA, et al. Insulin resistance and hyperinsulinemia in patients with thalassemia major treated by hypertransfusion. *N Engl J Med* 1988;318(13):809-14.
[126] Dmochowski K, Finegood DT, Francombe W, Tyler B, Zinman B. Factors determining glucose tolerance in patients with thalassemia major. *J Clin Endocrinol Metab* 1993;77(2):478-83.
[127] Cavallo-Perin P, Pacini G, Cerutti F, et al. Insulin resistance and hyperinsulinemia in homozygous beta-thalassemia. *Metabolism* 1995;44(3):281-6.
[128] Pappas S, Donohue SM, Denver AE, Mohamed-Ali V, Goubet S, Yudkin JS. Glucose intolerance in thalassemia major is related to insulin resistance and hepatic dysfunction. *Metabolism* 1996;45(5):652-7.
[129] Sougleri M, Labropoulou-Karatza C, Paraskevopoulou P, Fragopanagou H, Alexandrides T. Chronic hepatitis C virus infection without cirrhosis induces insulin resistance in patients with alpha-thalassaemia major. *Eur J Gastroenterol Hepatol* 2001;13(10):1195-9.
[130] Arrigo T, Crisafulli G, Meo A, et al. Glucose tolerance, insulin secretion and peripheral sensitivity in thalassaemia major. *J Pediatr Endocrinol Metab* 1998;11 Suppl 3:863-6.
[131] Cario H, Holl RW, Debatin KM, Kohne E. Insulin sensitivity and beta-cell secretion in thalassaemia major with secondary haemochromatosis: assessment by oral glucose tolerance test. *Eur J Pediatr* 2003;162(3):139-46.
[132] Diagnosis and classification of diabetes mellitus. *Diabetes Care* 2004;27 Suppl 1:S5-S10.
[133] Whitehead JP, Soos MA, Jackson R, Tasic V, Kocova M, O'Rahilly S. Multiple molecular mechanisms of insulin receptor dysfunction in a patient with Donohue syndrome. *Diabetes* 1998;47(8):1362-4.
[134] Tritos NA, Mantzoros CS. Clinical review 97: Syndromes of severe insulin resistance. *J Clin Endocrinol Metab* 1998;83(9):3025-30.
[135] Kadowaki T, Bevins CL, Cama A, et al. Two mutant alleles of the insulin receptor gene in a patient with extreme insulin resistance. *Science* 1988;240(4853):787-90.
[136] Maassen JA, Tobias ES, Kayserilli H, et al. Identification and functional assessment of novel and known insulin receptor mutations in five patients with syndromes of severe insulin resistance. *J Clin Endocrinol Metab* 2003;88(9):4251-7.
[137] Longo N, Wang Y, Smith SA, Langley SD, DiMeglio LA, Giannella-Neto D. Genotype-phenotype correlation in inherited severe insulin resistance. *Hum Mol Genet* 2002;11(12):1465-75.
[138] Moller DE, Flier JS. Insulin resistance--mechanisms, syndromes, and implications. *N Engl J Med* 1991;325(13):938-48.
[139] Ten S, Maclaren N. Insulin resistance syndrome in children. *J Clin Endocrinol Metab* 2004;89(6):2526-39.

[140] Garg A. Acquired and inherited lipodystrophies. *N Engl J Med* 2004;350(12):1220-34.
[141] Misra A, Garg A. Clinical features and metabolic derangements in acquired generalized lipodystrophy: case reports and review of the literature. *Medicine* (Baltimore) 2003;82(2):129-46.
[142] Bolan C, Oral EA, Gorden P, Taylor S, Leitman SF. Intensive, long-term plasma exchange therapy for severe hypertriglyceridemia in acquired generalized lipoatrophy. *J Clin Endocrinol Metab* 2002;87(1):380-4.
[143] Haque WA, Shimomura I, Matsuzawa Y, Garg A. Serum adiponectin and leptin levels in patients with lipodystrophies. *J Clin Endocrinol Metab* 2002;87(5):2395.
[144] Williams DG, Bartlett A, Duffus P. Identification of nephritic factor as an immunoglobulin. *Clin Exp Immunol* 1978;33(3):425-9.
[145] Mathieson PW, Peters K. Are nephritic factors nephritogenic? *Am J Kidney Dis* 1994;24(6):964-6.
[146] Mathieson PW, Wurzner R, Oliveria DB, Lachmann PJ, Peters DK. Complement-mediated adipocyte lysis by nephritic factor sera. *J Exp Med* 1993;177(6):1827-31.
[147] Garg A. Lipodystrophies. *Am J Med* 2000;108(2):143-52.
[148] Jasin HE. Systemic lupus erythematosus, partial lipodystrophy and hypocomplementemia. *J Rheumatol* 1979;6(1):43-50.
[149] Torrelo A, Espana A, Boixeda P, Ledo A. Partial lipodystrophy and dermatomyositis. *Arch Dermatol* 1991;127(12):1846-7.
[150] Bastard JP, Caron M, Vidal H, et al. Association between altered expression of adipogenic factor SREBP1 in lipoatrophic adipose tissue from HIV-1-infected patients and abnormal adipocyte differentiation and insulin resistance. *Lancet* 2002;359(9311):1026-31.
[151] Dube MP, Johnson DL, Currier JS, Leedom JM. Protease inhibitor-associated hyperglycaemia. *Lancet* 1997;350(9079):713-4.
[152] Temple ME, Koranyi KI, Nahata MC. Lipodystrophy in HIV-infected pediatric patients receiving protease inhibitors. *Ann Pharmacother* 2003;37(9):1214-8.
[153] Amaya RA, Kozinetz CA, McMeans A, Schwarzwald H, Kline MW. Lipodystrophy syndrome in human immunodeficiency virus-infected children. *Pediatr Infect Dis J* 2002;21(5):405-10.
[154] Bitnun A, Sochett E, Babyn P, et al. Serum lipids, glucose homeostasis and abdominal adipose tissue distribution in protease inhibitor-treated and naive HIV-infected children. *Aids* 2003;17(9):1319-27.
[155] Melvin AJ, Lennon S, Mohan KM, Purnell JQ. Metabolic abnormalities in HIV type 1-infected children treated and not treated with protease inhibitors. *AIDS Res Hum Retroviruses* 2001;17(12):1117-23.
[156] Lainka E, Oezbek S, Falck M, Ndagijimana J, Niehues T. Marked dyslipidemia in human immunodeficiency virus-infected children on protease inhibitor-containing antiretroviral therapy. *Pediatrics* 2002;110(5):e56.
[157] Pandit MK, Burke J, Gustafson AB, Minocha A, Peiris AN. Drug-induced disorders of glucose tolerance. *Ann Intern Med* 1993;118(7):529-39.
[158] Olefsky JM, Kimmerling G. Effects of glucocorticoids on carbohydrate metabolism. *Am J Med Sci* 1976;271(2):202-10.
[159] Long CN KB, Fry EG. The adrenal cortex and carbohydrate metabolism. *Endocrinology* 1940;26:309-44.

[160] Pagano G, Cavallo-Perin P, Cassader M, et al. An in vivo and in vitro study of the mechanism of prednisone-induced insulin resistance in healthy subjects. *J Clin Invest* 1983;72(5):1814-20.

[161] Yasuda K, Kitabchi AE. Decreased insulin binding of human erythrocytes after dexamethasone or prednisone ingestion. *Diabetes* 1980;29(10):811-4.

[162] Greenspan LC, Gitelman SE, Leung MA, Glidden DV, Mathias RS. Increased incidence in post-transplant diabetes mellitus in children: a case-control analysis. *Pediatr Nephrol* 2002;17(1):1-5.

[163] Al-Uzri A, Stablein DM, R AC. Posttransplant diabetes mellitus in pediatric renal transplant recipients: a report of the North American Pediatric Renal Transplant Cooperative Study (NAPRTCS). *Transplantation* 2001;72(6):1020-4.

[164] Johny KV, Nampoory MR, Costandi JN, et al. High incidence of post-transplant diabetes mellitus in Kuwait. *Diabetes Res Clin Pract* 2002;55(2):123-30.

[165] al-Asfari R, Hadidy S, Hadid I, Ramadan F. The prevalence of diabetes post kidney transplantation. *Transplant Proc* 1999;31(8):3230.

[166] Gillette PC, Hill LL, Starling KA, Fernbach DJ. Transient diabetes mellitus secondary to L-asparaginase therapy in acute leukemia. *J Pediatr* 1972;81(1):109-11.

[167] Pui CH, Burghen GA, Bowman WP, Aur RJ. Risk factors for hyperglycaemia in children with leukemia receiving L-asparaginase and prednisone. *J Pediatr* 1981;99(1):46-50.

[168] Turner GR, Marks JF, Buchanan GR. Relative hyperglucagonemia in L-asparaginase- and prednisone-induced glucose intolerance in management of acute lymphocytic leukemia. *Clin Pediatr (Phila)* 1983;22(5):363-7.

[169] Luef G, Abraham I, Haslinger M, et al. Polycystic ovaries, obesity and insulin resistance in women with epilepsy. A comparative study of carbamazepine and valproic acid in 105 women. *J Neurol* 2002;249(7):835-41.

[170] Wirrell EC. Valproic acid-associated weight gain in older children and teens with epilepsy. *Pediatr Neurol* 2003;28(2):126-9.

[171] Verrotti A, Basciani F, De Simone M, Trotta D, Morgese G, Chiarelli F. Insulin resistance in epileptic girls who gain weight after therapy with valproic acid. *J Child Neurol* 2002;17(4):265-8.

[172] Jacobsen LK, Walker MC, Edwards JE, Chappell PB, Woolston JL. Clozapine in the treatment of a young adolescent with schizophrenia. *J Am Acad Child Adolesc Psychiatry* 1994;33(5):645-50.

[173] Stigler KA, Potenza MN, Posey DJ, McDougle CJ. Weight gain associated with atypical antipsychotic use in children and adolescents: prevalence, clinical relevance, and management. *Paediatr Drugs* 2004;6(1):33-44.

[174] Kumra S, Jacobsen LK, Lenane M, et al. Childhood-onset schizophrenia: an open-label study of olanzapine in adolescents. *J Am Acad Child Adolesc Psychiatry* 1998;37(4):377-85.

[175] Malone RP, Cater J, Sheikh RM, Choudhury MS, Delaney MA. Olanzapine versus haloperidol in children with autistic disorder: an open pilot study. *J Am Acad Child Adolesc Psychiatry* 2001;40(8):887-94.

[176] Frazier JA, Biederman J, Tohen M, et al. A prospective open-label treatment trial of olanzapine monotherapy in children and adolescents with bipolar disorder. *J Child Adolesc Psychopharmacol* 2001;11(3):239-50.

[177] Ramankutty G. Olanzapine-induced destabilization of diabetes in the absence of weight gain. *Acta Psychiatr Scand* 2002;105(3):235-6; discussion 6-7.
[178] Ananth J, Venkatesh R, Burgoyne K, Gunatilake S. Atypical antipsychotic drug use and diabetes. *Psychother Psychosom* 2002;71(5):244-54.
[179] Lindenmayer JP, Nathan AM, Smith RC. Hyperglycaemia associated with the use of atypical antipsychotics. *J Clin Psychiatry* 2001;62 Suppl 23:30-8.
[180] Saito E, Kafantaris V. Can diabetes mellitus be induced by medication? *J Child Adolesc Psychopharmacol* 2002;12(3):231-6.

In: Insulin Resistance in Children and Adolescents ISBN 1-59454-215-5
Editors: D. Daneman and J. Hamilton, pp. 209-233 

*Chapter 9*

# THERAPEUTIC APPROACHES TO INSULIN RESISTANCE IN CHILDREN

*Michael Freemark*
Division of Pediatric Endocrinology and Diabetes,
Duke University Medical Center, Durham, USA

## ABSTRACT

Treatment of insulin resistance requires a multifaceted approach designed to reduce body fat mass and blood pressure, increase insulin sensitivity in target tissues, reduce serum lipids and the expression of inflammatory cytokines, and normalize vascular/endothelial function. This review appraises the success of diet, exercise and pharmacologic agents in achieving these objectives and provides recommendations regarding the management of insulin resistance in children.

## INTRODUCTION

The pancreatic hormone insulin is the linchpin in the control of mammalian intermediary metabolism. In concert with other hormones and growth factors, insulin regulates blood glucose and lipid concentrations, stimulates fat deposition, glycogen storage and muscle protein synthesis, promotes linear growth and weight gain, and facilitates normal sexual development and function. Defects in insulin action ("insulin resistance") may result from mutations in the insulin receptor or its signaling components or from acute or chronic illness (infection, acidosis, uremia, lipodystrophy and the polycystic ovary syndrome), heightened production of insulin antagonists (glucocorticoids, growth hormone, prolactin, catecholamines, thyroid hormone and sex steroids), or pharmacotoxicity (for example prednisone, medroxyprogesterone acetate, protease inhibitors and atypical antipsychotics such as clozapine, olanzapine and risperidone). However, the most common cause of insulin resistance in children and adults is obesity [1]. The accumulation of visceral and abdominal subcutaneous fat correlates strongly with insulin resistance [1-3]. In contrast, insulin sensitivity correlates less well with femoral and gluteal stores of subcutaneous fat.

The combination of visceral/abdominal obesity, insulin resistance, dyslipidemia, hepatic steatosis, and hypertension constitutes the "metabolic syndrome" (Figure 1). In advanced stages the metabolic syndrome is accompanied by dysregulation of basal insulin secretion, loss of first phase glucose-dependent insulin production, and altered insulin processing, revealed as an increase in the circulating ratio of proinsulin to insulin [4]. The defects in beta cell function and loss of insulin production prefigure the development of type 2 diabetes ([1, 3, 5-8] Figure 2). Obesity and insulin resistance, even in the absence of type 2 diabetes, predispose to ovarian hyperandrogenism and reproductive dysfunction, cardiovascular disease, stroke, and malignancy ([9-19], Figure 1); however, the emergence of diabetes compounds the risks of vascular complications.

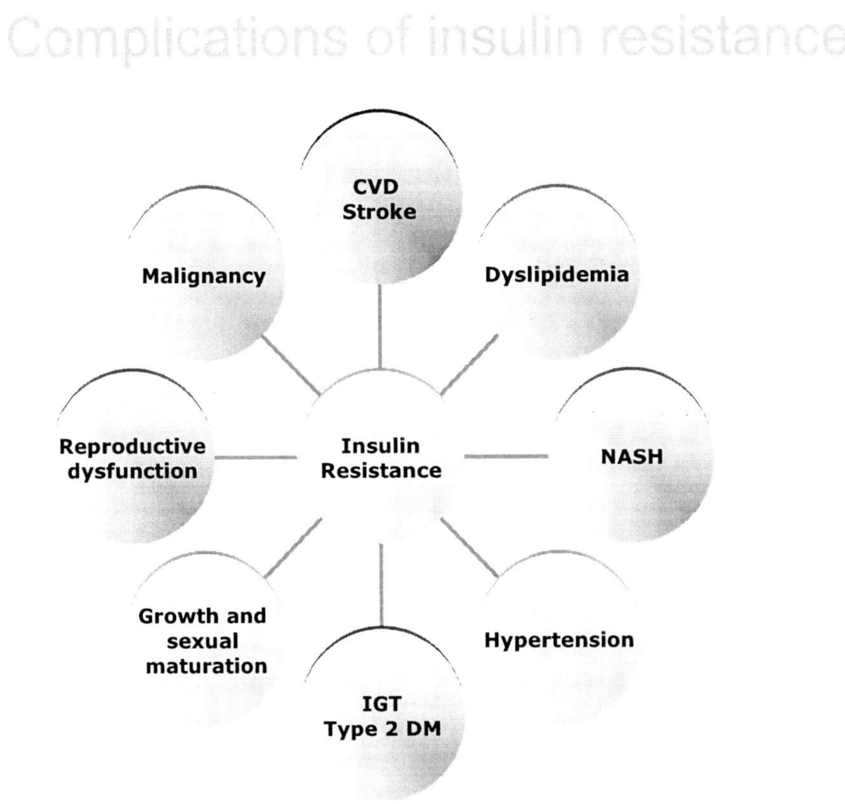


Figure 1. Complications of insulin resistance and the metabolic syndrome. CVD, cardiovascular disease; NASH, non-alcoholic steatohepatitis; IGT, impaired glucose tolerance; Type 2 DM, type 2 diabetes mellitus.

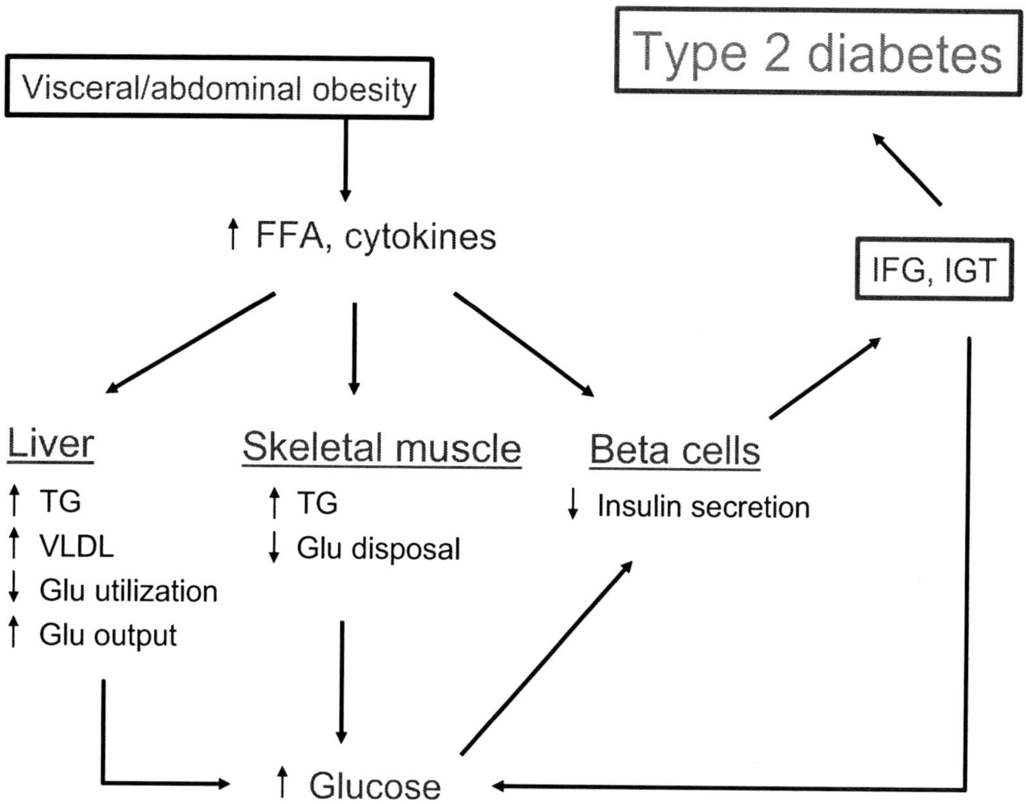


Figure 2. The deposition of visceral fat is accompanied by adipose tissue resistance to insulin action and heightened sensitivity to catecholamines (1-3). Adipose tissue uptake of glucose and FFA are reduced, rates of lipolysis are increased and triglyceride clearance is impaired because of down-regulation of lipoprotein lipase. The insulin resistance in adipose tissue is mediated by cytokines such as TNF alpha and IL-6 and by a fall in adiponectin. FFA released from visceral fat gain direct access to the liver via the portal vein, leading to hepatic triglyceride (TG) accumulation, very low density lipoprotein (VLDL) synthesis, decreased hepatic glucose (glu) utilization and increased glucose production. When fatty acid availability exceeds the rate of fatty acid oxidation, TG and their metabolites (long-chain fatty acyl coA, diacylglycerol) accumulate within skeletal muscle cells, reducing muscle insulin sensitivity and decreasing glucose disposal. Chronic elevations of glucose and FFA, in concert with inflammatory cytokines (5-8), induce beta cell dysfunction, loss of glucose-dependent insulin secretion, and ultimately, impaired fasting glucose (IFG), impaired glucose tolerance (IGT) and type 2 diabetes.

The pathogenetic mechanisms by which obesity and insulin resistance cause glucose intolerance and vascular insufficiency remain poorly understood. Nevertheless, emerging evidence suggests a complex web involving hyperinsulinemia, dyslipidemia, hyperglycaemia, hypertension, oxygen radicals, inflammatory cytokines, vascular growth and adhesion factors, and prothrombotic agents ([20-29], Figure 3). In theory, the therapy of insulin resistance requires a multifaceted approach (Figure 4) designed to: (a) reduce body mass index and visceral fat mass in obese patients; (b) increase the sensitivity of skeletal muscle and adipose tissue to insulin action, decrease circulating insulin concentrations, decrease hepatic glucose production, and reduce fasting and post-prandial glucose concentrations; (c) reduce circulating free fatty acid and triglyceride concentrations and normalize plasma lipids; (d) decrease blood pressure; (e) reduce the expression of inflammatory cytokines; and (f) normalize vascular and endothelial function. These objectives can be achieved in some instances through intensive lifestyle intervention involving caloric restriction and regular exercise. Pharmacologic agents may reinforce the effects of diet and exercise and reduce the risk of, or even reverse, complications. In all cases, the social milieu functions as a critical determinant of therapeutic success.

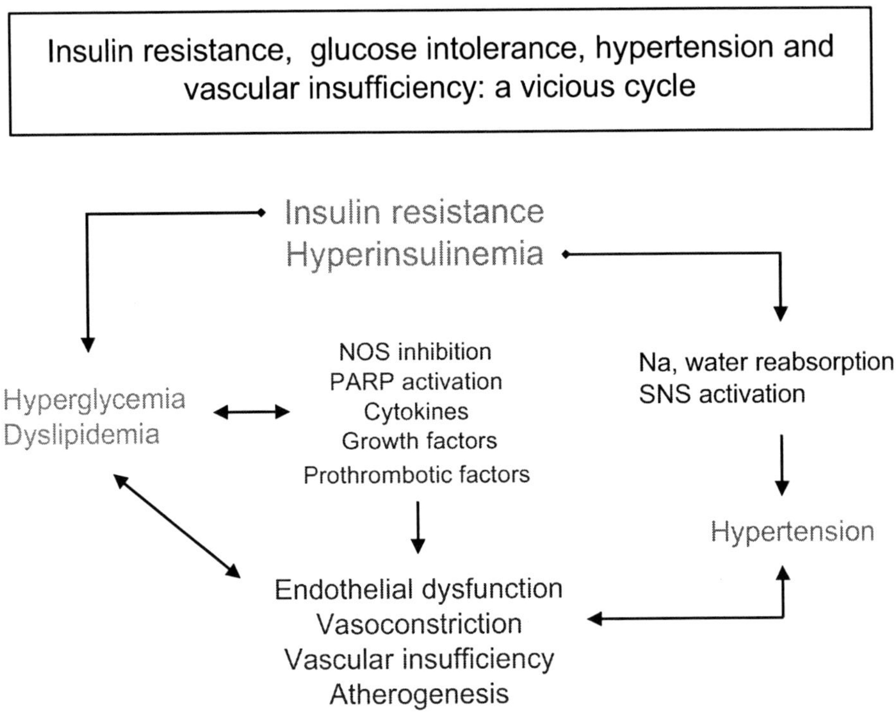


Figure 3. Under normal conditions insulin stimulates vasodilatation through induction of nitric oxide synthase (NOS), which generates NO in vascular endothelial cells. In obesity and other states associated with insulin resistance, the function of NOS is disrupted, leading to vasoconstriction and loss of tissue perfusion. The pathogenesis of vascular insufficiency is complex. Hyperinsulinemia causes sodium and water reabsorption and activation of the sympathetic nervous system (SNS), predisposing to hypertension (20-23). Hyperglycaemia contributes to endothelial dysfunction through generation of superoxide radicals; reactive oxygen species inhibit NOS and activate poly(ADP ribose) polymerase (PARP). Activation of PARP inhibits glyceraldehyde phosphate dehydrogenase activity and thereby promotes the formation of polyols, glucosamine, and advanced glycation endproducts and the activation of protein kinase C (24-27). Glucose-dependent expression of growth factors (such as vEGF and EGF) and cytokines (IL-1, IL-6 and TNF alpha) and a reduction in plasma adiponectin concentrations aggravate these effects by stimulating migration and proliferation of smooth muscle cells and increasing leukocyte adhesion to endothelial surfaces. Reduction in NO availability enhances platelet aggregation and limits fibrinolysis, promoting the progression of atheromatous clots. Increases in the concentrations of the prothrombotic plasminogen activator-1, which is also overexpressed by adipose tissue in obesity, may contribute to fibrin deposition on luminal walls (24-29), and the production of endothelin-1 in terminal blood vessels is increased, promoting vasoconstriction. These effects are exacerbated by dyslipidemia. The consequent reductions in tissue perfusion limit insulin-mediated glucose disposal, creating a vicious cycle.

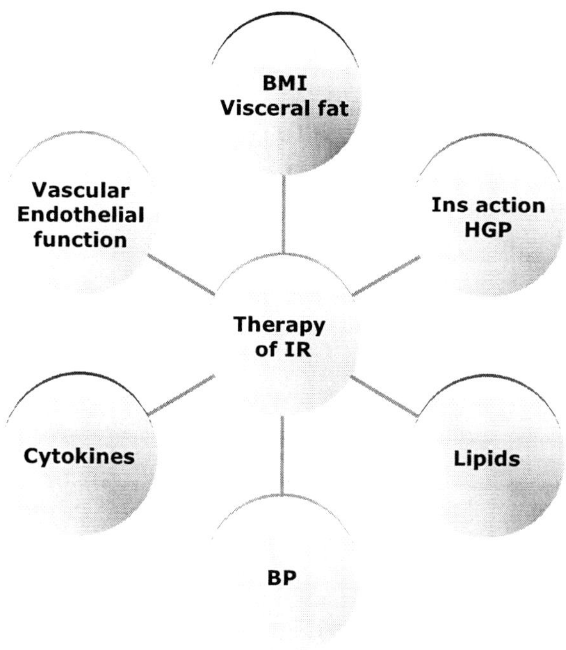


Figure 4. The therapy of insulin resistance requires a multifaceted approach designed to: (a) reduce body mass index (BMI) and visceral fat mass in obese patients; (b) increase the sensitivity of skeletal muscle and adipose tissue to insulin (Ins) action, decrease hepatic glucose production (HGP), and reduce fasting and post-prandial glucose concentrations; (c) decrease circulating insulin concentrations; (d) reduce circulating free fatty acid and triglyceride concentrations and normalize plasma lipids; (e) decrease blood pressure (BP); (f) reduce the expression of imflammatory cytokines; and (g) normalize vascular and endothelial function.

This chapter summarizes the potential benefits and risks of lifestyle intervention and pharmacotherapy in the treatment of insulin resistance and prevention of long-term complications.

## IDENTIFICATION AND SCREENING OF HIGH RISK PEDIATRIC PATIENTS

The first objective in preventing long-term complications is to identify populations at highest risk. Type 2 diabetes and the metabolic syndrome occur more commonly among African Americans, Hispanic Americans, Native Americans, Pacific Islanders and (possibly) Asian Americans than among those of Caucasian background and are far more prevalent among subjects with positive family histories [1,30]. The prevalence of type 2 diabetes increases with age but risk is modified by events that transpire before birth: the disease occurs more frequently in those born to diabetic mothers and in subjects born small for gestational age, particularly if there is rapid catch-up growth in early childhood [31,32]. Teenage girls and young women with polycystic ovarian syndrome (PCOS) are characteristically insulin resistant and hyperinsulinemic; by virtue of a heightened risk of PCOS in adolescence, girls with early adrenarche may also be vulnerable [33].

Given the high incidence of impaired glucose tolerance (IGT) and undisclosed diabetes among children with BMI z score exceeding 2 SDs for age and gender [34], the author recommends screening obese children who have one or more of the risk factors listed in **Table 1**. Alternatively, screening can be conducted in children with BMI > 85$^{th}$ percentile for age and gender with two or more associated risk factors [35]. Particular attention should be focused upon obese children with family histories of type 2 or gestational diabetes and those from high-risk ethnic groups. Progressive abdominal obesity is an ominous finding in any child or adult. The presence of acanthosis nigricans, which suggests insulin resistance, should also raise concern. Given the strong association of PCOS with insulin resistance, the author recommends screening all girls with ovarian hyperandrogenism, regardless of BMI.

**Table 1. Screening for Glucose Intolerance and the Metabolic Syndrome in Children and Adolescents. BMI, Body Mass Index; GDM, Gestational Diabetes Mellitus; 2 Hour Glucose, Fingerstick Glucose Two Hours following Administration of glucola; HbA1c, Hemoglobin A1c; FFA, Free Fatty Acids**

**High-risk children and adolescents:**

Obese (BMI z score > 95th percentile for age and gender), plus:

- a) High-risk ethnic group, and/or
- b) Family history of type 2 diabetes or GDM, and/or
- c) Acanthosis nigricans, and/or
- d) Prominent abdominal fat deposition

Ovarian hyperandrogenism

**Screening procedures:**

Blood pressure

Fasting glucose and insulin levels

Fasting lipid panel (+ FFA if possible)

2 hour glucose level (+ insulin if possible)

HbA1c (less useful)

For screening purposes some investigators recommend a fasting blood glucose level [35]; however, isolated measures of fasting blood glucose concentrations will miss a significant proportion of children with impaired glucose tolerance [34]. Others favor a formal glucose tolerance test [34]. In our clinic we have adopted a modified glucose challenge that better suits the need for population screening of obese children (Table 1). Our approach includes fasting measures of insulin, glucose and lipids, with a fingerstick glucose obtained 2 hours following the administration of glucola (1.75 gm/kg, max 75 gm). The blood pressure is obtained at the time of the initial blood sample. With this single venipuncture and one fingerstick sample, it is possible to identify patients with undisclosed diabetes, impaired fasting glucose (IFG, fasting glucose 111-125 mg%, 6.1-6.9 mmol/L), impaired glucose tolerance (IGT, 2 hour glucose 140-199 mg%, 7.8 – 11.0 mmol/L), dyslipidemia, and hypertension. Patients with insulin resistance but normal glucose tolerance can be identified by calculation of the quantitative insulin sensitivity check {QUICKI = 1/[log fasting insulin (uU/ml) + log fasting glucose (mg%)]}, which in obese adults correlates strongly with insulin sensitivity measured by insulin clamp techniques [36]. Measurement of free fatty acids in the fasting sample (revised QUICKI = 1/[log fasting insulin (uU/ml) + log fasting glucose (mg%) + log FFA (mmol)]}, permits detection of insulin resistance even in non-obese subjects [36].

## MANAGEMENT OF INSULIN RESISTANCE AND PREVENTION OF TYPE 2 DIABETES

Dietary and exercise counseling (*of the entire family*) are required for all obese or insulin resistant children and adolescents. However, those with IFG or IGT are at particularly high risk for developing type 2 diabetes; consequently, aggressive measures should be taken in this subgroup, regardless of age. There are two general approaches, not necessarily viewed in isolation: intensive lifestyle intervention and pharmacotherapy.

### Lifestyle Intervention

#### *Diet*

Mild caloric restriction can be safe and effective when obese children and their families are motivated and encouraged to change longstanding feeding behaviors. Significant reductions in weight are unusual and often transient unless caloric restriction is accompanied by increased energy expenditure. Diets severely restricted in calories produce more dramatic weight loss but cannot be sustained under free-living conditions. Very low calorie diets are potentially dangerous and may precipitate recurrent and futile cycles of dieting and binge eating.

The role of dietary macronutrients in the pathogenesis of obesity, insulin resistance and type 2 diabetes is highly controversial. Diets low in saturated fats reduce total energy intake, improve insulin sensitivity, and, in combination with exercise, can reduce significantly the risks of type 2 diabetes and cardiovascular disease in adults with impaired glucose tolerance (37 and below). Intake of polyunsaturated fat and long-chain omega-3 fatty acids, on the other hand, is associated with improved insulin sensitivity or glucose tolerance [37].

Yet recent investigations have shown that obese men and women lost more weight and had more significant reductions in plasma triglyceride concentrations on low-carbohydrate diets than on conventional low-fat diets [38,39]. A review of adult studies [40] suggests that the efficacy of low-carbohydrate diets may be related to caloric restriction and rather than to reduction in carbohydrate intake per se. Moreover, the effect of a low-carbohydrate diet may diminish with time. Adherence to low carbohydrate and low-fat diets is inconsistent without strong and continuing supervision and encouragement; drop-out rates in most studies are high.

Other macronutrients, vitamins and trace elements may contribute to diabetes risk. For example, intake of fiber (particularly whole grains and cereal) correlates inversely with the risks of type 2 diabetes and cardiovascular disease [41,42]. Insoluble and soluble fiber may limit fat absorption and thereby improve glucose tolerance. The intake of magnesium (from whole grains, nuts and green leafy vegetables) and dairy products containing Vitamin D and calcium may also correlate inversely with diabetes risk in young adults [43,44].

Limited evidence suggests that the nature or quality of ingested carbohydrate may modulate weight gain in childhood. The insulin secretory response to foods containing rapidly absorbed, concentrated carbohydrates (high glycemic index) exceeds the response to foods containing protein, fat and fiber. The rapid rise and subsequent fall in blood glucose following ingestion of sucrose may precipitate hunger [45], while fructose is lipogenic and delays the oxidation of fatty acids, facilitating fat storage [46]. Studies of the effects of glycemic index on weight gain in children are inconclusive. Still, a 19-month study [47] of Massachusetts school children found a positive correlation between BMI and the consumption of sugar-sweetened drinks, and a modified low-glycemic diet (45-50% carbohydrate, 30-35% fat) reduced BMI z score and fat mass in a pilot study of 7 obese adolescents [48]. Anecdotal evidence from our clinic suggests that simple elimination of concentrated soft drinks from the diet can reduce caloric intake in some obese adolescents by as much as 500-1000 kcal/d and thereby facilitate weight reduction.

From the available data, it seems reasonable to conclude that: (a) caloric restriction and weight reduction by any means will likely reduce the risk of type 2 diabetes and subsequent cardiovascular disease in obese children; (b) reduced intake of saturated fats will benefit obese adolescents as well as adults; (c) reduced consumption of high glycemic foods such as soda, fruit drinks, candy, white bread, pasta and potatoes will benefit obese children; and (d) a balanced diet containing vegetables, fruits, whole grains, fiber, lean meat, fish, and low-fat dairy products is best.

***Exercise***

A sedentary lifestyle increases the risk of diabetes, while exercise, in combination with caloric and fat restriction, reduces the rate of progression to diabetes in adults with IGT. The Malmo Feasability Study [49] and the DaQing study [50] demonstrated that lifestyle intervention reduced, by 63% and 36% respectively, the rate of progression to diabetes in adults with IGT. The Finnish Diabetes Prevention Study [51] randomized individuals with IGT and BMI >25kg/m$^2$ to a control group or an intensive intervention group, which was counseled to reduce total and saturated fat intake, increase fiber intake, reduce body weight and increase physical activity. No subjects who achieved target goals developed diabetes. In contrast, one third of those who failed to reach a single target developed diabetes. The primary determinant of diabetes prevention was an increase in insulin sensitivity associated with weight loss [52]. The Diabetes Prevention Program (DPP) [53] compared intensive to standard lifestyle recommendations. Intensive lifestyle changes, which included weight reduction, a decrease in saturated fat intake, and regular exercise (150 minutes per week) were accompanied by a 58% relative risk reduction in the prevalence of diabetes during a 3 year period.

The mechanisms by which exercise improves insulin sensitivity and glucose tolerance are complex, involving metabolic adaptations in adipose tissue, liver and skeletal muscle (Figure 5). Exercise has beneficial effects on fat storage and distribution, with losses of visceral fat depots exceeding those of subcutaneous fat stores [54]. Lean body mass increases, thereby augmenting resting energy expenditure. A reduction in visceral fat mass increases adipose tissue sensitivity to insulin; this explains in part the reductions in fasting and postprandial free fatty acid, LDL and triglyceride concentrations and the increase in plasma HDL levels in adults who adhere to a rigorous diet and exercise regimen [55]. The effect of exercise on plasma triglyceride is mediated through induction of lipoprotein lipase and reduction in triglyceride production [56].

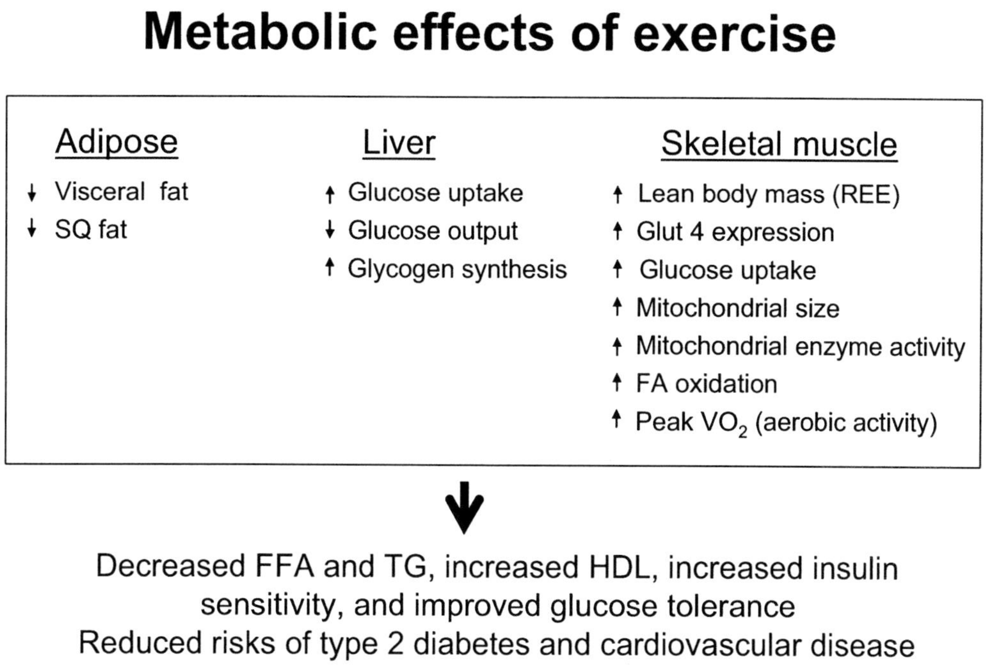


Figure 5. Effects of exercise on intermediary metabolism. REE, resting energy expenditure.

Exercise increases hepatic glucose uptake and glycogen synthesis and decreases hepatic glucose production [57], thereby reducing fasting glucose and insulin concentrations. In skeletal muscle, exercise stimulates insulin-dependent glucose uptake and thereby reduces post-prandial glucose levels; this action is mediated by increases in muscle GLUT-4 synthesis and induction of GLUT-4 translocation from intracellular pools to the plasma membrane [58]. The induction of GLUT-4 activity may be mediated in turn by an increase in cellular levels of AMP-activated protein kinase (AMPK) [59,60]. Activation of AMPK after an acute bout of exercise promotes increased cycling of existing GLUT-4 transporters in skeletal muscle as well as enhanced expression of hexokinase II and mitochondrial enzymes [60].

Several studies suggest that insulin action is related to the oxidative capacity of skeletal muscle. Insulin resistant individuals (including those with type 2 diabetes) have reduced activities of muscle oxidative enzymes [61]; aerobic exercise training increases muscle oxidative enzyme activity [62] and improves insulin sensitivity by 26-46% [58]. The effect of exercise on oxidative enzyme activity [60] may reflect in part an increase in mitochondrial size [62,63]. Interestingly weight loss alone may improve insulin sensitivity but does not alter fasting rates of lipid oxidation. In contrast, weight loss coupled with exercise increases fat oxidation [64].

Few studies have assessed the effects of exercise on insulin resistance in children. Nevertheless, a randomized, modified cross-over study [65] of 79 obese children (age 7-11 years) demonstrated that four months of exercise training (40 minutes of activity 5 days a week) decreased fasting insulin (10%) and triglyceride (17%) concentrations and reduced percent body fat (5%) even in the absence of dietary intervention. The effects on plasma insulin and body fat were reversed when training was discontinued. An 8 week trial of cycle ergometry and resistance training in obese adolescents reduced abdominal (7.0%) and trunk (3.7%) fat mass and normalized flow-mediated dilation of the brachial artery [66]. Though preliminary, these findings suggest that exercise has beneficial effects in obese children as well as adults. The capacity for voluntary exercise declines as BMI rises. It is therefore critical to begin regular exercise before the child becomes morbidly obese and functionally immobile.

Unfortunately, the long-term success of lifestyle intervention in adults has been disappointing, and rates of insulin resistance in children and adults continue to increase despite widespread recognition of the dangers of dietary indiscretion and a sedentary existence. This has stimulated interest in potential pharmacologic approaches to diabetes prevention and treatment of other insulin resistant states.

## Pharmacologic Approaches to Preventing Type 2 Diabetes

Emerging evidence suggests that a number of pharmacologic agents may reduce the risk of type 2 diabetes in high-risk patients. The majority of studies have focused on the biguanides (metformin) and the thiazolidinediones (Figure 6), but other agents, including acarbose, the statins and angiotension converting enzyme (ACE) inhibitors, are currently under evaluation. Only a few investigations have been performed in children, though initial findings are consistent with those in adults.

Metabolic effects of metformin and the thiazolidinediones (TZDs)

| | Metformin | TZDs |
|---|---|---|
| Hepatic glucose uptake | Increased | Variable increase |
| HGP | Decreased | Variable decrease |
| Adipose glucose uptake | Variable/negligible | Increased (SQ > Visc) |
| Lipolysis, FFA, and TG | Variable/negligible | Decreased |
| Fat stores | Decreased SQ > Visc | Decreased Visc, Incr SQ |
| Adiponectin | No effect | Increased |
| Skeletal mm glu uptake | No effect | Increased |
| Total insulin sensitivity | Variable | Increased |
| Food intake | Decreased | No effect |
| Body weight | Mild decrease | Mild-mod increase |
| Glucose tolerance | Improved | Improved |

Figure 6. Metabolic effects of metformin and the thiazolidinediones (TZDs). HGP, hepatic glucose production; FFA, free fatty acids; TG, triglycerides; glu, glucose; SQ, subcutaneous; Visc, visceral.

***Metformin***

Metformin is a bisubstituted, short-chain hydrophilic guanidine derivative that works through activation of AMP protein kinase [67]. Its major site of action is the liver: the drug increases hepatic glucose uptake, decreases gluconeogenesis, and reduces hepatic glucose production ([68,69], Figure 6). Metformin increases insulin-receptor binding [70-72] but has variable and often only minor effects on peripheral insulin sensitivity; there is no effect on skeletal muscle glucose uptake or plasma adiponectin concentrations [70-73]. Major advantages of the drug include decreased food intake, weight loss [73,74], decreased fat stores (subcutaneous > visceral), and improved lipid profiles. Of even greater importance, long term studies suggest that metformin reduces cardiovascular morbidity and mortality in diabetic adults [75,76].

Given that most children and adults with insulin resistance or IGT are obese, the effects of metformin on food intake, body weight, and plasma lipid concentrations are of particular interest. In obese adults with normal glucose tolerance, treatment with metformin reduced daily food intake, body weight, body fat and plasma leptin concentrations, and downward trends were noted in LDL and total plasma cholesterol [77,78].

Metformin also has beneficial effects on body weight and intermediary metabolism in women with PCOS [79,80]. In trials lasting 6-12 months, metformin reduced BMI, waist circumference, plasma leptin concentrations, and stores of subcutaneous and visceral adipose tissue. Fasting glucose and C-peptide levels and glucose-stimulated insulin levels declined, as did serum testosterone and PA-1 levels.

Non-obese women with PCOS, like their obese counterparts, are at increased risk for insulin resistance and type 2 diabetes. In normal weight (BMI ≤ 25), post-menarchal young (13.6-22 yr old) women with ovarian hyperandrogenism, hyperinsulinemia and normal glucose tolerance, metformin increased insulin sensitivity and reduced plasma insulin, triglyceride, and testosterone levels and the ratio of LDL to HDL. The addition of flutamide, an androgen antagonist, potentiated the effects of metformin on triglyceride, LDL/HDL and adrenal androgen concentrations and markedly reduced hirsutism scores. The combination of metformin and flutamide reduced abdominal and total body fat mass and increased lean body mass despite reductions in plasma GH and IGF-1 levels [81-83].

There have been two randomized, double-blind, placebo-controlled studies of metaformin in obese adolescents with insulin resistance, normal glucose tolerance, and a positive family history of type 2 diabetes. In the first trial (n=29), metformin reduced BMI z score (3.6% relative to placebo controls), plasma leptin, and fasting glucose (-9.8 mg%) and insulin (-12 uU/ml), even in the absence of dietary intervention [84]. Since increases in BMI and fasting glucose and insulin concentrations predict the development of type 2 diabetes in target populations [1,85,86], these findings suggested that metformin might prove useful in the prevention of glucose intolerance in high risk adolescents.

In the second trial (n=24), the combination of a low calorie diet (1500-1800 calorie/day for girls and boys, respectively) and metformin reduced weight by 6.5%; diet alone caused a 3.8% weight loss [87]. Patients treated with metformin had greater decline in body fat (-6% vs. -2.7% in the placebo group), a decrease in plasma leptin levels, a 50% decrease in plasma insulin concentrations, and increased insulin sensitivity as determined by fasting and 2 hour glucose and insulin levels. Plasma cholesterol and triglyceride levels also declined by 22% and 39%, respectively. These findings suggested that metformin and diet may act synergistically to limit weight gain and increase glucose tolerance in obese, insulin resistant adolescents.

The recently-completed Diabetes Prevention Program [53] established the efficacy of metformin in delaying or preventing the onset of type 2 diabetes in adults (age $\geq$ 25 yr) with impaired glucose tolerance (IGT). 3234 subjects were randomly assigned to one of three interventions. These included: a placebo group that received standard lifestyle recommendations; a metformin (850-1700 mg/d)-treated group that received standard lifestyle recommendations; and a group that received an intensive program of lifestyle modification. A fourth, troglitazone-treated group was disbanded after the development of severe hepatotoxicity in a small number of subjects. The experimental groups were studied for 1.8-4.6 years.

Daily energy and fat intake decreased only in the group randomized to intensive lifestyle modification. Nevertheless patients in the metformin group also lost weight, though not as much as those in the intensive lifestyle group. In both groups, weight loss was most significant in the first 6-12 months of the study. The changes in body weight were accompanied by reductions in the rates of progression from IGT to type 2 diabetes. The 3 year cumulative incidence of diabetes was 28.9% in the placebo group, 21.7% in the metformin-treated group, and 14.4% in the intensive lifestyle group. Overall, therefore, intensive lifestyle intervention was more effective than metformin.

Of note, certain subgroups responded preferentially to the various interventions. Metformin was as effective as lifestyle change in subjects with BMI exceeding 34.9 and in those with highest fasting glucose concentrations (Figure 7); these subgroups are at greatest risk for progression to type 2 diabetes. Metformin was also as effective as lifestyle intervention in younger adults aged 25-44 years. On the other hand, treatment effects did not vary according to gender, race or ethnic group.

In addition to reducing the risk of development of type 2 diabetes, intensive lifestyle intervention and metformin also had favorable, albeit small, effects on blood pressure and serum lipids. Systolic and diastolic blood pressures were reduced by 1.1 and 3.3 mm Hg, respectively, in the metformin and intensive lifestyle groups, while total cholesterol, LDL and triglyceride concentrations declined by 5 and 8 mg%, 4.0 and 4.3 mg%, and 6 and 23 mg%, respectively, and HDL levels increased slightly (0.5 and 0.8 mg%, respectively).

Metformin was well tolerated by the majority of subjects, though many patients had transient abdominal discomfort which can be prevented by taking the medication with food. There were no instances of hepatic dysfunction or lactic acidosis; nevertheless, the drug should not be administered to patients with underlying cardiac, hepatic, renal or gastrointestinal disease.

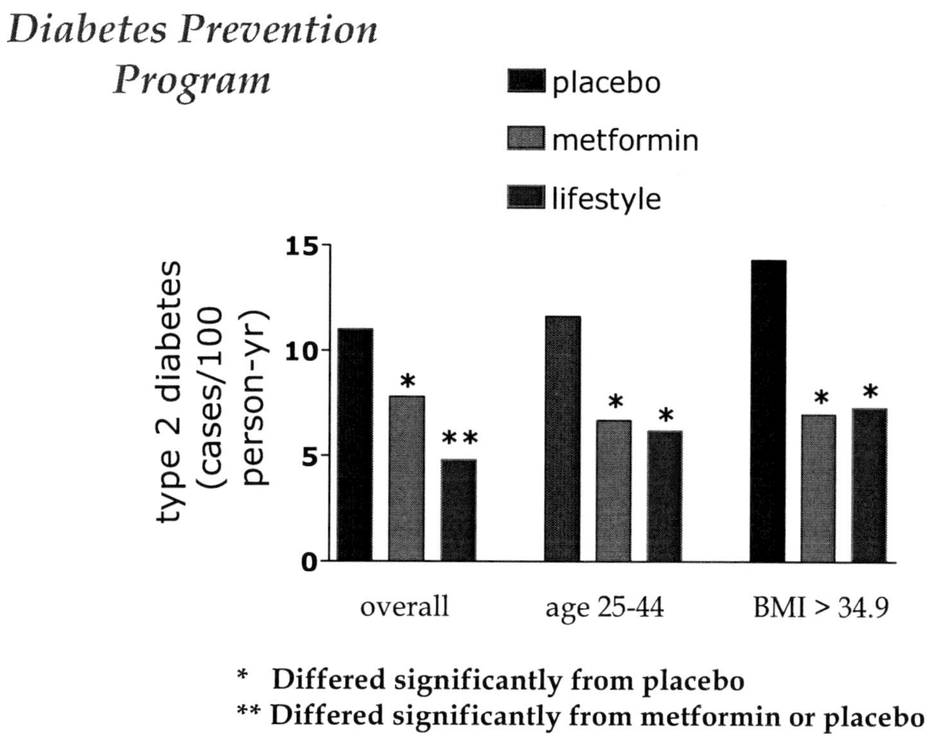


Figure 7. Effects of metformin and intensive lifestyle intervention on rates of type 2 diabetes in adults with IGT. Data adapted from Knowler et al. Diabetes Prevention Program [53] with permission.

The major effects of lifestyle intervention and metformin were exerted within the first 12-18 months of the study. After the first year, fasting blood glucose concentrations, HbA1c concentrations and rates of diabetes increased in both the intensive lifestyle and metformin groups, and the slopes of the intervention and treatment curves after the first year appeared to parallel the slope of the placebo group. This finding suggests that the interventions may delay, rather than truly prevent, the development of type 2 diabetes. Nevertheless, studies performed in non-diabetic subjects 1-2 weeks after the trial's conclusion showed that the protective effect of metformin persisted in three-fourths of the drug-treated subjects even after discontinuation of medication [88]. The duration of this protective effect is unknown; prolonged treatment with metformin might be necessary to reduce the rate of progression to diabetes in high risk subjects.

***Thiazolidinediones***

The thiazolidinediones (TZDs) regulate lipid and carbohydrate metabolism through binding to peroxisome proliferator-activated receptor (PPAR)-γ. When activated by TZDs, PPAR-γ heterodimerizes with the retinoid X receptor and binds to the promoters of target genes including lipoprotein lipase, fatty acid transport protein, acetyl coA-synthase, and aP2 [89]. The major effects of the TZDs are exerted in adipose tissue and skeletal muscle [3,89-91], (Figure 6). The drugs induce the differentiation of small insulin-sensitive adipocytes, increase adipose insulin receptor number, adiponectin expression and adipose tissue glucose uptake, and reduce expression of TNF alpha and, in mice, resistin. Rates of lipolysis and FFA release are reduced, triglyceride clearance is enhanced, and hepatic VLDL synthesis decreases. Circulating triglyceride levels decline during treatment with pioglitazone and to a lesser extent with rosiglitazone. With adipogenic and anti-lipolytic actions, the TZDs increase total body fat mass and body weight, though fat may be re-distributed from visceral to subcutaneous stores [91-94]. TZDs potentiate the effects of insulin on skeletal muscle glucose uptake through induction of glucose transporters (GLUTs) 1 and 4 [91]. These actions, which may be mediated indirectly through effects on adipose gene expression [94], require the presence of insulin and may be mediated by activation of phosphatidylinositol (PI) 3-kinase [95]. Glucose tolerance improves in type 2 diabetic patients treated with TZDs; plasma insulin concentrations decline while plasma adiponectin levels rise. The rise in adiponectin, in concert with direct anti-inflammatory effects of the TZDs on the vascular endothelium [96], reduces carotid intimal medial thickness and increases arterial distensibility. TZDs also reduce plasma C-reactive protein concentrations in diabetic patients and the percentage of small dense LDL levels in diabetic and non-diabetic hypertensive adults [97,98]. In theory, these changes reduce the risk of development and/or progression of atheromatous lesions.

A few studies have examined the effects of the TZDs on glucose tolerance, lipid profiles and other cardiovascular risk factors in nondiabetic adults and in women with PCOS. No such investigations have been performed in children or adolescents. Nolan et al demonstrated that troglitazone decreases insulin resistance and improves glucose tolerance in obese non-diabetic patients [99]. Rates of glucose disposal and the insulin-sensitivity index increased while glycemic responses to oral glucose declined. The mean fasting insulin concentrations decreased by 48% and the plasma insulin responses to oral glucose and mixed meals decreased by 40 and 41 % respectively. Other investigators noted that TZDs reduce blood pressure in nondiabetic obese adults [90,100]. In women with PCOS, a three month trial of troglitazone reduced fasting glucose and insulin concentrations and improved, but did not normalize, whole body insulin sensitivity [101]. Troglitazone also improved endothelial function as measured by leg blood flow.

The results of these studies indicate that the TZDs increase insulin sensitivity, improve glucose tolerance and reduce cardiovascular risk in insulin resistant adults and in women with PCOS. That the TZDs, like metformin, can reduce the risk of type 2 diabetes in target populations was established in the TRIPOD study [102], a randomized, placebo-controlled, double-blinded investigation of women with impaired glucose tolerance (IGT). The experimental group consisted of Latino women with a history of gestational diabetes and IGT at the time of initiation of the study. During the 30 month investigation, annual diabetes incidence rates were 12.1% in the placebo group and 5.4% in the troglitazone group. Those with an initial increase in whole body insulin sensitivity were most likely to benefit from troglitazone. Interestingly, protection from diabetes persisted for at least 3-8 months after the drug was discontinued. This finding suggests that the drug may have altered the natural progression of diabetes and not simply masked progression through a pharmacologic action. As with metformin, the duration of this protective action is currently unknown.

Unfortunately, troglitazone was removed from the commercial market because the drug caused fatal hepatic failure in a small number of subjects. Non-lethal hepatotoxicity has also been reported with other currently available TZDs [103], though at far lower frequencies than with troglitazone. Hepatic dysfunction must be excluded before TZD therapy is initiated and liver function tests should be measured monthly for the first 6 months of treatment, every 2 months for the remainder of the first year, and at regular intervals thereafter [103]. Other potential complications of TZD therapy include anemia, edema, and as noted previously, weight gain.

***Other Potentially Useful Pharmacologic Agents***

Acarbose, an alpha glucodase inhibitor, may reduce progression to type 2 diabetes by limiting gastrointestinal absorption of carbohydrate. The STOP-NIDDM trial [104] demonstrated a 25-36% reduction in type 2 diabetes in obese adults (mean age 55 yr, mean BMI 31) with impaired glucose tolerance. Post-prandial glucose and insulin concentrations were reduced and weight declined slightly in patients treated with acarbose (100mg tid) for a mean of 3.3 yr. In addition, the rate of development of cardiovascular events (coronary heart disease, cardiovascular death, congestive heart failure, stroke and peripheral vascular disease) was only one-half that in the placebo group [105]. However, the drop-out rate in the acarbose group was 24% and the gastrointestinal side effects of the medication, which include flatulence and diarrhea, limit its acceptability in children and adolescents.

A post-hoc analysis of the HOPE study showed a 40% reduction in newly diagnosed diabetes in patients treated with the angiotensin converting enzyme (ACE) inhibitor Ramipril [106]. And a post-hoc analysis of the West of Scotland Coronary Prevention Study [107] demonstrated a 25% reduction in the incidence of newly diagnosed diabetes in patients treated with Pravastatin. The effects of these medications on rates of development of diabetes have not yet been demonstrated in a prospective study.

***New Approaches: Metabolic Inhibitors, and Cytokine Therapy***

Pharmacologic agents currently in use target the complications of insulin resistance indirectly. Animal studies suggest that approaches that target metabolic signaling and cytokine production directly may prove useful in the prevention of type 2 diabetes and cardiovascular disease.

An appealing therapeutic candidate is the adipocytokine adiponectin. Adiponectin levels decline in obesity and other states accompanied by insulin resistance but rise following treatment with thiazolidinediones. Administration of recombinant adiponectin to obese mice reduces blood glucose and insulin concentrations, increases insulin sensitivity and hepatic fatty acid oxidation, reduces hepatic fatty acid synthesis, reverses hepatic steatosis, and decreases body weight [108-111]. Targeting of poly (ADPribose) polymerase (PARP) also shows promise. Activation of PARP by glucose-induced oxidative stress inhibits glyceraldehyde phosphate dehydrogenase activity and may thereby promote the formation of polyols, glucosamine, and advanced glycation endproducts and the activation of protein kinase C [27,112]. These metabolites mediate glucose-dependent endothelial dysfunction. In an animal model of diabetes, the pharmacological inhibition of poly (ADPribose) polymerase improves endothelial function [113]. It is likely that future investigations will identify new targets and pharmacotherapeutic agents that will prevent long-term complications in high-risk patients.

## Balancing Lifestyle Intervention and Pharmacotherapy in Diabetes Prevention

In theory, intensive lifestyle intervention should benefit all pediatric patients who are at high risk for developing type 2 diabetes. But lifestyle intervention is difficult, time-consuming and, in many cases of childhood obesity, ineffective. Treatment failure may prolong or exacerbate insulin resistance, dyslipidemia, and glucose intolerance, leading to irreversible beta cell dysfunction, overt type 2 diabetes and progressive cardiovascular disease.

The physician is thus faced with a difficult dilemma: the efficacy of traditional lifestyle approaches has not yet been demonstrated in populations of obese children, and failure to correct defects in insulin sensitivity and glucose tolerance in obese patients with glucose intolerance may have irreversible adverse consequences. Yet the long-term safety and efficacy of pharmacologic agents have not yet been established.

In the opinion of the author, pharmacotherapy should be considered for treatment of adolescents at highest risk for the development of type 2 diabetes; these include obese patients with IGT or IFG. Prior to initiation of drug therapy, such children should undergo a trial of intensive lifestyle intervention. If 6-12 months of lifestyle intervention proves unsuccessful despite a good-faith effort on the part of the patient, a trial of medication can be justified. "Good faith effort" means that the patient has attempted to follow a low saturated fat/low calorie diet recommended by a dietary counselor and has increased his or her energy expenditure through regular exercise. "Unsuccessful" means that the elevations of fasting or post-prandial glucose persist or worsen despite lifestyle intervention.

Given its long-term track record of safety in men and women, the reversibility of its complications, its proven efficacy in treating insulin resistant as well as diabetic adolescents and adults and women with PCOS, and its ability to limit weight gain, the author considers metformin the drug of choice for treating the obese child with IFG or IGT. The decision to initiate drug therapy relieves neither the child nor the physician of the commitment to long-term lifestyle change; thus diet and exercise regimens should be maintained, even if they had not proven effective in the absence of medication. Given the lack of studies of TZDs in insulin-resistant children or adolescents, their potential, albeit rare, for severe hepatic complications, and their tendency to cause weight gain, the author would limit the use of TZDs to adolescents who fail to respond to, or cannot tolerate, metformin. Since the danger of hepatic dysfunction with combined therapy in pediatric patients is unknown, the TZDs should not be used in conjunction with metformin in non-diabetic children pending demonstration in long-term studies that the drug combination is safe.

It is not possible at this time to provide firm or uniform guidelines regarding the duration of pharmacologic intervention. A trial off medication may be warranted if glucose tolerance is normalized, particularly if there has been a decline in BMI z score. If IGT persists despite compliance with the medical/pharmacologic regimen, it may be necessary to intensify lifestyle intervention and/or to increase the dose of medication. If glucose tolerance declines or the patient develops overt diabetes, he/she may require the addition of insulin or another pharmacologic agent.

In contrast to children with IGT or IFG, obese children with normal fasting and 2 hour (or post-prandial) glucose concentrations should at the present time be managed with lifestyle intervention alone. The use of metformin or other pharmacologic agents in such children must at this time be considered experimental.

## A Multifaceted Approach to Prevention of Complications

The major causes of death in adults with IGT or type 2 diabetes are myocardial infarction and stroke [10-17]. Although cardiovascular risk in patients with IGT and type 2 diabetes varies with glycemic control, other factors may play equal or more important roles in disease pathogenesis. These include obesity, hypertension, smoking, dyslipidemia, ethnic background and family history. In theory, aggressive lifestyle intervention in children and adolescents should include reduction in BMI z score and abolition of smoking. Pharmacologic therapy may be necessary to reduce blood pressure, control microalbuminuria, and treat dyslipidemia. A multifactorial approach that combined dietary counseling, statins, angiotensin converting enzyme inhibitors, and low-dose aspirin reduced by 50-60% reductions the long-term (8 yr) risks of nephropathy, retinopathy, autonomic neuropathy and cardiovascular end-points (myocardial disease and stroke and amputation) in diabetic adults with microalbuminuria [114]. Such an approach may be necessary in the management of obese, insulin-resistant and glucose-intolerant adolescents, who are commonly hypertensive and hyperlipidemic. The age and intensity of intervention may depend upon the family history of cardiovascular disease as well as the magnitude of problems in the individual teenager under the physician's care.

## Closing Thoughts

This discussion of diabetes prevention has focused on the medical model by which the physician and health care team manage risks and complications of an individual patient or his or her family. But diabetes prevention necessitates a collaboration between the medical and lay communities to address societal conditions that nurture and sustain childhood obesity and the development of type 2 diabetes.

For example, a major effort should be undertaken to eliminate soda and candy from school cafeterias and vending machines. School boards could solicit competitive bids for distributors of "healthy foods", reviewed by committees of local health experts, and could require price reductions for nutritious foods and milk. Schools could also require periods of mandatory exercise for school children of all ages, with facilities to make that exercise participatory and exciting. There should be expansion of community opportunities for exercise and energy expenditure, including development of bike and hiking trails, open and park space, pedestrian walkways, and public transportation. Second-hand smoke, which may increase the risk of cardiovascular disease, should be reduced by eliminating smoking in public places. Finally, federal and local PR campaigns should publicize the risks of type 2 diabetes in minority populations and those with positive family histories, the hazards of excessive weight gain in childhood, and the benefits of daily exercise and of limits in consumption of concentrated sweets and high-fat foods.

## REFERENCES


[1] Freemark, M. Pharmacologic approaches to the prevention of type 2 diabetes in high risk pediatric patients. *J Clin Endocrinol Metab* 2003; 88: 3-13.

[2] Arner, P. Regional adipocity in man. *J Endocrin* 1997; 155: 191-192.

[3] Arner, P. The adipocyte in insulin resistance: key molecules and the impact of the thiazolidinediones. *Trends in Endocrin and Metab* 2003; 14:137-145.

[4] Bergman, RN, Finegood, DT, Kahn, SE. The evolution of β-cell dysfunction and insulin resistance in type 2 diabetes. *Eur J Clin Invest* 2002; 32:35-45.

[5] Yu C, Chen Y, Cline GW, Zhang D, Zong H, Wang Y, Bergeron R, Kim JK, Suchman SW, Cooney GJ, Atcheson B, White MF, Kraegen EW, Shulman GI. Mechanism by which fatty acids inhibit insulin activation of insulin receptor substrate-1-associated phosphatidyl 3-kinase activity in muscle. *J Biol Chem* 2003; 277: 50230-50236.

[6] Kashyap S, Belfort R, Gastaldelli a, Pratipanawatr T, Berria R, Pratipanawatr W, Bajaj M, Mandarino L, DeFronzo R, Cusi K. A sustained increase in plasma free fatty acids impairs insulin secretion in nondiabetic subjects genetically predisposed to develop type 2 diabetes. *Diabetes* 2003; 52: 2461-2474.

[7] Kern, PA, Di Gregorio, GB, Lu, T, Rassouli, N, Ranganathan, G. Adiponectin expression from human adipose tissue: relation to obesity, insulin resistance, and tumor necrosis factor-alpha expression. *Diabetes* 2003; 52:1779-1785.

[8] Oyadomari S, Takeda K, Takiguchi M, Gotoh T, Matsumoto M, Wada I, Akira S, Araki E, Mori M. Nitric oxide-induced apoptosis in pancreatic beta cells is mediated by the endoplasmic reticulum stress pathway. *Proc Natl Acad Sci U S A*. 2001 Sep 11;98(19):10845-50.

[9] Sam S, Dunaif A. Polycystic ovary syndrome: Syndrome XX? *Trends Endo Metab* 2003; 14: 365-370.

[10] Haffner SM, Lehto S, Ronnemaa T, Pyorala K, Laasko M. Mortality from coronary heart disease in subjects with type 2 diabetes and in nondiabetic subjects with and without prior myocardial infarction. *N Engl J Med* 1998; 339: 229-234.

[11] Kuller LH, Velentgas P, Barzilay J, Beauchamp NJ, O'Leary DH, Savage PJ. Diabetes mellitus: subclinical cardiovascular disease and risk of incident cardiovascular disease and all-cause mortality. *Arterioscler Thromb Vasc Biol* 2000; 20:823-829.

[12] Berenson, GS, Srinivasan SR, Bao W, Newman WP III, Tracy RE, Wattigney WA. Association between multiple cardiovascular risk factors and atherosclerosis in children and young adults. *N Eng J Med* 1998; 338: 1650-1656.

[13] McGill HC Jr, McMahan CA, Herderick, EE, Zieske AW, Malcom GT, Tracy RE, Strong JP. Pathological Determinants of Atherosclerosis in Youth (PDAY) Research Group. Obesity accelerates the progression of coronary atherosclerosis in young men. *Circulation* 2002; 105: 2712-2718.

[14] Tominaga M, Eguchi H, Manaka H, Igarashi K, Kato T, Sekikawa A. Impaired glucose tolerance is a risk factor for cardiovascular disease, but not impaired fasting glucose: the Funagata Diabetes Study. *Diabetes Care* 1999; 22: 920-924, .

[15] Temelkova-Kurktschiev TS, Koehler C, Henkel E, Leonhardt W, Fuecker K, Hanefield M. Postchallenge plasma glucose and glycemic spikes are more strongly associated

with atherosclerosis than fasting glucose or HbA1c level. *Diabetes Care* 2000; 23: 1830-1834.

[16] Bonora E, Kiechl S, Willeit J, Oberhollenzer F, Egger G, Bonadonna RO, Muggeo M. Carotid atherosclerosis and coronary heart disease in the metabolic syndrome: prospective data from the Bruneck Study. *Diabetes Care* 2003; 26: 1251-1257.

[17] deMarco R, Locatelli F, Zoppini G, Verlato G, Bonora E, Muggeo M. Cause-specific mortality in type 2 diabetes: the Verona Diabetes Study. *Diabetes Care* 1999; 22: 756-761.

[18] Calle, EE, Rodriguez, C, Walker-Thurmond, K, Thun, MJ. Overweight, obesity, and mortality from cancer in a prospectively studied cohort of U.S. adults. *N Engl J Med* 2003; 348:1625-1638.

[19] Must, A, Jacques, PF, Dallal, GE, Bajema, CJ, Dietz, WH. Long-term morbidity and mortality of overweight adolescents. A follow-up of the Harvard Growth Study of 1922 to 1935. *N Engl J Med* 1992; 327:1350-1355.

[20] Montani, JP, Antic, V, Yang, Z, Dulloo, A. Pathways from obesity to hypertension: from the perspective of a vicious triangle. *Int J Obesity* 2002; 26:s28-s38.

[21] Taittonen, L, Uhari, M, Nuutinen, M, Turtinen, J, Pokka, T, Akerblom, HK. Insulin and blood pressure among healthy children. *Am J Hypertens* 1996; 9: 193-199.

[22] Burke, GL, Webber, LS, Srinivasan, SR. Fasting plasma glucose and insulin levels and their relationship to cardiovascular risk factors in children: Bogalusa Heart Study. *Metabolism* 1986; 35:441-446.

[23] Tack CJ, Smits P, Willemsen JJ, Lenders JW, Thien T, Lutterman JA. Effects of insulin on vascular tone and sympathetic nervous system in NIDDM. *Diabetes* 1996; 45:15-22.

[24] Vincent MA, Montagnani M, Quon MJ. Molecular and physiologic actions of insulin related to production of nitric oxide in vascular endothelium. *Curr Diab Reports* 23 : 279-288 .

[25] Caballero AE, Arora S, Saouaf R, Lim SC, Smakowski P, Park JY, King GL, LoGerfo FW, Horton ES, Veves A. Microvascular and macrovascular reactivity is reduced in subjects at risk for type 2 diabetes. *Diabetes* 1999; 48: 1856-1862.

[26] Nishikawa T, Edelstein D, Du XL, Yamagishi S, Matsumura T, Kaneda Y, Yorek MA, Beebe D, Oates PJ, Hammes HP, Giardino I, Brownlee M. Normalizing mitochondrial superoxide production blocks three pathways of hyperglycemic damage. *Nature* 2000; 404: 787-790; .

[27] Du XL, Matsumura T, Edelstein D, Rossetti L, Zsengeller Z, Szabo C, Brownlee M. Inhibition of GAPDH activity by poly (ADPribose) polymerase activates three major pathways of hyperglycemic damage in endothelial cells. *J Clin Invest* 2003; 112: 1049-1057.

[28] Deedwania PC. Mechanisms of endothelial dysfunction in the metabolic syndrome. *Curr Diab Reports* 2003; 3: 289-292.

[29] Ouchi N, Kihara S, Arita Y, Maeda K, Kuriyama H, Okamoto Y, Hotta K, Nishida M, Takahashi M, Nakamura T, Yamashita S, Funahashi T, Matsuzawa Y. Novel modulator for endothelial adhesion molecules: adipocyte-derived plasma protein adiponectin. *Circulation* 1999; 100:2473-2476.

[30] Goldfine AB, Bouche C, Parker, RA, Kim C, Kerivan A, Soeldner JS, Martin BC, Warram JH, Kahn CR. Insulin resistance is a poor predictor of type 2 diabetes in

individuals with no family history of disease. *Proc Natl Acad Sci USA* 2003; 100:2724-2729.

[31] Veening, MA, van Weissenbruch, MM, Heine, RJ, Delemarre-van de Waa, HA. Beta-cell capacity and insulin sensitivity in prepubertal children born small for gestational age: influence of body size during childhood. *Diabetes* 2003; 52:1756-1760 .

[32] Hypponen E, Power C, Smith GD. Prenatal growth, BMI, and risk of type 2 diabetes by early midlife. *Diabetes Care* 2003; 26: 2512-2517.

[33] Silfen ME, Manibo AM, McMahon DJ, Levine LS, Murphy AR, Oberfield SE. Comparison of simple measures of insulin sensitivity in young girls with premature adrenarche: the fasting glucose to insulin ratio may be a simple and useful measure. *J Clin Endocrinol Metab* 2001; 86:2863-2868.

[34] Sinha R, Fisch G, Teague B, Tamborlane WV, Banyas B, Allen K, Savoye M, Rieger V, Taksali S, Barbetta G, Sherwin RS, Caprio S. Prevalence of impaired glucose tolerance among children and adolescents with marked obesity. *N Engl J Medicine* 2002; 346:802-810.

[35] American Diabetes Association. Type 2 diabetes in children and adolescents. *Diabetes Care* 2000; 23: 381-389.

[36] Lhoret-Rabasa R, Bastard J-P, Jan V, Ducluzeau P-H, Andreelli F, Guebre F, Bruzeau J, Louche-Pellissier C, Maitrepierre C, Peyrat J, Chagne J, Vidal H, Laville M. Modified quantitative insulin sensitivity check index is better correlated to hyperinsulinemic glucose clamp than other fasting-based index of insulin sensitivity in different insulin-resistant states. *J Clin Endocrinol Metab* 2003; 88: 4917-4923.

[37] Lovejoy JC. The influence of dietary fat on insulin resistance. *Curr Diab Reports* 2002; 2: 435-440.

[38] Foster GD, Wyatt HR, Hill JO, MCguckin BG, Brill C, Mohammed BS, Szapary PO, Rader DJ, Edman JS, Klein S. A randomized trial of a low-carbohydrate diet for obesity. *N Eng J Med* 2003; 348: 2082-2090.

[39] Samaha FF, Iqbal N, Seshadri P, Chicano KL, Daily DA, McGrory J, Williams T, Williams M, Gracely EJ, Stern L. A low-carbohydrate as compared with a low-fat diet in severe obesity. *N Engl J Med* 2003; 2074-2081.

[40] Bravata DM, Sanders L, Huang J, Krumholz HM, Olkin I, Gardner CD. Efficacy and safety of low-carbohydrate diets: a systematic review. *JAMA* 2003; 289: 1837-1850.

[41] Montonen J, Knekt P, Jarvinene R, Aromaa A, Reunanen A. Whole-grain and fiber intake and the incidence of type 2 diabetes. *Am J Clin Nutr* 2003; 77: 622-629.

[42] Salmeron J, Manson JE, Stampfer MJ, Colditz GA, Wing AL, Willett WC. Dietary fiber, glycemic load, and risk of non-insulin-dependent diabetes mellitus in women. *JAMA* 1997; 277: 472-477.

[43] Rodriguez-Moran M, Guerrero-Romero F. Oral magnesium supplementation improves insulin sensitivity and metabolic control in type 2 diabetic subjects: a randomized double-blind controlled trial. *Diabetes Care*. 2003; 26:1147-52.

[44] Pereira MA, Jacobs DR, Van Horn L, Slattery ML, Kartashov AI, Ludwig DS. Dairy consumption, obesity and the insulin resistance syndrome in young adults: the CARDIA Study. *JAMA* 2002; 287: 2081-2089.

[45] Warren JM, Henry CJ, Simonite V. Low glycemic index breakfasts and reduced food intake in preadolescent children. *Pediatrics* 2003; 112(5):e414.

[46] Elliott SS, Keim NL, Stern JS, Teff K, Havel PJ. Fructose, weight gain, and the insulin resistance syndrome. *Am J Clin Nutr*. 2002; 76:911-22.

[47] Ludwig DS, Peterson KE, Gortmaker SL. Relation between consumption of sugar-sweetened drinks and childhood obesity: a prospective, observational study. *Lancet* 2001; 357: 505-508.

[48] Ebbeling CB, Leidig MM, Sinclair KB, Hangen JB, Ludwig DS. A reduced glycemic load diet in the treatment of adolescent obesity. *Arch Pediatr Adolesc Med* 2003; 157: 773-779.

[49] Eriksson, KF, Lingarde, F. Prevention of type 2 (non-insulin dependent) diabetes mellitus by diet and physical exercise. The 6 year Malmo feasibility study. *Diabetologia* 1991; 34:891-898.

[50] Pan, X. R, Li, G. W, Hu, Y. H, Wang, J. X, Yang, W. Y, An, Z. X, Hu, Z. X, Lin, J, Xiao, J. Z, Cao, H. B, Liu, P. A, Jiang, X. G, Jiang, Y. Y, Wang, J. P, Zheng, H, Zhang, H, Bennett, P. H and Howard, B. V. The Da Qing IGT and Diabetes Study: effects of diet and exercise in preventing NIDDM in people with impaired glucose tolerance. *Diabetes Care* 1997; 20: 537-544 .

[51] Uusitupa M, Louheranta A, Lindstrom J, Valle T, Sundvall J, Eriksson J, Tuomilehto J. The Finnish Diabetes Prevention Study. *Brit J Nutr* 2000; 83:s137-s142 .

[52] Uusitupa M, Lindi V, Louheranta A, Salopuro T, Lindstrom J, Tuomilehto J. Long-term improvemernt in insulin sensitivity by changing lifestyles of people with impaired glucose tolerance. 4-year results from the Finnish Diabetes Prevention Study. *Diabetes* 2003; 52: 2532-2538.

[53] Knowler, W. C, Barrett-Connor, E, Fowler, S. E, Hamman, R. F, Lachin, J. M, Walker, E. A and Nathan, D. M. Reduction in the incidence of type 2 diabetes with lifestyle intervention or metformin. *N Eng J Med* 2002; 346: 393-403, and presentation by Dr. Steven Kahn at the 62nd Annual Meeting of the American Diabetes Association, San Francisco.

[54] Mourier A, Gautier JF, De Kerviler E, Bigard AX, Villette JM, Garnier JP, Duvallet A, Guezennec CY, Cathelineau G. Mobilization of visceral adipose tissue related to the improvement in insulin sensitivity in response to physical training in NIDDM : Effects of branched-chain amino acid supplements. *Diab Care* 1997; 20:385-391.

[55] Tuomilehto, J, Lindstrom, J, Eriksson, J. G, Valle, T. T, Hamalainen, H, Ilanne-Parikka, P, Keinanen-Kiukaanniemi, S, Laakso, M, Louheranta, A, Rastas, M Salminen, V and Uusitupa, M. Pevention of type 2 diabets mellitus by changes in lifestyle among subjects with impaired glucose tolerance. *N Eng J Med* 2001; 344: 1343-1350.

[56] Simonelli, C, Eaton, RP. Reduced triglyceride secretion: a metabolic consequence of chronic exercise. *Am J Physiol* 1978; 234:E221-227.

[57] Angus, DJ, Febbraio, MA, Hargreaves, M. Plasma glucose kinetics during prolonged exercise in trained humans when fed carbohydrate. *Am J Physiol Endocrinol Metab* 2002; 283: E573-E577.

[58] Short KR, Vittone JL, Bigelow ML, Proctor DN, Rizza RA, Coenen-Schimke JM, Nair KS. Impact of aerobic exercise training on age-related changes in insulin sensitivity and muscle oxidative capacity. *Diabetes* 2003; 52: 1888-1896.

[59] Ryder, JW, Chibalin, AV, Zierath, JR. Intracellular mechanisms underlying increases in glucose uptake in response to insulin or exercise in skeletal muscle. *Acta Physiol Scand* 2001; 171:249-257.

[60] McGee SL, Howlett KF, Starkie RL, Cameron-Smith D, Kemp BE, Hargreaves M. Exercise increases nuclear AMPK in human skeletal muscle. *Diabetes* 2003; 52:926-928.

[61] Simoneau, JA, Kelley, DE. Altered glycolytic and oxidative capacities of skeletal muscle contribute to insulin resistance and NIDDM. *J Appl Physiol* 1997; 83:166-171.

[62] Santoro C, Cosmas A, Forman D, Morghan A, Bairos L, Levesque S, Roubenoff R, Hennessey J, Lamont L, Manfredi T. Exercise training alters skeletal muscle mitochondrial morphometry in heart failure patients. *J Cardiovascular Risk* 2002; 9:377-381.

[63] Holloszy, JO. Adaptation of skeletal muscle to endurance exercise. *Med Sci Sports* 1975; 7:155-164.

[64] Goodpaster, BH, Katsiaras, A, Kelley, DE. Enhanced fat oxidation through physical activity is associated with improvements in insulin sensitivity in obesity. *Diabetes* 2003; 52:2191-2197.

[65] Ferguson MA, Gutin B, Le NA, Karp W, Litaker M, Humphries M, Okuyama T, Riggs S, Owens S. Effects of exercise training and its cessation on components of the insulin resistance syndrome in obese children. *Int J Obes* 1999; 22:889-895.

[66] Watts K, Beye P, Siafarikas A, Davis EA, Jones TW, O'Driscoll G, and Green DJ. Exercise training normalizes vascular dysfunction and improves central adiposity in obese adolescents. J Amer Coll Cardiol 2004, in press. A parallel study in obese pre-teens is in press in the *Journal of Pediatrics*. .

[67] Zhou, G, Myers, R, Li, Y, Chen, Y, Shen, X, Fenyk-Melody, J, Wu, M, Ventre, J, Doebber, T, Fujii, N, Musi, N, Hirshman, M. F, Goodyear, L. J and Moller, D. E. Role of AMP-activated protein kinase in mechanism of metformin action. *J Clin Invest* 2001; 108: 1167-74.

[68] Hundal RS, Krssak M, Dufour S, Laurent D, Lebon V, Chandramouli V, Inzucchi SE, Schumann WC, Petersen KF, Landau BR, Shulman GI. Mechanism by which metformin reduces glucose production in type 2 diabetes. *Diabetes* 2000; 49:2063-2069.

[69] Mitheux, G, Guignot, L, Bordet, JC, Wiernsperger, N. Intrahepatic mechanisms underlying the effect of metformin in decreasing basal glucose Production in Rats Fed a High-Fat Diet. *Diabetes* 2002; 51:139-143.

[70] Cusi, K, Consoli, A and DeFronzo, RA. Metabolic effects of metformin in non-insulin dependent diabetes mellitus. J Clin Endocrinol Metab 1996; 81: 4059-4067.

[71] DeFronzo, RA. Pharmacologic therapy for type 2 diabetes mellitus. *Ann Int Med* 1999; 131: 281-303.

[72] Song, S, Andrikopoulos, S, Filippis, C, Thorburn, A. W, Khan, D, and Proietto, J. Mechanism of fat-induced hepatic gluconeogenesis: effect of metformin. *Am J Physiol Endocrinol Metab* 2001; 281: E275-E282.

[73] Hallsten K, Virtanen KA, Lonnqvist F, Sipila H, Oksanen A, Viljanen T, Ronnemaa T, Viikari J, Knuuti J, Nuutila P. Rosiglitazone but not Metformin enhances insulin-and exercise-stimulated skeletal muscle glucose uptake in patients with newly diagnosed type 2 diabetes. *Diabetes* 2002; 51: 3479-3485.

[74] Virtanen KA, Hallsten K, Parkkola R, Janatuinen T, Lonnqvist F, Viljanen T, Ronnemaa T, Knuuti J, Huupponen R, Lonnroth P, Nuutila P. Differential effects of

rosiglitazone and metformin on adipose tissue distribution and glucose uptake in type 2 diabetic subjects. *Diabetes* 2003; 52:283-290.

[75] Effect of intensive blood-glucose control with metformin on complications in overweight patients with type 2 diabetes (UKPDS 34). UK Prospective Diabetes Study (UKPDS) Group. *Lancet.* 1998; 352:854-65.

[76] Mather, KJ, Verma, S, Anderson, TJ. Improved endothelial function with metformin in type 2 diabetes mellitus. J Am Coll Cardiol 2001; 37: 2131-2132.

[77] Paolisso, G, Amato, L, Eccellente, R, Gambardella, M, Tagliamonte, MR, Varricchio, G, Carrella, C, Giugliano, D, D'Onofrio, F. Effect of metformin on food intake in obese subjects. *Eur J Clin Invest* 1998; 28 (6): 441-446.

[78] Glueck, CJ, Fontaine, RN, Wang, P, Subbiah, MTR, Weber, K, Illig, E, Streicher, P, Sieve-Smith, L, Tracy, TM, Lang, JE, McCullough, P. Metformin reduces weight, centripetal obesity, insulin, leptin, and low-density lipoprotein cholesterol in nondiabetic, morbidly obese subjects with body mass index greater than 30. *Metabolism* 2001; 50: 856-861.

[79] Pasquali, R, Gambineri, A, Biscotti, D, Vicennati, V, Gagliardi, L, Colitta, D, Fiorini, S, Cognigni, GE, Filicori, M, Morselli-Labate, AM. Effect of long-term treatment with metformin added to hypocaloric diet on body composition, fat distribution, and androgen and insulin levels in abdominally obese women with and without the polycystic ovary syndrome. J. *Clin. Endocrin. Metab* 2000; 85: 2767-2774.

[80] Moghetti P, Castello R, Negri C, Tosi F, Perrone F, Caputo M, Zanolin E, Muggeo M. Metformin effects on clinical features, endocrine and metabolic profiles, and insulin senstivity in polycystic ovary syndrome: a randomized, double-blind, placebo-controlled 6 month trial, followed by open, long-term clinical evaluation. *J Clin Endocrinol Metab* 2000; 85:139-146.

[81] Ibanez, Valls, Potau N, Marcos MV, deZegher F, Sensitization to insulin in adolescent girls to normalize hirsutis, hyperandrogenism, oligomenorrhea, dyslipidmeia and hyperinsulinism after precocious pubarche. *J Clin Endocrinol Metab* 2000; 85: 3526-3530.

[82] Ibanez L, Valls C, Ferrer A, Ong K, Dunger DB, DeZegher F. Additive effects of insulin-sensitizing and anti-androgen treatment in young, nonobese women with hyperinsulinism, hyperandrogenism, dyslipidemia, and anovulation. *J Clin Endocrinol Metab* 2002; 87: 2870-2874.

[83] Ibanez L, Ong K, Ferrer A, Amin R, Dunger D, deZegher F. Low-dose flutamide-metformin therapy reverses insulin resistance and reduces fat mass in nonobese adolescents with ovarian hyperandrogenism. *J Clin Endocrinol Metab* 2003; 88: 2600-2606.

[84] Freemark, M, Bursey, D. The effects of metformin on body mass index and glucose tolerance in obese adolescents with fasting hyperinsulinemia and a family history of type 2 diabetes. *Pediatrics* 2001; 107 (4): e55 .

[85] McCance DR, Pettitt DJ, Hanson RL, Jacobsson LTH, Bennett PH, Knowler WC. Glucose, insulin concentrations and obesity in childhood and adolescence as predictors of NIDDM. *Diabetologia* 1994; 37: 617-623.

[86] Martin BC, Warram JH, Krolewski AS, Bergman RN, Soeldner JS, Kahn CR. Role of glucose and insulin resistance in development of type 2 diabeges mellitus: results of a 25 year follow-up study. *Lancet* 1992; 340: 925-929.

[87] Kay, JP, Alemzadeh, R, Langley, G, D'Angelo, L, Smith, P and Holshouser, S. Beneficial effects of metformin in normoglycemic morbidly obese adolescents. *Metabolism* 2001; 50: 1457-1461.

[88] Diabetes Prevention Program Research Group. Effects of withdrawal from metformin on the development of diabetes in the diabetes prevention program. *Diabetes Care* 2003; 26: 977-980.

[89] Spiegelman, BM. PPAR-gamma: adipogenic regulator and thiazolidinedione receptor. *Diabetes* 1998; 47:507-514.

[90] Gurnell M, Savage DB, Chatterjee KK, O'Rahilly S. The metabolic syndrome: PPAR gamma and its therapeutic modulation. *J Clin Endocrinol Metab* 2003; 88: 2412-2421.

[91] Hauner H. The mode of action of thiazolidinediones. *Diab Metab Res Rev* 2002; 18 Suppl 2: S10-S15.

[92] Kelly, IE. Han, TS, Walsh, D, Lean, ME. Effects of thiazolidinedione compound on body fat and fat distribution of patients with type 2 diabetes. *Diabetes Care* 1999; 22:288-293.

[93] Ciaraldi TP, Kong AP, Chu NV, Kim DD, Baxi S, Loviscach M, Plodkowski R, Reitz R, Caulfield M, Mudaliar S, Henry RR. Regulation of glucose transport and insulin signaling by troglitazone or metformin in adipose tissue of type 2 diabetic subjects. *Diabetes* 2002; 51: 30-36 .

[94] Norris AW, Chen L, Fisher SJ, Szanto I, Ristow M, Jozsi AC, Hirshman MF, Rosen ED, Goodyear LJ, Gonzalez FJ, Spiegelman BM, Kahn CR. Muscle-specific PPAR$\gamma$-deficient mice develop increased adiposity and insulin resistance but respond to thiazolidinediones. *J Clin Invest* 2003; 112:608-618 .

[95] Kim YB, Ciaraldi TP, Kong A, Kim D, Chu N, Mohideen P, Mudaliar S, Henry RR, Kahn BB. Troglitazone but not metformin restores insulin-stimulated phosphoinositide 3-kinase activity and increases p110 (beta) protein levels in skeletal muscle of type 2 diabetic subjects. *Diabetes* 2002; 51:443-448.

[96] Rajala MW, Scherer PE. Minireview: The adipocyte – At the crossroads of energy homeostasis, inflammation, and atherosclerosis. *Endocrinology* 2003; 144: 3765-3773.

[97] Satoh N, Ogawa Y, Usui T, Tagami T, Kono S, Uesugi H, Sugiyama H, Sugawara A, Yamada K, Shimatsu A, Kuzuya H, Nakao K. Antiatherogenic effect of pioglitazone in type 2 diabetic patients is irrespective of the responsiveness to its antidiabetic effect. 2003. *Diab Care* 2003; 26:2493-2499.

[98] Freed MI, Ratner R, Marcovina SM, Kreider MM, Biswas N, Cohen BR, Brunzell JD. Effects of rosiglitazone alone and in combination with atorvastatin on the metabolic abnormalities of type 2 diabetes mellitus. *Am J Cardiol* 2002; 90:947-952.

[99] Nolan, JJ, Ludvik, B, Beerdsen, P, Joyce, M, Olefsky, J. Improvement in glucose tolerance and insulin resistance in obese subjects treated with troglitazone. *N Engl J Med* 1994; 331:1188-1193.

[100] Parulkar AA, Pendergrass ML, Granda-Ayala R, Lee TR, Fonseca VA. Nonhypoglycemic effects of thiazolidinediones. *Ann Int Med* 2001; 134: 61-71.

[101] Paradisi, G, Steingberg, HO, Shepard, MK, Hook, G, Baron, AD. Troglitazone therapy improves endothelial function to near normal levels in women with polycytic ovary syndrome. *J Clin Endocrinol Metab* 2003; 88:576-580.

[102] Buchanan TA, Xiang AH, Peters RK, Kjos SL, Marroquin A, Goico J, Ochoa C, Tan S, Berkowitz K, Hodis HN, Azen SP. Preservation of pancreatic (beta)-cell function and

prevention of type 2 diabetes by pharmacological treatment of insulin resistance in high-risk Hispanic women. *Diabetes* 2002; 51:2796-2803.

[103] Tolman, KG, Chandramouli, J. Hepatoxicity of the thiazolidinediones. *Clin Liver Dis* 2003; 7:369-379.

[104] Chiasson JL, Josse RG, Gomis R, Hanefeld M, Karasik A, Laakso M; STOP-NIDDM Trial Research Group. Acarbose for the prevention of type 2 diabetes mellitus: the STOP-NIDDM randomized trial. *Lancet* 2002; 359:2072-2077.

[105] Chiasson, J-L, Josse, RG, Gomis, R, Hanefeld, M, Karasik, A, Laakso. Acarbose treatment and the risk of cardiovascular disease and hypertension in patients with impaired glucose tolerance. The STOP-NIDDM Trial. *JAMA* 2003; 290: 486-494.

[106] Yusuf S, Gerstein H, Hoogwerf B, Pogue J, Bosch J, Wolffenbuttel BH, Zinman B; HOPE Study Investigators. Ramipril and the development of diabetes. *JAMA* 2001; 286: 1882-1885.

[107] Freeman DJ, Norrie J, Sattar N, Neely RD, Cobbe SM, Ford I, Isles C, Lorimer AR, Macfarlane PW, McKillop JH, Packard CJ, Shepherd J, Gaw A. Pravastatin and the development of diabetes mellitus: evidence for a protective treatment effect in the West of Scotland Coronary Prevention Study. *Circulation* 2001; 103:357-362.

[108] Yamauchi, T, Kamon J, Waki H et al. The fat-derived hormone adiponectin reverses insulin resistance associated with both lipoatrophy and obesity. *Nat. Med.* 2001. 7:941-946.

[109] Fruebis, J, Tsao TS, Javorschi S, Ebbets-Reed D, Erickson MR, Yen FT, Bihain BE, Lodish HF. Proteolytic cleavage product of 30-kDa adipocyte complement-related protein increases fatty acid oxidation in muscle and causes weight loss in mice. *Proc. Nat. Acad. Sci. U. S. A.* 2001; 98:2005-2010.

[110] Berg, AH, Combs TP, Du X, Brownlee M, Scherer PE. The adipocyte-secreted protein Acrp30 enhances hepatic insulin action. *Nat. Med.* 2001; 7:947-953.

[111] Xu, A, Wang Y, Keshaw H, Xu LY, Lam KSL, Cooper, GJS. The fat-derived hormone adiponectin alleviates alcoholic and nonalcoholic liver diseases in mice. *J Clin Invest* 2003; 112: 91-100.

[112] Reusch JEB. Diabetes, microvascular complications, and cardiovascular complications: what is it about glucose? *J Clin Invest* 2003; 112: 986-988.

[113] Soriano FG, Pacher P, Mabley J, Liaudet L, Szabo C. Rapid reversal of the diabetic endothelial dysfunction by pharmacological inhibition of poly (ADPribose) polymerase. *Circ Res* 2001; 89: 684-691.

[114] Gaede P, Vedel P, Larsen N, Jensen GV, Parving HH, Pedersen O. Multifactorial intervention and cardiovascular disease in patients with type 2 diabetes. *N Engl J Med* 2003; 348:383-393.

# INDEX

## A

## B

## C

## D

## E

## F



## G

## I

## M

## N



## O



## P

## Q



## R



## S

## T

## U



## V